THE 24-HOUR PHARMACIST

HONEST ADVICE AND AMAZING CURES FROM AMERICA'S MOST TRUSTED PHARMACIST®

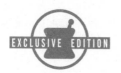
EXCLUSIVE EDITION

SUZY COHEN, RPh

AUTHOR OF THE SYNDICATED COLUMN "DEAR PHARMACIST®"

RODALE

To my loyal readers and patients: You have put your faith

and trust in me to offer guidance and improve your health—

this book and my prayers are for you.

© 2008, 2007 by Suzy Cohen

Printed in the United States of America

Rodale Inc. makes every effort to use acid-free ♾, recycled paper ♻.

Interior illustration credits: pages 1, 63, 203, and 293 ©CartoonStock; and page 137 ©Tribune Media Services, Inc. All Rights Reserved. Reprinted with permission.

Book design by Jaime Putorti

The information in this book was previously published by HarperCollins Publishers in 2007. Rodale Inc. direct mail edition is published in 2008 under license from HarperCollins Publishers.

Library of Congress Cataloging-in-Publication Data

Cohen, Suzy, R. Ph
    The 24-hour pharmacist : honest advice and amazing cures from America's most trusted pharmacist / Suzy Cohen.
        p.   cm.
    "Previously published by HarperCollins Publishers in 2007."
    Includes bibliographical references and index.
    ISBN-13 978–1–59486–961–7 direct mail hardcover
    ISBN-10 1–59486–961–8 direct mail hardcover
    1. Pharmacology—Popular works.   2. Drugs—Popular works.   3. Medicine, Popular.   4. Dietary supplements.   I. Title.
RM301.15.C62 2008
615'.1—dc22   2008023891

4 6 8 10 9 7 5 3   direct mail hardcover

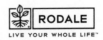

RODALE
LIVE YOUR WHOLE LIFE™

We inspire and enable people to improve their lives and the world around them
For more of our products visit **rodalestore.com** or call 800-848-4735

Contents

A Word of Caution to the Reader

The information presented in this book is based on the training and professional experience of the author. The treatments, herbs, vitamins, and supplements recommended in this book should not be taken without consulting your physician to be sure they are right for you with your particular medical condition. Appropriate laboratory and clinical monitoring is essential, even when using relatively safe and natural treatments. This book was written for informational and educational purposes only and is not intended to treat, diagnose, or cure your condition. It is just intended to open your eyes so you can explore all potential options for health and wellness. The author and the publisher expressly disclaim all liability for any injury that may arise from the use of the information contained in this book.

Introduction

You always remember those pivotal points in your life. I had been working in nursing homes for about seven years where I was responsible for monitoring the medication of about 1,000 patients. I was frustrated by the job because, although I was able to be helpful to these elderly people, I wished I could have helped them avoid the state they were in—to help them be healthier in the first place—so they wouldn't end up needing so much medication.

One evening, my husband burst into the house, and instead of his typical hello, he said, "Suzy, I was stuck in traffic and I got this great idea!" I imagined two tickets to Vail for a romantic getaway. Instead, he said, "I saw it! I had a vision and saw your picture in the newspaper . . . you are going to write health articles and help lots of people!" He went on for a few minutes, throwing in concepts such as TV, radio, and lecturing.

That's nice. "Do you want gravy with your mashed potatoes?" I was certain that by dessert he would be over the whole idea. After all, I barely knew how to work our new computer and I'd never written anything except Christmas cards and my To Do list. Write for newspapers? He must have had too much coffee. Aside from all that, the idea of public speaking sent shockwaves through my body, and suddenly I got my own vision, something along the lines of a Valium and smelling salts. But then I thought about it.

Since I have an open mind and my loving parents taught me that if I put my mind to something I could achieve it, I decided to try. I was already deeply entrenched in the medical profession as a clinically trained pharmacist, and I knew the power of pills—their virtues and their dangers—and I wanted to share that information, as well as all the great news about natural cures. It took two years and a bunch of respectful "no thanks," but eventually an editor gave me my first big break. I wrote one column each week for his paper, *The Lake City Reporter*, for about ten thousand readers. Today, my column circulates to over 24 million readers a week and is sold internationally. I routinely do TV, radio, and lectures—and it's fun! I am passionate about health care, and my mission is to get you as healthy as possible. No matter what happens or how bad you feel today, there is always hope. You are holding this book for a reason. Medications can be valuable to your health, but you must keep your mind open to all your options. Listen to the quiet inner voice that guides you, and thank you for letting me be your 24-hour pharmacist.

part I

Above the Waist

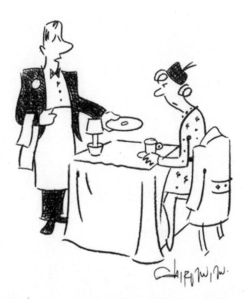

"We're sorry we served you caffeinated coffee.
Please accept this sleeping pill with compliments
of the management."

1

Overcoming Fatigue

From Stupor Woman to Super Woman

The most frequent question I get as a pharmacist is "What can I take for more energy?" The answer isn't two cans of Red Bull or a NoDoz tablet! C'mon, ladies, we're only fooling ourselves if we think these temporary pick-me-ups will cure us. They won't, although I confess my personal favorite is a caramel macchiato with whipped cream. But seriously, coffee, caffeine tablets, soda pop, and energy drinks all eventually worsen your condition because they lift you temporarily but further exhaust you in the long run. If you're tired, your body is telling you something—so let's figure out what it's saying.

Drained or Depressed?

If you tell your doctor that you're tired and overwhelmed, you may be found "Zoloft deficient." I've taken to calling "depression" a Pez dispenser diagnosis because it's dumped out so frequently. Maybe you're just spent, not sad. Of course, sometimes fatigue and depression go hand in hand—but not *always*. In a moment, I'll outline the many faces of fatigue so you can see who you identify with.

But most importantly, don't let your doctor prescribe antidepressants until you've ruled out other causes of fatigue, particularly low thyroid hormone, adrenal burnout, imbalanced hormones, or side effects from medication.

If you are already on antidepressants and don't think you need to be, DON'T stop taking them abruptly; work with your doctor to taper off. You could face serious withdrawal reactions if you stop suddenly.

The Many Faces of Fatigue

✳ **Working Wanda**—She stays up late, works too much, and simply has to cross off every single item on her To Do list—no wonder she's tired! Though her general health is still fine, she's headed for trouble if she doesn't learn to curl up like a noodle sometimes. She needs to put the word "NO" in her vocabulary sometimes.

✳ **Morning Mary**—She's almost always tired in the morning (and maybe other times, too). She holds onto weight because there's a breakdown somewhere in her thyroid gland that lowers circulating hormone levels.

✳ **Juggling Janet**—This busy lady has run herself ragged, and now her adrenal glands just can't pump out any more of the "stress hormones" that used to rev her up and help her meet life's challenges. She's tired in the morning and okay by midday—but crashes hard between 3 P.M. and 5 P.M. Some Juggling Janets catch a second wind at night, but the true hallmark of this type is that fatigue is unrelieved by sleep or rest.

✳ **Stupor Woman**—She's tired morning, noon, and night—the result of low thyroid hormone, imbalanced hormones, *and* low adrenal hormone! Her fantasy? To hook herself up to an IV drip of amphetamines! All kidding aside, many gals with all-day fatigue (and of course people suffering with Chronic Fatigue Syndrome and fibromyalgia) have both thyroid and adrenal imbalances.

✳ **Sleepy Sally**—This poor woman is tired because she suffers from insomnia, which could be the result of low thyroid hormone, low adrenals, medications, depression, anxiety, or diet. She should finish this chapter just in case, then jump to Chapter 9 on Insomnia.

Did You Get Mugged by a Drug?

Hundreds of popular medications are "drug muggers," stripping your cells of the energizing nutrients you need. As a result, you turn into an exhausted "medication mummy." The good news: When you know which nutrients are depleted by medications, you can replenish them and start enjoying your life again!

Oral Contraceptives and Hormone Replacement Therapy (HRT)

Drugs that contain estrogen mug your body of precious B vitamins, magnesium, tyrosine, vitamin C, and zinc, turning you into a Morning Mary or Juggling Janet because of the thyroid and adrenal compromise. This is so common, I can't tell you how frequently I dispense a birth-control pack along with a 30-day supply of thyroid meds. Incidentally, you could be dealing with low testosterone because birth control pills deplete this hormone too. You won't get pregnant while on birth control, but without testosterone, you don't feel like doing it! Other drug-mugging effects of contraception and HRT include: fatigue, cervical dysplasia, PMS, skin problems, moodiness, gastrointestinal (GI) problems, cardiovascular problems, weak bones, depression, and infections. See Chapter 12 (Monthly Madness) to find out how to feel better while taking these medications.

Statin Cholesterol Reducers

Medications in the "statin" class work by blocking an enzyme that creates cholesterol in the liver. These statins are the top-selling drugs in the world, and they go by brand names such as Lipitor, Zocor, Mevacor, Crestor, Pravachol, and Vytorin. Unfortunately, statins rob you of a powerful antioxidant and energizer called Coenzyme Q10, also called CoQ10, which you need so that your heart can beat, your muscles can work, and your energy can flow. So when cholesterol meds mug your CoQ10, you get those terrible muscle aches. You may feel fatigued, weak, and short of breath, and, ironically, you may develop heart problems—even though these drugs are intended to fight heart disease!

There are probably millions of people walking around in a tired funk because their heart and muscles are starving for CoQ10, a nutrient needed for life, and for energy. Statin-induced CoQ10 deficiency—and the subsequent fatigue, heart rhythm abnormalities, and shortness of breath—is completely preventable by supplementing with CoQ10, a nutrient that is extremely well tolerated. There are dozens of well-controlled studies that support the use of CoQ10 for patients with heart problems, and in light of the current congestive heart failure epidemic, I see no reason to dismiss this powerful nutrient. In an article published in *Biofactors* in 2003, Doctors Peter and Ali Langsjoen said it best with, "As physicians, it is our duty to be absolutely certain that we are not inadvertently doing harm to our patients by creating a widespread deficiency of a nutrient critically important for normal heart function."

CoQ10 lowers your cholesterol, and it gets your blood flowing. A randomized double-blind study published in the *European Heart Journal* (September 2007) found that CoQ10 supplementation (100 mg three times daily) improved blood flow to the heart by relaxing blood vessels in patients with coronary artery disease (CAD). Recent research also supports this heart-healthy benefit in people with diabetes.

If you suspect that you're taking a Drug Mugger of CoQ10, see Chapter 26 (Drug Muggers), then to be on the safe side, take *a minimum of 100 mg* of Coenzyme Q10 every morning, and if you can afford it, and it's okay with your doctor, take 100 mg two or three times daily. Check out Chapter 2 for more on this wonder supplement.

Blood Pressure Medications

These drug muggers also steal CoQ10, as well as calcium, potassium, magnesium, and melatonin (a hormone that helps us sleep and maintain mood). The result? Fatigue, muscle weakness, water retention in the hands and feet, asthma, cramps, and insomnia. The remedy? Take Coenzyme Q10 (*100 mg every morning*), magnesium chelate or glycinate (*200 mg twice daily*), and melatonin (about *1 mg at bedtime*). You can also add potassium to your diet in the form of bananas, orange juice, figs, bran, apricots, raisins, squash, beans, baked potato with skin, watermelon, or spinach. (Don't take the liquid laxative form of magnesium sold in the green bottles unless you need a laxative; you'll find lots of brands of "magnesium oxide" sold in most pharmacies, but I think another form is better tolerated—"magnesium chelate or glycinate"—and that's why I suggest that you pick up this supplement from your health-food store.)

Other Medications

Look in your medicine cabinet because these drugs can make you feel like a medication mummy too!

* allergy, cough, and cold remedies that contain an anti-histamine

* calcium supplements

* migraine meds

* muscle relaxers and painkillers

* SERMs (Evista, tamoxifen)

* tri-cyclic antidepressants

* supplements for sleep or anxiety containing GABA (gamma-aminobutyric acid)

> *If you think you're taking an "exhausting" medication that I haven't mentioned, ask your pharmacist to look it up and see whether fatigue is a possible side effect. Then ask a pharmacist or your doctor to help you find an alternative medication or supplement.*

Our Amazing Adrenals

One of these glands sits on top of each kidney, each one weighing less than a grape. Adrenal glands use vitamins, enzymes, and cholesterol to create about a dozen hormones that rejuvenate and energize our bodies, including cortisol (a stress hormone); DHEA (which makes sex hormones and balances cortisol); estrogen, progesterone, and testosterone (the sex hormones); and, of course, adrenaline, a.k.a. epinephrine (which gives us that burst of energy to overcome challenges and cope with stress). In fact, during extreme stress, the adrenals help us "power up" in the famous "fight or flight" reaction that sharpens our senses (so we know how to maneuver our car quickly), increases our heart rate (so we can run faster if a Rottweiler is chasing us), and slows our digestion (if our kayak flips over, we don't need to digest food).

If you're a Juggling Janet, you keep your adrenal pilot light burning 24/7 because you're dealing with a collection of stressful issues like debt, work challenges, illness, an insensitive spouse—or little things like traffic jams! Eventually your pilot light blows out and your adrenals come very close to stopping production. As the years go by, you end up with almost no coping chemicals left in your system. Instead of being able to handle the little things the way you used to, you're overcome with exhaustion, mood swings, panic attacks, depression, and irritability.

One terrific solution is to check out the work of one of the world's leading authorities on adrenal burnout, Dr. James Wilson. Not only is he the author of *Adrenal Fatigue: The 21st Century Stress Syndrome* (Smart Publications, 2001), but he also has a website, www.adrenalfatigue.org. Take the "Adrenal Questionnaire" on his website (or in his book) to determine if you have mild, moderate, or severe fatigue. Dr. Wilson offers a tailor-made line of supplements to help you, based on the results of your questionnaire, but you have to go to www.futureformulations.com for those.

> Symptoms of adrenal burnout include early-morning fatigue, afternoon exhaustion, low sex drive, anxiety, depression, confusion, memory loss, brain fog, blood sugar problems, PMS, hot flashes, slow recovery from illness, achy joints, and insomnia. People with adrenal burnout also tend to crave salty snacks and drive themselves harder with caffeine.

Don't Mess with My Water Molecules!

Stress affects our cells even on a molecular level. A Japanese researcher, Masaru Emoto, took pictures of water crystals that were "charged" with prayer or music and compared them with those that had been "stressed" with negative emotions or polluted with dirt. In his fascinating book *Messages from Water* (Hado Publishing, 1999), you can see for yourself the toll stress takes on your body. You'll see images of shattered water molecules, and after all, we are 70 to 80 percent water. Check out Emoto's World of Water website, www.hado.net. And then the next time someone stresses you out, take a deep breath, forgive the person, and walk away because he or she is literally messing up your water molecules! It's better to be happy than to be right!

Hormone Testing

If you want to find out whether your stress hormones are running on overdrive, or totally depleted, Genova Diagnostics offers a great saliva test, the "Adreno-cortex Stress Profile," which accurately measures cortisol and DHEA and gives you a morning DHEA level along with a complete 24-hour analysis of how your cortisol levels fluctuate. The test is done at home but your doctor needs to be a provider for Genova Diagnostics. To become a provider, all your physician has to do is fax them his or her license. Find out more at www.gdx.net. Another terrific option for people who want hormonal testing like this but can't easily convince their physician to become a Genova provider is to take their health into their own hands. That's why I like the laboratory called ZRT Labs. They work with consumers (as well as physicians) directly, and they conduct similar tests to Genova (including tests for levels of estrogen, testosterone, DHEA, cortisol, thyroid, and others). You can call them at 866-600-1636 or visit www.zrtlab.com and order the hormonal test that you'd like. They will mail a kit to your home so you can do the test, and then you mail back your samples in a sealed, prepaid envelope. It's so easy, and I've done it myself. Within a week or two, they mail the results of your test to your home, along with a short write-up about what it all means. You can then go to your doctor and hand over a complete hormonal workup for him or her to review. Some insurance plans will pay for this.

The Care and Feeding of Your Adrenals

Stimulants like caffeinated drinks, sugar, soda, carbs, and fast food may pick you up temporarily, but they'll give you a bigger letdown later. So if you're feeling fatigued, avoid white flour, white pasta, and white rice (okay, a little sushi is fine). But otherwise, cut out the refined flours and grains, which are nutritionally void and contribute to adrenal burnout. And stop skipping meals because you don't have the time to eat! That's the fastest way to create blood sugar imbalances (like diabetes), and you will eventually pay a price.

I would also like you to very lightly sauté or steam greens every single day (chard, mustard and turnip greens, kale, asparagus, or broccoli)—they're high in B vitamins, and will leave you feeling energized and relaxed. These veggies are very sensitive, so make sure they're vivid green; if you cook them until they turn muddy green, you'll lose the precious nutrients. Eat some seafood, too, which is rich in minerals and omega-3s. Get seafood that isn't too high in mercury contamination, such as Norwegian sardines and Arctic char. I also like wild-caught salmon, cod, mackerel, and herring—not the farm-raised fish. Finally, drink plenty of fresh water every day—don't let your lips get dry.

Suzy's Secrets from Behind the Counter

Test Yourself for Adrenal Burnout

Here's a quick home test to see whether you have adrenal fatigue. Sit in a dark room in front of a mirror for about 5-10 minutes to make sure your pupils are fully dilated. Shine a flashlight into your eyes for about a minute. Normally your pupils will shrink to the size of a pinpoint and stay small. With adrenal fatigue, they will likely go to pinpoint size first, dilate, shift back and forth for a few seconds, and then just stay dilated.

Going from Stupor Woman to Super Woman—Adrenally Speaking

There isn't a fast way to repair those tired achy glands that you have taken for granted for so long. But over several months—maybe a year—you can enjoy a great payoff if you take adaptogenic herbs, plant-derived substances that create balance (a.k.a. homeostasis) in your body. I love adaptogenic herbs because they're so smart: They automatically correct what's "high" or "low" while not changing anything that's at a normal level—how cool is that?! I recommend buying combinations of the following adaptogens, which are sold in multitasking formulas. You can buy them individually and try one at a time. Or, if you'd prefer, give one herb a month's trial before moving on.

＊ *Cordyceps sinensis*—Also called "caterpillar fungus," this mushroom extract calms you down, helps you sleep, lowers your blood pressure, and helps with impotence. It's great for energy, which is why Olympic athletes take it. *Dosage: 300–400 mg twice daily.*

＊ **Rhodiola rosea**—This herb from Siberia calms you down, protects your heart, eases depression, enhances your work performance, beats fatigue, and might even help you sleep better. A Soviet study using Russian cadets, published in a 2003 issue of *Phytomedicine,* showed that rhodiola could ease fatigue, improve short-term memory, and control blood pressure and pulse during times of stress. *Dosage: 50–100 mg twice daily.*

✳ **Ashwagandha**—Also called Indian ginseng and "winter cherry," this Ayurvedic herb from India helps you sleep; reduces anxiety, restlessness, and insomnia; and eases arthritis pain and inflammation. Studies have shown that it can even boost thyroid function and control blood sugar and cholesterol. *Warning:* You may want to avoid in peptic ulcer disease, and do not combine this with prescribed tranquilizers. *Dosage: 400–500 mg two or three times daily.*

✳ **Panax ginseng**—Also known as Korean ginseng, this herb improves adrenal function and sex drive; stabilizes blood pressure and energy; and brings your ratios of cortisol and DHEA into a healthy range. You're taking too much if you get acne or facial hair, but side effects are unusual with normal dosing. *Dosage: 200 mg two or three times daily.*

✳ **Licorice root**—Also known as "glycyrrhiza," this herb wakes up your adrenal glands, boosts immunity, and clears up eczema and psoriasis. Only "whole licorice root" supports the adrenal glands, whereas another popular version, "DGL," only supports gastric health. *Dosage: 500–1,000 mg before meals and at bedtime, 4 days a week.* Note: excessive use can cause heart problems.

The following are some other nutrients needed to build up your energy reserves. You can find them in various combinations or buy them individually. You don't need to take them all, so I've listed them in the order that I would try them. Check out the first few, and if they don't work or if you feel you need something more, move on to the next—let your instincts be your guide. When building a regimen for yourself, it's best to bring in one new supplement each week to make sure you feel well on everything.

✳ **Pantethine or B$_5$**—The perfect B vitamin, it works specifically for adrenal health, preventing infection, normalizing cholesterol, and overcoming fatigue, whereas low levels of B$_5$ can cause exhaustion, low appetite, burning hands and feet, and hair loss. Grains, nuts, beans, rice, and yeast are rich in B$_5$, or supplement with *500–1,000 mg per day.* Cost: $20–$30.

❋ **Magnesium chelate or glycinate**—You need magnesium to make adrenal hormones and fight fatigue. These types of magnesium are easier to absorb and easier on the stomach. It's also fabulous for leg cramps, depression, and fibromyalgia pain—but be careful; too much magnesium can cause diarrhea, especially if you buy the "sulfate" or "citrate" form of magnesium. Get the capsules or tablets of magnesium, not that liquid laxative in the green bottle that pharmacies carry! Solaray, Solgar, and Now are three great capsule/tablet brands. Try *200–300 mg once or twice a day.* Cost: $10–$20.

❋ **Vitamin C**—You need C to restore cortisol levels to normal after a stressful incident, or during periods of prolonged stress. The better Cs are either buffered or sustained-release with a ratio of 2:1 ascorbic acid: bioflavonoids. Take about *500 mg twice daily.* Cost: $15–$20.

❋ **DHEA (dehydroepiandrosterone)**—You might be low on this steroid if you're fatigued, so taking a supplement may boost your energy levels, but it's important to have your levels tested before taking this particular supplement because it sparks production of estrogen and testosterone. If you are low, try it for eight weeks, then take four weeks off so that your body can learn to produce its own DHEA again. You can repeat the cycle once if necessary. I also like DHEA creams; some are sold OTC (like Life Extension or Life-Flo), while others are prescribed by your doctor and compounded in specific dosages to custom-fit your needs. Remember, DHEA is a steroid hormone, so don't fool around with it. Too little DHEA may cause fatigue, low sex drive, bone loss, and depression. Too much can cause hair loss, not to mention that it might also promote hormone-driven cancers. So please, test to find out if you really need it, and if that's not possible, take only a low dose for a short time and only with the blessings of your doctor. There is a newer safer version of DHEA sold now called 7-Keto and this does not increase growth of hormone-driven cancers. Cost: $15–$20.

❋ **R-lipoic acid**—This super antioxidant helps mitochondria—the cell's motor—generate energy. It's terrific for people with blood sugar imbalances, pesticide exposure, and peripheral neuropathy pain. *50–100 mg every morning.* Alpha lipoic acid is similar and just fine as an alternative if you prefer, but take a higher dosage: *100–200 mg every morning.*

✻ **Essential fatty acids**—Fish oils that contain the essential fatty acids EPA/DHA help reduce inflammation and pain. *Dosage: 1,000 mg twice daily with meals.* You'll get more benefit from them if you also eat lots of colorful fruits and veggies, or else take an antioxidant supplement.

Remember, it's not the amount of stress in your life that matters; we all have stress in our lives to some degree. It's how you decompress. No matter what we're dealing with, we still need to get enough sleep, relax more, catch a funny movie, watch the sunset, or get a massage. Anything that nourishes our spirits helps ease fatigue, but walks in nature, exercise, meditation, and hobbies that we love are great ways to decompress and energize the soul. "Working Wandas," pay attention to this because you are the type of woman that can especially benefit.

Thyroid Exhaustion

Your thyroid is a butterfly-shaped gland located at the base of your throat. It produces the thyroid hormone, which regulates energy and body temperature, among other things.

If you think you're a "Morning Mary," you might have low thyroid, a condition known as hypothyroidism, which means you feel sluggish, tire easily, are sensitive to cold, and look pale. You may have lost the outer edges of your eyebrows; have trouble shedding weight; and struggle with low blood pressure, low body temperature, constipation, high cholesterol, and nighttime cramps. You may get dizzy when you get up; feel depressed; or have puffy eyes, thin brittle fingernails, dry skin and hair, hair loss, or ringing in your ears (tinnitus). And of course, you'll feel little or no desire for sex. Sometimes, nourishing your adrenal glands is all it takes to correct thyroid imbalances, so please balance your adrenals before taking thyroid medication.

Low thyroid is primarily a women's problem, so it's safe to say that estrogen—the female hormone—plays a role somehow. That's because estrogen is a drug mugger that steals tyrosine and zinc from our bodies, and we need both of those to make enough thyroid hormone. Estrogen also regulates our use of zinc and copper, which in turn regulate thyroid function, sex drive, and mood. Minerals such as these have serious overdose consequences so don't just supplement with them indiscriminately unless you are sure you are deficient.

A high copper-zinc ratio could produce hypothyroidism. (A low copper-zinc ratio produces the opposite condition, hyperthyroidism—characterized by nervousness, hand tremors, palpitations, insomnia, weight loss, light periods, fatigue, and sensations of feeling hot.) A *New England Journal of Medicine* study has also confirmed that estrogen can increase protein binding of thyroxine, a precursor to active thyroid hormone, which leaves less "free" thyroid hormone floating around where you need it. The result? Again, fatigue in the form of hypothyroidism.

Typical blood tests taken at your doctor's office don't always reveal low thyroid because they only measure certain types of thyroid hormone. If a blood test does prove your thyroid hormone to be low, you will probably be prescribed thyroid medication containing precursor hormones that your body has to activate. These drugs include Synthroid, Levoxyl, and Levothyroxine. Armour Thyroid is a combination and contains both active hormone and precursor hormones, making it a more effective prescription choice for most people.

Unfortunately, many people with low thyroid slip through the cracks because their condition is "subclinical"—not detectable by regular tests. People who regularly have a low pulse or low metabolic temperature are usually hypothyroid, so if you think you've got low thyroid and your doctor can't find evidence of it, I have a clever idea for you. One thing you can do is take your underarm (axillary) temperature.

Use a regular glass thermometer and shake it down before falling asleep. In the morning, when you first start to rouse, reach for the thermometer and put it deep in your armpit. Lie still in your bed (you can read if you want) for about ten minutes, or fifteen minutes if you're overweight (since in that case, your body needs more time to reach its metabolic temperature). Glass thermometers are hard to find these days. It's okay to use a digital one if that's all you have. When it beeps, you have your temperature. If your temp ranges between 97.8 and 98.2 degrees F, thyroid isn't your problem, but readings less than 97.8 generally indicate either hypothyroidism or hypoadrenalism (adrenal burnout). Also, a hypothyroid temperature is generally stable and low, while a hypoadrenal temperature varies.

Because the thyroid is connected chemically with the adrenals, many people have both conditions—hello, Stupor Woman! I suggest keeping a two-week record of your morning temp and sharing it—and your con-

It's best to take your thyroid medications and supplements first thing upon arising in the morning, on an empty stomach, thirty to sixty minutes before breakfast.

cerns—with your doctor so he or she can find out which of your body's systems are actually affected. You'll need lab tests for conclusive evidence. Genova and ZRT offer home testing kits to help uncover the cause of your fatigue.

Feed Your Thyroid

Cigarette smoke lowers your production of thyroid hormone, so try to avoid it. And stick to limited servings—one or two per day—of grapefruit, soybean products, broccoli, and cabbage. The breast- and prostate-protective supplement known as Indole-3 Carbonil (I3C), derived from cruciferous veggies, might also lower thyroid levels, so keep your dosage to *200 mg once daily if you have hypothyroidism.* Keep these foods to a minimum, because they can lower thyroid too: turnips, peanuts, pine nuts, and millet.

When cooking, choose olive, grape seed, and coconut oil rather than soy oil. Buy certified organic foods because pesticides and xeno-biotics (see Chapter 12) harm the thyroid gland and lower production of thyroid hormone.

A very good resource for people with thyroid disease is The Broda O. Barnes, M.D. Research Foundation (www.brodabarnes.org).

On the other hand, meats, dairy, eggs, beans, nuts, bananas, and avocados are great sources of tyrosine, which boosts thyroid hormone. Seafood and seaweed are excellent sources of iodine and some other minerals needed to make thyroid hormone. Nothing beats seaweed when it's served up as wakame, or my favorite—a tuna roll with spicy mayo and ginger!

Going from Stupor Woman to Super Woman—Thyroidally Speaking

You can kick-start your thyroid gland with any of the OTC products I list below—no doctor required! Buy them separately and see how you feel for a month or two; or for a serious kick-start, get a combination formula. One good combo is Enzymatic Therapy's Thyroid & L-Tyrosine; another is Thorne Research's Thyrocsin.

  * **Natural salt**—This type of salt contains naturally occurring trace minerals such as iodine, magnesium, potassium, and iron. The cool

thing about these salts is that they're very similar to the salt in our bodies and they haven't been heavily refined, heated, or bleached as has common white table salt (sodium chloride). Our bodies absorb natural sea salts easily, and the minerals they contain support thyroid health. I like RealSalt (www.realsalt.com), or you can find amazing gourmet salts taken from the Himalayas, Peru, and Hawaii at www.seasalt.com. It's important to realize that this type of healthy salt sustains life and promotes health, whereas chemically adulterated or bleached salts are harmful. Please switch your saltshaker!

✳ **Selenium**—This is the best mineral you can take if you have low thyroid (or if you're a man with low sperm count). Selenium content in the soil varies greatly from state to state, so you probably can't tell whether your fruits or veggies contain it or not—but count on bleached white-flour foods being deficient. Selenium can ease thyroid disorders, especially those that are autoimmune-related, and it helps lower your mercury burden. Its best friend is vitamin E, with whom it works to produce energy and reduce the risk of cancer and inflammation. Look for "selenium citrate" or "selenium picolinate" and *take 100–200 mcg every morning.* You can add a 3 P.M. dose if necessary, to feel more normal and energetic throughout the day.

✳ **Tyrosine**—You need this natural amino acid in order to make thyroid hormone, but flooding your body with it isn't helpful because it needs to be in balance with other elements in the body, such as iodine. However, I do recommend a *little* tyrosine because it makes two brain chemicals that ease depression and keep you energized, passionate, and focused—dopamine and norepinephrine. Avoid it if you have uncontrolled high blood pressure or experience heart palpitations. Otherwise, *try 100–500 mg once or twice daily.*

✳ **Iodine**—This trace mineral is not produced in the body, and it is necessary for thyroid, breast, and prostate health. I think that most Americans are deficient because they don't get enough in their diets. Iodine used to be added to baked goods, but forty years ago, laws changed and now baked goods contain the additive bromine. Many scientists consider bromine to be toxic, plus it can deplete iodine, leading to deficiency. Soils are often deficient in iodine too, so iodine levels in Americans have steadily declined over the last few decades. Studies have made a connection to iodine deficiency and an enlarged thyroid (goiter), breast and prostate cancer, hypothyroidism, Reynaud's disease, and fibrocystic breast disease. Low iodine could also cause dry eyes, inability to sweat, dry skin, ovarian cysts, and decreased acid production in the stomach (see Chapter 4 for more on that one).

If you think you have low iodine levels, it's easy to check with a urine test; just ask your doctor. You could supplement with over-the-counter Iodoral tablets sold in health-food stores or online. I like that brand because it's a tablet and contains both iodine and iodide, so it is particularly helpful. Iodine supplements should only be taken when iodine testing shows a genuine deficiency.

A physician can write a prescription for you for the same substance sold as a liquid drug called Lugol's Solution. Unfortunately, iodine is radically misunderstood and feared, so getting your doctor's blessings about this could take perseverance. Studies show that it's generally safe in dosages 100 times higher than the United States Recommended Daily Allowances suggest, and I personally took 50 mg each day for 2 months to correct my own deficiency. That's 333 times the U.S. RDA, but again, I was deficient. Most people do not need doses that high, but I share my story to illustrate the mineral's safety for those who genuinely need it. If you're deficient in iodine, you're at risk for serious illnesses, so it's important to find out your levels, especially if you identified with "Morning Mary" or "Stupor Woman" explained earlier in this chapter.

✳ **Zinc**—This antioxidant mineral is crucial if you take acid blockers, HRT, or birth control pills—or if you're a man (it's essential to the production of testosterone). Typical signs of low zinc include hair loss, low appetite, inability to taste foods, and mental fatigue; in men, add erectile dysfunction to the list; and in children, lack of zinc can stunt growth.

You can find out if you're zinc-deficient in ten seconds. Buy zinc in the liquid form at your health-food store and swish a teaspoon around your mouth. If it registers as bitter and nasty, consider yourself lucky—your zinc levels are in a good range! If you don't taste the zinc, or if it's slightly sweet, you are likely deficient. Foods rich in zinc include meats, liver, oysters, eggs, and whole wheat. Supplement with liquid zinc but start with low doses because this mineral (like any other) is harmful in excessive dosages. Keep track of your progress and stop when you taste the bitterness. Another simple way to supplement is with zinc lozenges, sold widely at pharmacies in the cough/cold aisle. *Typical dosage: 5–25 mg with dinner, or follow the directions on the label.*

To "B" or Not to "B"

Without such B vitamins as folate, B_6, B_{12}, riboflavin, and pantethine, you're going to feel tired—no two ways about it. You want *all* the Bs, too: Think of B vitamins as a concert in which all the instruments just sound better together. A high-quality B-complex once daily will do for most women, about *50 mg each morning;* back off if you get bad dreams, which can be caused by too much B_6. But do take *1 tablet of "body ready" 5-MTHF* (FolaPro by Metagenics), a supplement that can compensate for any inability to activate folic acid, a genetic

Clinical Trials for the Curious

Rhodiola rosea has been used for centuries in Arctic and Alpine regions to help people cope with the cold and stressful environments found there. In a 2003 study of Russian cadets, scientists concluded that the Arctic herb had anti-stress effects and could ease fatigue and boost mental performance. The Soviet study, which was published in *Phytomedicine* that same year, involved 121 healthy Russian male cadets ages 19 to 21. The well-designed double-blind, placebo-controlled study found that those men who took Rhodiola showed increased short-term memory and improved mental capacity (measured by having the men memorize or arrange numbers). We are talking about improved quality, not quantity, of work. And during physiological stress and fatigue, those who took Rhodiola maintained a lower blood pressure and pulse than those who took a placebo. Though the cadets were given dosages of Rhodiola ranging from 370 to 555 mg, the lower dose worked as well or better than the higher dose. If the fatigue-beater works for Russian cadets, it will probably work for you! In case you are sensitive, stick to lower doses, such as 50 to 100 mg two times daily.

condition that occurs in about 25 to 30 percent of the population. I call these people "Folate Misbehavers" because they can't convert folic acid to 5-MTHF. They have a higher risk of fatigue, depression, cervical dysplasia, and cancers of the breast, ovaries, and cervix. Men who are Folate Misbehavers are at higher risk for prostate cancer.

You may also be taking a "drug mugger" medication that is stealing your Bs (see Chapter 26). So "B" on the safe side and supplement with adequate B vitamins. A standard multivitamin won't do it; you will need a full range of B-complex, plus the additional 5-MTHF.

5-MTHF is harder to find, but worth the hunt. It is the active form of folic acid and is natural to the human body. It is the best form to use because it can circulate in the blood and get transported to tissues all over the body.

More specifically, it gets into the brain, so it improves mood, slows down kids with ADHD, and supports many neuropsychiatric conditions that depend on this B vitamin.

Just don't overdo the folate (5-MTHF), because too much can be as harmful as too little.

2

Straight from the Heart

Don't Let Your Ticker Become a Time Bomb

Okay, folks, now here's a lifesaving fact you may not realize: The symptoms of heart disease are everyday things that you easily might never think about—until it's too late. For example, possible symptoms include getting short of breath while exerting yourself; spider veins; unexplained fatigue; swollen ankles; and even bleeding gums (the dreaded gingivitis). Conventional medicine can't promise to prevent heart disease, either; if it could, then heart disease wouldn't be the number one killer of women in the United States—and someone somewhere in the world wouldn't die of it every thirty-four seconds.

Today, most American physicians try to prevent heart disease by using diet, drugs, and exercise to lower blood pressure, cholesterol, and weight. Sure, that's important, but the development of heart disease depends on a number of other complex factors, including inflammation, free-radical assault, nutrient deficiency, "thick" blood, and even your ability to activate B vitamins. The good news? Inexpensive nutrients can help address all these factors and can also reinforce the precious blood vessel walls leading to your heart and brain. Just give me ten precious minutes—they might save your life.

The Problem with Plaques

Consider Sue, a 58-year-old woman complaining of occasional chest pain (she has angina pectoris). Sue's angina is caused by gunk—okay, the technical term is "atherosclerotic plaques"—stuck in the blood vessels that lead to her heart. (Atherosclerosis is also known as "hardening of the arteries.") Sue's blood vessels are probably three-quarters clogged by now, and her cells can't breathe because they aren't getting enough oxygen or nutrients. In fact, the chest pain she gets is the suffocation cry of millions of dying heart cells. She has suffered a long time with fatigue and weakness from an impaired heart and poor circulation, which also explains the swelling in her legs. If the portion of her heart cells devoted to creating and conducting electricity die too, she'll get irregular heartbeats—a pounding sensation in her chest.

Sue is headed down a long, dreary path of drugs or bypass surgery. Her angina pain may be new, but the blockage inside has been building since she was a teenager.

Circulation 101

Let's see how Sue got herself into this condition. Like all of us, Sue has a meshwork of veins, arteries, and tiny capillaries spread throughout her body, which when stretched out would cover half an acre. Think of these blood vessels as your body's pipeline, made up of "connective" tissue that is composed primarily of two substances—collagen and elastin. Vitamin C helps create this connective tissue, which is why a shortage of C weakens your pipeline—and, therefore, your heart. It may also be why, way back in 1985, researchers discovered that high doses of vitamin C mimic the cholesterol-lowering action of a statin drug—but without the side effects!

According to research by Dr. Matthias Rath, when deprived of C, weakened vessels start to form lesions—they actually crack, so that minute amounts of blood begin to leak out. One of the first signs of damage is gingivitis. So if the capillaries in your mouth are inflamed and bleeding, what do you think the other vessels in your body are doing? That's exactly right—they're leaking too. Now, if that process starts in your teenage years, imagine how, over the decades, millions of these microscopic cracks have been weakening your pipeline. But don't worry; your body will try to intervene in an effort to

> Atherosclerotic plaques are nature's plaster cast, protecting a chronically weakened blood vessel. When these plaques break free and get lodged in vessels leading to the heart, it's called a heart attack. Strokes, by contrast, are caused by blood clots that lodge in the arteries leading to the brain.

heal you. Cholesterol sticks to the cracks in an effort to "seal" the weakened blood vessel and repair it. So I like to think of cholesterol as an indicator—a red flag—alerting you to your damaged arteries, rather than the serious health risk that overzealous pharmaceutical campaigns would have you believe.

That said, cholesterol *should* be kept under control—keep working with your physician on that one. But your priority for preventing heart disease and stroke should be stabilizing your pipeline to prevent cracks in the first place. So read the rest of this chapter to find out a number of ways you can support your heart and pipeline. If you're interested in learning more about vitamin C and your heart, read *Why Animals Don't Get Heart Attacks—But People Do* (MR Publishing, 2003), by Dr. Rath. He is a cardiologist and world-famous scientist best known for his groundbreaking work in the field of heart disease.

Suzy's Secrets from Behind the Counter

Chocolate Is Good for Your Heart and Soul!

Okay, here's the best secret I'm ever going to give you: Chocolate is actually good for your heart. That's right. Researchers studied people eating chocolate—where was I?!—and they found that two hours after a yummy dark-chocolatefest, levels of a heart-healthy nutrient called pro-cyanidins went up by a factor of 20. Sweet! Best of all, they noticed that harmful leukotrienes—substances that cause blood clots—went down! If you have no allergies or sugar issues, you could easily justify two squares of dark chocolate a day. Choose the kind that contains at least 70 percent cocoa—just enough to boost your procyanidins, but not enough to torpedo your diet. Read the labels of the chocolate you are drooling for, since the percent of cocoa varies from brand to brand.

Crucial Tests to Ask Your Doctor For

If you think you're at risk for heart disease, I urge you to ask your doctor for the following tests and then to work with him or her to address these conditions. Don't let your doctor jump right to prescribing meds—as I explain below, there are often other steps you can take.

* **Levels of Lipoprotein A**—A blood test can measure how much gunky Lipoprotein A, or Lp(a), is stuck to your arteries, making this test a better predictor than measuring cholesterol levels for sure. If you measure high, try taking Dr. Matthias Rath's formula Epican Forte, which contains the perfect proportions of vitamin C, L-lysine, and L-proline to address this condition. You can find Epican Forte in health-food stores and at www.drrathresearch.org. *Take 2 capsules 3 times a day.*

✳ **Levels of "high sensitivity" C-reactive protein (CRP)**—This is different than a regular C-reactive protein test because it measures how inflamed your body is. The more inflammation, the higher your risk for heart disease and other potentially fatal conditions. You can lower CRP levels with *natural vitamin E (400 IU), fish oil (2,000 mg taken with food twice daily), B-complex (50 mg daily), folic acid (800 mcg daily), Coenzyme Q10 (100 mg daily),* and *fresh grated ginger on your foods.*

✳ **Homocysteine levels**—Testing for homocysteine levels measures inflammation, a major contributing factor to heart disease. Your homocysteine levels also tell you whether you're activating folic acid—important, since insufficient folic acid may also contribute to your risk of heart disease. If your homocysteine levels are high, you'll need to bring them down by taking more folic acid plus vitamin B$_{12}$—these two Bs work together to reduce inflammation. I like Thorne's Methyl-Guard—a combination B formula—but there are many other fabulous products sold OTC. Garlic works, too; *try eating a clove daily or take Kyolic's Aged Garlic,* which is actually patented for its ability to reduce homocysteine levels.

✳ **Fibrinogen levels**—This test checks to see how thick your blood is, since thicker blood puts you at higher risk for heart disease, stroke, and cancer. (Your cancer risk goes up, too, because thick blood means stagnation.) To lower your fibrinogen levels, use worms! Savvy scientists extract a substance called "lumbrokinase" from Japanese silkworms—this stuff actually dissolves clots and thins the blood. Be picky with brands, though, or you'll wind up with nothing more than ground-up earthworms. Eeew! Boluoke is one good brand that was used in clinical research trials, and it's sold to patients from doctors' offices even though it doesn't require a prescription. Your physician should be able to acquire it for you by calling the wholesaler, Canada RNA, at 866-287-4986 (www.canadarna.com). A bottle costs about $95. But you can also go to a health-food store yourself and buy a similar clot buster called nattokinase, a natural enzyme derived from soy reported to reduce blood clotting and therefore reduce your risk of stroke. I like Enzymedica's brand, Natto-K, which I take myself as part of my health routine. Other quality companies that produce nattokinase include Solaray, Allergy Research, Enzymatic Therapy, and Vitamin Research. (For more on how to find these products, see Resources.)

Hormones and Your Heart

It's so confusing! First they told us hormone replacement therapy (HRT) would protect us against heart disease—now they think those drugs are dangerous to our pipelines and our hearts. So what are we to do?

The confusion was heightened in the wake of a huge landmark study sponsored by the National Institutes of Health called the Women's Health Initiative (WHI), which followed some 161,000 women for fifteen years and is still ongoing. One part of the WHI came to a screeching halt a few years ago when researchers realized that women taking various combinations of synthetic estrogen or progestin drugs were suffering higher death rates due to breast cancer, stroke, and heart attack. The take-home message to doctors and women alike is that synthetic prescription hormones, specifically those like Premarin and Prempro that contain horse-derived estrogen, or man-made progestins may do your pipeline more harm than good. On the other hand, natural, bioidentical hormones seem to have far fewer risks to your heart and circulatory system and in some cases protect against cancer. So, ladies, you *must* get in the driver's seat of your own health and find out more about bioidentical versus synthetic hormones. Check out Chapters 10–13, for a start.

Medicine That Can Break Your Heart

Some medications list cardiac arrest as a potential side effect: painkillers containing codeine (Tylenol #3), hydrocodone (Lortab, Vicodin), or oxycodone (Percocet, OxyContin); Viagra (sildenafil); triptan drugs for migraines (Imitrex); and diuretics that deplete potassium levels (such as furosemide). True, cardiac arrest is infrequent—but it's possible, so if you have a history of heart disease, see if your doctor can suggest some alternate choices. ***Never stop taking a prescription med without your doctor's supervision.***

Cholesterol: The Misunderstood Substance

Today, we tend to blame cholesterol for our risk of heart disease and commit to slashing it at all costs. We need to be careful, though: Not all cholesterol is "bad"—only the form known as LDL, part of the gunk that sticks to your arteries [with the help of Lp(a)]. High cholesterol may reflect poor health, or it might be a totally innocent bystander of other destructive forces that you may be overlooking. Of course, it's important to lower your cholesterol, but it's become an American obsession, even though approximately one-half of all heart attack victims don't even have high cholesterol levels!

Now, here's the upside of cholesterol: It helps make pregnenolone, our "Mother Hormone," which then turns into many important hormones such as DHEA (our "youth" hormone), testosterone (the male sex hormone), cortisol (our coping hormone), and estrogen and progesterone (two primary female sex hormones). So if our cholesterol levels ever got too *low*, we'd be more prone to allergies, infections, fatigue, confusion, memory loss, incontinence, and depression. We'd also lose interest in sex and—are you sitting down?—we might even have put ourselves at a *higher* risk for certain types of heart disease.

Suzy's Secrets from Behind the Counter

Sex Is Good for Your Heart!

According to some recent research, enjoying regular and enthusiastic sex—about three times a week—reduces a man's risk for heart attack or stroke by half. They haven't done comparable research for women—but why wait until they do? Tell your partner about this new heart-healthy activity—and explain that you're just carrying out doctor's orders!

Statins: Will They Save Your Heart?

Today's most common statin drugs include Lipitor (atorvastatin), Mevacor and Altocor (both of which contain lovastatin), Zocor (simvastatin), Crestor (rosuvastatin), and Pravachol (pravastatin). Some medications such as Advicor and Caduet are combination drugs that contain a statin along with some other medications to control blood pressure.

Statins work by blocking a natural liver enzyme called HMG-CoA Reductase. Since cholesterol is made primarily in the liver, statin action stops cholesterol production at its source, but it won't affect the dietary cholesterol that you ingest in the form of, say, a cheeseburger.

Statins rank among the top ten drugs sold each year and have brought in billions of dollars for their makers. These drugs may reduce cardiovascular disease for some people, and in 2006, statins were even shown to possibly protect your heart after a heart attack. In 2008, a shocking study came out regarding two popular cholesterol-reducing drugs, Vytorin and Zetia. Even though millions of dollars are spent to pitch these specialty drugs to folks, neither one slowed the buildup of arterial plaques any better than a cheap generic statin.

The problem with statins is that they never truly address one major cause of heart disease, which is a weakened heart muscle and leaky arteries. Plus, these cholesterol-busters are known to cause liver damage, which explains why your doctor starts monitoring your liver as soon as you start taking them. Symptoms such as itchy yellowing skin, dark urine, or abdominal pain need to be addressed by your doctor as they could indicate liver damage.

Statin drugs are likely to cause lots of other side effects, including memory loss, muscle weakness, pain, depression, weakness and cramping in arms and legs, nausea, fatigue, and joint pain. Statins also have some potentially fatal side effects, including pancreatitis, a dangerous and painful inflammation of your pancreas; and rhabdomyolysis, a serious deterioration of your muscles that leads to kidney damage. So if you take one of these drugs, please make sure you are taking the lowest effective dosage and do yourself a favor by cleaning up your diet and taking natural safer supplements that could help you reduce your statin dosage or eventually get off it. Be sure to always supplement with CoQ10 if you take a statin drug to mitigate some of the side effects, such as muscle weakness, fatigue, and cardiac irregularities.

Suzy's Secrets from Behind the Counter

Timing Is Everything

Our bodies make the most cholesterol in the wee hours of the morning, so take your cholesterol meds after dinner or at bedtime.

CoQ10: The Miracle Nutrient?

Clinical research has documented the effectiveness of statins to manage elevated cholesterol, but ironically these drugs may *harm* your heart by depleting a valuable nutrient, Coenzyme Q10 (CoQ10), which prevents heart failure. Yes, statins are drug muggers for CoQ10. The mechanism by which statins lower cholesterol also causes a reduction in heart-healthy CoQ10, which could explain the rising incidence of statin-induced weakening of the heart, a condition termed "cardiomyopathy." Drug manufacturers know about the nutrient depletion effect and how it could damage both the liver and heart. Merck filed 2 patents (in 1989, and again in 1990) on the combination of their drug Mevacor (lovastatin) plus CoQ10 which they have yet to manufacture. If you take a statin, watch out for these signs of cardiac compromise: Shortness of breath, fatigue, fluid buildup in the hands or feet—you may notice your shoes are tight; coughing or wheezing, memory loss, no appetite or butterflies in your chest (increased heart rate). Supplementation with CoQ10 should help you to reverse some of these problems by replenishing what the drug mugger stole.

CoQ10 is vital to our survival—and it's also been shown to help people who suffer from hypertension, migraine, Parkinson's, AIDS, diabetes, and cancer. Better yet, CoQ10 can also lower Lp(a), that icky, sticky stuff that clogs your arteries. Our CoQ10 levels decline as we age and can also be depleted by chronic illness and certain medications—including statins, diabetic medications, and many blood pressure medications.

Our greatest concentration of CoQ10 is in the heart, so when CoQ10 gets "mugged" by our drugs, millions of heart cells die. Possible results of CoQ10 depletion include congestive heart failure, high blood pressure, angina, mitral valve prolapse, cardiac rhythm problems, and stroke—even though your cholesterol ratios are perfect. Depleted CoQ10 levels can also lead to muscle cramps and pain, which, by the way, is a very common side effect of statins that CoQ10 supplementation can relieve.

So if you want to really protect your pipeline, your heart, and your brain, *please* take CoQ10! I recommend *50–100 mg once or twice daily in the morning and/or midday.* If you take a statin drug, then I recommend at least *100 mg twice daily. Don't take it too late in the day because it's energizing and you don't want it to interfere with your sleep.*

Real CoQ10 is bright orange, so make sure your product has the color of quality. I prefer softgels over capsules because you get better uptake into your bloodstream. Some good brands of CoQ10 that are sold in pharmacies and health-food stores include Jarrow, Country Life, Healthy Origins, and Vitamin World. Cost: $30–$40 for a month's supply.

Nature's Best Cholesterol Busters

What if you can't tolerate or afford statins, or choose not to take them? Here's a list of natural alternatives that may work for you.

✳ **Policosanol**—Derived from the wax of such plants as sugar cane and yams, this nutrient can lower your LDL levels, and, with your doctor's permission, you can use it as an alternative to aspirin for anti-platelet therapy. Take *10 mg each evening with dinner.* Since your doctor routinely tests your cholesterol levels, you'll know how well you're responding within a few months. You can always increase your dose to *20 mg each evening* for additional benefit. This supplement is sold in natural health-food stores and online. Cost: $10–$25 per month.

✳ **Red yeast rice (RYR)**—This is nature's statin. It works exactly the same way as prescribed statins, but it's weaker. Since it behaves like a statin, it has the capacity to steal CoQ10 from your reserves, so when you take your *600 mg once or twice daily,* add *100 mg of CoQ10 each morning.* RYR may be able to normalize cholesterol ratios but—unlike statins—with little or no damage to the liver. If you're not already on a statin drug, you can try RYR so long as your doctor says it's okay. Just as with statins, you should get baseline liver tests before you start RYR and while you're taking it—ask your doctor. (It's safer than statins—but anything that involves cholesterol ultimately involves your liver, so your doctor will want to be extra careful.) If you already take a statin, your doctor will need to lower your medication dose or even stop it while you gradually increase your dosage of RYR. You should see effects within three months. Get it at health-food stores. Cost: $25–$35 per month.

Note: Not all RYR supplements contain the active statin to lower cholesterol. After the FDA applied some pressure to the manufacturers of this dietary supplement, some discontinued their products; others removed the statin component, and still others just removed the statin name reference, which seems to have satisfied the pharmaceutical giants. So look on your bottle and see if it has a percentage of mevinolinic acid on it, also called "monacolins." These terms mean that your RYR contains the active statin ingredient needed to lower cholesterol.

✳ **Pantethine**—This B vitamin increases your good cholesterol (HDL) and lowers the bad kind (triglycerides and LDL) as well as bringing your total number down. It also helps produce an all-over sense of well-being and energy as well as mental clarity, so it's terrific for adrenal fatigue. (See Chapter 1.) You can try *200–250 mg once or twice a day.* Cost: $30–$60 per month.

Note: High doses of pantethine are usually okay for a few weeks to really boost the body's metabolism, however, it would be ideal to reduce the dosage to about 50–100 mg every morning for maintenance. Be aware that too much pantethine can cause insomnia.

✳ **Fiber**—Binds cholesterol in the gut. You can eat such high-fiber foods as oatmeal, whole grains, apples, carrots, pears, berries, cabbage, and the like. Or you can take psyllium, a common ingredient in over-the-counter fiber supplements and laxatives, which are often prescribed along with statins. I recommend two high-fiber foods a day, or follow the directions on your psyllium bottle, which you'll find at any pharmacy or health-food store. Consume fiber at least two hours away from your medications.Cost: $10–$15 per month.

Note: Don't abuse the fiber. Taking too much, especially when you don't drink enough water, will cause severe constipation. If that happens, you may need an enema (or two!) and mineral oil to eliminate the hard, dry, impassable stool.

Going the Alternate Route

If you are on a statin or other medication, ask your doctor if you can lower that dosage and bring in something like policosanol for a three-month trial (of course, improve your diet, too!). Your doctor may be so impressed by the results that he or she will keep lowering your dosage or even take you off meds altogether. Work with your doctor to decide whether to punch up the policosanol dose or switch to red yeast rice.

It's okay to eat fiber and to take pantethine and fish oils while taking either policosanol or red yeast rice—or statins, for that matter. My rule with supplements in general is to "start low and go slow," bringing in one new supplement each week, rather than beginning various new supplements all at once. This helps you identify any possible side effects.

How do you know which supplement to start first? Use your intuition. You might give each supplement a 90-day trial and have your levels tested. It is also safe to combine these supplements to enhance their effects. Your body knows.

The Rainbow Diet

Another terrific heart-healthy suggestion is to eat more colorful foods—and I don't mean M&Ms! Intensely colored fruits and veggies are packed with antioxidants, especially vitamin C, and they give you a nutritional punch in the fight against heart disease and cancer. A recent study published in *The American Journal of Clinical Nutrition* actually proved that eating healthy foods can lower your cholesterol levels just as well as some prescribed statin anticholesterol drugs. So try the following ideas—or create your own Rainbow Diet:

* **Orange**—Oranges, a great source of vitamin C, which prevents cracking of your arteries

* **Red**—Pomegranates, a terrific source of potassium and B_6 to lower cholesterol and blood pressure. Don't eat too much if you take statins, antiarrhythmics, or calcium-channel blockers. It can spike levels.

* **Yellow**—Corn provides fiber and folic acid, which reduce inflammation and cholesterol.

* **Green**—Broccoli offers you I3C, a nutrient that lowers your risk of cancer.

* **Blue**—Blueberries contain resveratrol, which slows the aging process and heart damage, and protects against cancers, especially female types.

✳ **Purple**—Eggplant is loaded with B vitamins, copper, and potassium, which controls blood pressure and may lower cholesterol.

✳ **White**—Coconut. Surprise! You thought I was going to say oatmeal for its fiber content, and, yes, that's true—but what you probably didn't know is that coconut oil contains lauric acid, which destroys all kinds of dangerous organisms that might cause inflammation or heart-related infections. Avoid processed coconut oil; instead, use about 1 tablespoon of the unprocessed kind instead of olive or vegetable oil. Spectrum and Jarrow are two brands of organic coconut oil sold at health-food stores and online.

When it comes to drinking healthy, the color I want you to remember is green. That's because the one beverage that will do more to protect your heart than any other is that old health-food standby, green tea. It contains catechins, including EGCG (epigallocatechin-gallate), which lowers LDL and, even better, prevents gunk from sticking to your artery walls and forming clots. Now, you may have heard that red wine does the same task, and it does—but green tea is safer because it doesn't damage your liver, interfere with your driving, or become addictive.

Other Heart-Smart Nutrients

✳ **D-ribose** is a relatively unheard of but well-researched natural sugar that makes our energy molecule, ATP, so it's great for people who are fatigued or have congestive heart failure and coronary artery disease. It gives your heart more oomph with every beat and helps relieve muscle aches, weakness, and fibromyalgia pain. A 2001 study in the *Journal of Molecular and Cellular Cardiology* demonstrated D-ribose's ability to improve symptoms of heart failure. And in 2003, similar positive results were echoed in the *European Journal of Heart Failure*. That journal published an interesting story that didn't make too much news in the United States, but I'm going to tell you about it right now. Scientists designed a randomized placebo-controlled study to see if D-ribose could improve heart function, and it did. Fifteen people were given 5 grams three times a day of either D-ribose or a placebo. After only three weeks of treatment, the echocardiograph measured enhanced heart function.

One terrific source is Morningstar Minerals' Energy Boost Plus (www.msminerals.com). Follow the dosage on the bottle. Cost: $50–$80 per month.

✳ **Magnesium** and **calcium** help balance your pH and lower blood pressure. You can buy terrific combinations of these at any pharmacy. Follow the dosage on the bottle. Cost: $15 per month.

✳ **Vitamin E** keeps blood platelets from sticking together and clotting, similar to blood-thinning drugs but without side effects. It works well alongside vitamin C to prevent buildup of gunk. Take *400–800 IU daily natural d-alpha tocopherol.* Even better, try *a combination form of E that contains both tocopherols and tocotrienols.* Cost: $10 per month.

✳ **L-carnitine** helps you maintain energy, prevents leg cramps, and breaks down fats, especially triglycerides. When you look for this nutrient, you may also see Acetyl-L-carnitine on the shelf. That one is related: It's a specific type of carnitine that is terrific for people with memory disorders. But regular L-carnitine is what I suggest for your heart and muscles. Try *250 mg three or four times daily with meals.* Cost: $30 per month.

✳ **Flaxseed** is for vegetarians who don't want fish products. It's a weaker but still excellent source of essential fatty acids. Buy the ground-up seeds, not the oil, because the oil is so unstable that it goes rancid quickly. Then sprinkle some on oatmeal, salads, yogurt, cereal, baked goods, and smoothies. It's so easy and good *for* you, too!

✳ **L-arginine** keeps your arteries flexible. People with congestive heart failure, angina, and intermittent claudication may benefit. Doses vary widely, so ask your doctor about this one and try not to pay attention to that unfavorable study that came out a couple of years ago, which in my opinion was flawed and biased. I like Thorne's Perfusia SR, a long-acting brand, or CVS's Arginine TR. Morningstar Minerals makes a great-tasting liquid, and of course pharmacies and health-food stores carry other terrific brands. Arginine is easy to find.

 People prone to herpes infections should avoid excessive arginine or else balance it with lysine to prevent an outbreak. You

can supplement with lysine, or eat lysine-rich foods such as beef, chicken, turkey, cottage cheese, yogurt, and milk.

✳ **Fish oil**—This amazing substance comes from fish that swim around the coldest oceans on earth, such as those around Antarctica. Since our own bodies can't produce the essential fatty acids found in fish, we have to eat it, or take supplements like cod-liver oil or omega-3 fish oil. The active ingredients in fish oils are EPA (eicosapentaenoic acid) and DHA (docosahexaenoic acid). These help people with heart disease by normalizing heart rhythm, blood pressure, cholesterol ratios, and inflammatory chemicals. Essential fatty acids also lift depression, relieve arthritis, improve memory, moisten dry eyes, improve blood sugars and allergies, and help slow down hyperactive people and balance mood in bipolar disorder. That's the tip of the iceberg. Take about *1,000 mg EPA/DHA with food*; or if you have established heart disease, take *at least 2,000 to 4,000 mg per day in divided doses with your doctor's blessings*. This may slightly thin your blood—which is a good thing for most people, but do talk to your doctor if you take blood thinners.

Over the years, I've heard people say they get "fish burp" after taking their supplement. If this happens to you once in a while, it's no big deal; don't sweat it. You can try placing the whole bottle of gel caps in your refrigerator to chill them. Swallow each dose cold. You don't have to freeze them; that's not recommended for fresh oils.

The plot thickens if you get a fishy backlash with every dose, even daily. It could be that:

✳ Your product was made with oils that were rancid

✳ You have stashed your formula too long (or near heat) and it deteriorated

✳ You are not digesting fats in a normal, healthy way

By and large, the last is the most frequent cause for those awkward fish burps—which always occur at inopportune times, like during a dental exam or the silent prayer at church. Definitely not inspirational.

It's safe to say that many Americans have lost the ability to properly digest fats. You can improve digestion and stop fish burp with a digestive enzyme supplement, particularly one that contains pancreatic enzymes. It's that easy, and painless. Some people just need a hand to break down the foods they eat. Thorne Research makes a first-class brand called B.P.P., and Enzymedica produces one called Digest.

Take your fish oil supplement and your enzyme while you are eating. Enzymes can be taken at each meal, but one caution: Avoid enzymes if you have a gastric or duodenal ulcer.

Consider krill oil—it's all the rage now, for good reason. Krill are just tiny, shrimplike creatures that provide the same essential fatty acids

Clinical Trials for the Curious

A widely publicized 2004 report by researchers at Johns Hopkins University School of Medicine regarding vitamin E frightened consumers into thinking that vitamin E would increase their risk of dying. The report was a meta-analysis, which is not a true clinical trial, but rather a conclusion drawn by researchers who analyze older studies. The problem is that the researchers sorted and sifted the studies, basing their fear-provoking conclusions on the most infirm and most malnourished participants. In other words, those who would have been more naturally apt to die, with or without vitamin E.

It's a fact that statistics for studies can be skewed in such a way that interpretations become misleading. The Johns Hopkins researchers did point out that their conclusion on vitamin E would not pertain to younger people seeking to reduce their risk of heart disease. Also, the form of vitamin E matters. Synthetic forms of E (like "alpha" tocopherols) do not support heart health, whereas natural forms of E consisting of alpha, beta, delta, and gamma do.

A study can be interpreted many ways, and there are many well-designed trials that have documented vitamin E's safety and efficacy in reducing a person's risk for heart disease, cancer, Parkinson's, Alzheimer's, and even the common cold. The nutrient has proven itself to be a powerful antioxidant, able to sweep up damaging substances in the heart and circulatory system. Therefore, in my opinion, the Johns Hopkins report completely contradicted current medical consensus. If you wish to take vitamin E for cardiac support, take 400–800 IU daily of the mixed tocopherols and tocotrienols of vitamin E in their natural form.

as fish oil, as well as antioxidant protection—but without the fish burp. Krill oil slips into our cells a little easier than fish oil does, and you can find this at your local health-food store, online, at Thorne Research, or at Swanson Vitamins (see Resources).

Beware of some new-fangled brands that are enteric-coated. On the surface, the idea is good because the fish oils dissolve deeper down in your GI tract, and this completely eliminates fish burp. But enteric coatings may interfere with absorption of essential fatty acids, and worst of all, an enteric coating would camouflage the fact that your formula contains impure oils. Most companies producing fish oil are not slimy like that, but as your 24-hour pharmacist, I promise to warn you about unscrupulous behavior in the industry. Now, one more thing. In 2006, the FDA approved a drug version of omega-3s called Omacor, which had a name change to Lovaza in 2007. I don't think it holds any major advantage over high-quality OTC versions, and it's very expensive. However, if you prefer FDA-approved medications over dietary supplements, Lovaza is available. Personally, I have experimented with many OTC brands over the years, always with good results. I especially enjoy Nordic Natural's products. The company avoids excessive heat during manufacturing, and they actually *guarantee* their products to be free of toxins. They are fruit-flavored with strawberry or lemon essence. Nordic's products are often used in human clinical trials that are double-blind and placebo-controlled: www.nordicnaturals.com. Other terrific brands of fish oils are easily found at health-food stores and pharmacies nationwide, costing about $10–$20 for a month's supply. Take them with a meal.

A Broken Heart Can Really Kill You

A study conducted at Johns Hopkins in 2005 and published in *The New England Journal of Medicine* discovered that emotional shock such as the death of a loved one or a breakup can trigger sudden, reversible heart failure, a condition termed "stress cardiomyopathy." The physical cause is the surge of adrenaline and other hormones released from the emotional stress. The metaphysical cause is . . . just a broken heart.

3

Strong Bones and Straight Bodies

Ways to Keep Things Healthy Under the Skin

One of the most frequent questions I get from older readers of my syndicated column is "How can I protect my bones from breaking? I am losing height and scared of a hip fracture."

If I asked, you might say that your own bones aren't the least bit fragile, right? Well, you might want to rethink that. The scary truth is that osteoporosis is a major public health threat and can affect anyone, even women in their thirties. The good news is that it's 100 percent preventable—but you need the facts to arm yourself. So take the following little true-false quiz to find out how much *you* know about osteoporosis, a disease that the U.S. Surgeon General says affects 10 million Americans over the age of fifty, with about 34 million more currently at risk.

Myths and Facts About Osteoporosis

❁ *Only women get osteoporosis.*

False. Women are at greater risk than men, but as of 2006, 2 million men also have osteoporosis, and 12 million more are at risk. Medications are partly to blame, including oral steroid use, and so is the excessive consumption of alcohol. Low levels of testosterone are also a risk factor, so aging men who go through andropause will naturally lose bone mass.

✺ *I drink lots of milk and eat lots of dairy, so I don't have to worry about osteoporosis.*

False. Those dairy ads may sound convincing, but according to *The American Journal of Clinical Nutrition,* your calcium absorption rate is higher from vegetables such as Brussels sprouts, mustard greens, broccoli, turnip greens, and kale than it is from milk.

✺ *My mother was stooped over, so I'm bound to get this disease too.*

False. Family history does not guarantee your destiny. Remember, bone is a living organ. Throughout your lifetime, old bone is removed (a process known as "resorption") and new bone is added to the skeleton (a process known as "formation"). Sure, genetics plays a role, but you have control over many risk factors—and I'm going to help you, too!

✺ *Osteoporosis isn't such a big deal—its worst-case scenario is a broken bone.*

False. Osteoporosis is a *very* big deal because the disease involves a quiet and pervasive deterioration of your bones that eventually causes your vertebrae to collapse or your hip to fracture. Osteoporosis accounts for more than 1.5 million fractures every year, and you might even die if you hit your head while falling from that hip fracture—which, by the way, may give no notice. Or if you're one of the "lucky" ones, you may get earlier notice of impending trouble with back pain, loss of height, or increased kyphosis—that "hump" on your back that signals a weakness in the spinal column.

✺ *Drinking fluoridated tap water will strengthen my bones.*

Well, this one is both true *and* false. Drinking fluoridated tap water has been shown to cause slight increases in bone mass—but some really solid studies also show that too much fluoride can make your bones brittle.

Suzy's Secrets from Behind the Counter
Better to "B" Safe Than Sorry

Osteoporosis is associated with inflammation, measured by our levels of homocysteine. But B vitamins like folic acid, B_6, and B_{12} can help reduce our homocysteine levels, so shield your bones with a 50 mg B-complex each morning–and know that since homocysteine levels are also associated with heart disease, you're protecting your heart as well.

Don't Pig Out on Protein

Here's the number one thing I want you to remember about osteoporosis: It's all about what you eat! For example, too much animal protein in your diet actually robs your bones of calcium—especially red meat, but also poultry, eggs, and dairy.

It works like this: Meat-eaters load their bodies with a large burden of protein, which sometimes contains phosphates. Your body converts these phosphates into organic acids, which get into your blood. Your body has to neutralize the acid with its chemical opposite, alkaline—and guess what the best way to do that is? You guessed it, with calcium that is most often pulled from your bones—a process that, over time, can make your bones brittle.

Granted, what I'm telling you is controversial, because studies are conflicting, and some experts say animal proteins do not affect the development of osteoporosis. But there are lots of studies out there that I personally find more persuasive. For example, in 2001, *The American Journal of Clinical Nutrition* published a study that tightened the connection between meat-eaters and osteoporosis. The seven-year study, funded by the National Institutes of Health, followed more than 1,000 elderly women, comparing those with a meat-heavy diet, a balanced diet, and a primarily vegetable diet. Women who ate the most meat suffered the most hip fractures. You should also know that countries in which people eat less meat have lower rates of osteoporosis and fewer hip fractures.

Open your mind and your mouth to more sea vegetables such as seaweed in the form of wakame or hijiki—terrific sources of calcium, potassium, phosphorus, magnesium, iodine, and other bone-building nutrients.

I'm not saying you can't enjoy prime rib anymore, just tilt your diet in favor of vegetables rather than meats and consider fish as your primary source of animal protein, especially since seafood is rich in other bone-building nutrients, such as essential fatty acids, vitamins, and minerals. You can also take the whey protein supplements sold in health-food stores, adding them to your smoothies for a bone-healthy boost.

You Are What You Drink

Sticks and stones aren't the only things that break your bones . . . certain drinks might too! Did you know that coffee and soda pop can actually weaken your skeleton? Fizzy drinks are loaded with phosphoric acid—and do you remember what I said about acid? It has to be neutralized by your body, which drains calcium from your bones. So teenagers, beware—you may be setting yourselves up for osteoporosis by chugging too much soda.

To make matters worse, caffeine-loaded beverages such as coffee, tea, and soda act like diuretics in the body, flushing out bone-healthy minerals and nutrients. Today's teens are consuming too much soda, which is high in phosphorus and low in calcium. A recent study in the *Archives of Pediatrics and Adolescent Medicine* looked at high school girls who drank carbonated beverages. The authors found that girls who drank soda pop ran a risk of bone fractures that was about three times higher than girls who didn't drink the fizzy cola stuff. The soft drink industry denies that soda weakens the bones. In light of soda's contribution to obesity and tooth decay, it's probably a good idea to limit intake of cola beverages to no more than three servings a week and to drink more fresh water, tea, and juice.

So instead of loading up on calcium supplements that may constipate you, why not conserve the calcium you've already got? Vegetable juice, tomato juice, orange juice, apple juice, and milk might be more bone-healthy beverages. They all contain lots of potassium, which neutralizes acid. And with potassium on the job, your body doesn't have to yank precious calcium out of your bones.

Suzy's Secrets from Behind the Counter
Balance Those Blood-Pressure Meds

If you're taking blood-pressure meds or diuretics (also called "water pills"), you may be losing potassium, which, in turn, puts a strain on your stores of calcium: As we just saw, if potassium doesn't neutralize the acids in your bloodstream, calcium leaves your bones to do the job. To boost potassium naturally, eat some figs, bran, apricots, raisins, squash, beans, baked potato with skin, watermelon, or spinach—or take an over-the-counter supplement, especially one combined with magnesium. Normalizing potassium not only helps your bones but it helps make your heart beat properly too. Make sure you get your doctor's and pharmacist's blessings for oral potassium supplements because the nutrient interacts with a slew of medicines. Supplementing is usually safe and well-tolerated, but I want you to be 100 percent sure it's right for you.

Go Nuts!

Nuts like almonds, Brazil nuts, chestnuts, and hazelnuts are rich in calcium, potassium, and essential fatty acids, so chop some up and drop them into your oatmeal, cold cereals, and salads. Seeds, especially sesame seeds, are also loaded with calcium, so find places to sprinkle them toasted or raw.

Don't Cry over Spilled Milk . . .

Calcium is one of our best lines of defense against osteoporosis. Most Americans get it from cow's milk, but there are lots of other ways to get it. The best way to get it is to bone up on fruits, veggies, nuts, and seeds. By now you may be thinking, "But shouldn't I eat more dairy?" Well, consider that residents of the United States, Finland, Sweden, and England all have diets that are extremely high in cow's milk and dairy products—and yet these are the very countries with the *highest fracture rates in the world*! I don't think that dairy products cause osteoporosis, but I simply can't dismiss a few sound studies that correlate a declining calcium balance with increased dairy intake.

> If you're at risk for osteoporosis, cut back on foods made with bleached white flour or sugar, both of which cause you to increase insulin—which, in turn, can cause you to pee out your precious calcium and magnesium.

Now consider that the National Dairy Council itself funded a study in which postmenopausal women drank enough skim milk each day to provide an additional dose of 1,500 mg of calcium—and yet they were still losing calcium from their bones, according to a study published in *The American Journal of Clinical Nutrition*. The Framingham study also proved that high intake of fruits and vegetables can protect your bones. Switch from animal to vegetable protein as often as you can, relying on vegetables, grains and beans, nuts, and seeds rather than meat, chicken, or dairy. Your bones will thank you!

Suzy's Basic Building Blocks for Better Bone Mass— No Doctor Required!

SUPPLEMENT	DOSE
B-complex	*50 mg each morning*
Calcium citrate	*400–600 mg twice daily*

SUPPLEMENT	DOSE
Magnesium chelate or glycinate	*200–300 mg twice daily (about half the dose of the calcium)*
Vanadium	*100 mcg*
Zinc glycinate or picolinate	*2–10 mg*
Copper gluconate	*1–3 mg*
Manganese	*1 mg*
Vitamin C	*500–1,000 mg per day in divided doses*

You'll probably find these ingredients in your multivitamin formula, but it's highly unlikely that you'll get the proper amounts from a multivitamin. That's why I suggest you buy all these on your own, or even better, simplify your life by taking a combination formula that contains several "bone-building" nutrients. There are many terrific brands sold widely at health-food stores and pharmacies, such as Nature's Way's Calcium Complex Bone Formula. You can also order Thorne Research's Oscap by phone. When you get a dedicated formula for bones, you don't have to take as many pills per day, but you might also have to take a B-complex or some vitamin C separately, since they aren't generally part of bone-building formulas. Read the labels to be sure.

To "D" or Not to "D"? That Is the Question

Vitamin D promotes better absorption of calcium into the bones, and you get vitamin D from sunlight. But Americans are running scared, staying out of the sun for fear of skin cancer. So it's no accident that vitamin D deficiency is at an all-time high—just as the rates of osteoporosis are climbing.

Ideally, you'd get at least fifteen minutes of warm sunlight per day. If you can't get a few minutes of sun, or you take a medication that depletes your body's vitamin D (see Part V), then get some additional D into you. You can eat sardines, fresh wild-caught salmon, and other cold-water fish such as mackerel and cod. Even canned tuna fish has some benefit. If you don't like those or if you're concerned about excessive mercury from fish, take Nordic Natural's Arctic Cod Liver Oil because of the surprisingly acceptable orange flavor. I think supplementing is

In 2006, Harvard researchers found that secondhand smoke from one smoker in the house doubles the risk of osteoporosis in premenopausal women. Two or more smokers, and your risk triples!

ideal because it's so easy to get healthy levels of essential fatty acids in a single gelcap. Nordic exceeds standards for purification on their products, and many research trials have been conducted using their brands.

You can also supplement (yes, in addition to the nutrients outlined above): *1,000–2,000 IU vitamin cholecalciferol (sold as vitamin D₃) per day taken with a meal.*

Stress Affects Your Skeleton

Here's something most people don't realize: Everyday hassles and nonstop pressure can cause your body to jack up production of such "stress" chemicals as cortisol. And if your production of cortisol seriously surpasses your levels of another hormone called DHEA, your body weakens—bones included. One solution is to check out Chapter 1 and find out how to nourish your adrenal glands, which will help balance your production of stress hormones.

Everything You Need to Know About Osteoporosis Meds

Miacalcin and Calcimar

These drugs—prescribed for osteoporosis—are derived from fish (usually salmon). Their active substance is calcitonin, which we make in our thyroid to regulate bone construction. We can also get some from fish—but these potent meds contain more. Allergic reactions are common with these medications. Side effects from Calcimar include nausea, vomiting, and headache, while Miacalcin nasal spray's side effects include runny nose, nosebleed, joint pain, and—can you believe it?—bone pain. In a strange twist of fate, these and most other osteoporosis meds actually *lower* calcium levels in your bloodstream, so you will probably have to supplement with calcium whenever taking them.

Estrogens

We know that after the loss of estrogen caused by menopause, bones have a hard time hanging on to their calcium. That's one reason why doctors prescribe estrogen replacement drugs such as estradiol, Estratest, Premarin, and FemHRT, to name a few. But these drugs aren't the best choice for protecting your bones because studies have shown that synthetic estrogens (and progestin drugs) may compromise your heart and increase your incidence of stroke and breast cancer. In my book, natural and bioidentical hormones are a safer bet—check out Chapter 12 for a complete look at your options. And don't forget soy and flaxseed, two natural safer sources of estrogen.

SERMs

SERMs is short for "selective estrogen receptor modulators." These drugs mimic the effect of estrogens in many ways, except that they trigger hot flashes rather than relieve them. Side effects may include leg cramps, muscle aches and pain, weight gain, hot flashes, rash, leg swelling, blood clots, and possibly uterine cancer (especially with tamoxifen). So if you're taking a SERM, ask your doctor if it's okay to take my Hormone Helpers listed in Chapter 10 and if you can also supplement with calcium and vitamin D as I explained earlier in this chapter.

Bisphosphonates

The three most popular ones in the U.S. today are Boniva (ibandronate), Fosamax (alendronate), and Actonel (risedronate), which in August 2006 got a thumbs-up from the FDA to treat male osteoporosis. I hate to tell you that bisphosphonates have also traditionally been used in the textile and fertilizer industry to prevent corrosion, but pharmaceutical companies have patented them as medicine for people with weak bones.

Bisphosphonates do decrease the rate of bone loss, but while you're on these drugs, your bones don't experience the natural loss and replenishment normally experienced by all living human tissue—and we don't really know what the long-term effects of that will be. I have been asked hundreds of times in my syndicated column whether or not these bone-building drugs are safe because the media has reported dangerous stories. More specifically, some people who've taken a bisphosphonate drug have experienced bone death in the jaw, a condition called osteonecrosis, in which bone tissue dies. The makers of these drugs want to assure people that their medication is not entirely to blame (if at all) and that other factors (such as radiation) may have played a negative role. In any case, don't panic if you're on a bisphosphonate drug because this condition is rare and millions of people have taken the medication safely over the years.

As your 24-hour pharmacist, I will tell you the most commonly reported side effects happen in the stomach and esophagus. If you don't follow the specific instructions on the package, or if you're especially sensitive, the medication can literally bore a tiny hole in those delicate esophageal tissues. Please make sure that you take your medication first thing in the morning and do not lie down for at least thirty minutes after swallowing your dose. These medications can also cause joint pain and muscle aches.

Making Sense of Your Calcium

Calcium is crucial to strong healthy bones, but it's not entirely the answer—you also need magnesium, boron, zinc, copper, vitamin D, and other minerals to incorporate calcium properly. That's why many people buy multitasking combination supplements—the ideal way to go. But let's zoom in on the top-selling forms of calcium in most pharmacies: calcium carbonate and calcium citrate.

The carbonate form of calcium is a salt that comes in grades. Lower grades are used for chalk; higher pharmaceutical-grade calcium carbonate is used for human supplementation. Some readers have jokingly asked if they can just eat chalk (!) for heartburn, but I say no, it doesn't taste nearly as good as Viactiv, Oscal, Caltrate, and Tums. No, chewing chalk is definitely not an option for heartburn or for bone-building. Carbonate is my least favorite form of calcium because after the supplement is gone, your body kicks into gear and makes a lot of acid. As a result, calcium carbonate does help with heartburn temporarily—but then actually makes it worse. Plus, you don't get good absorption out of the gut and into your bones, so it's not that helpful for osteoporosis. I prefer calcium citrate (sold as Citracal) or another type of calcium called calcium "hydroxyapatite" (I like Vitamin Research's brand). Both of these forms are better tolerated and don't depend on stomach acid for their effect, so they can be taken by people who take acid blockers. These forms are less likely to cause kidney stones compared to calcium carbonate, which has been found to increase the risk of kidney stones. One thing about calcium, though: It may cause bloating, cramps, constipation, and gas, so your bones might be strong, but you could be banished to the basement! All three forms of calcium cost about $10–$20 for a month's supply.

Calcium Supplements That I Usually Don't Recommend

✳ **Dolomite, oyster shell, and bone meal** are naturally occurring sources of calcium carbonate. They may contain trace toxins like lead or cadmium, which can cause serious health problems in sensitive people.

✳ **Calcium phosphate, calcium lactate, and calcium gluconate** contain only very small amounts of absorbable calcium in each tablet.

✳ **Coral calcium** comes from the ocean, but it's just a pricey form of calcium carbonate mined from dead coral beds (which are mainly lime-stone). Some patients have told me that they get digestive upset and gas with this form, so it's not my favorite type of calcium.

How to Take Your Calcium

It's helpful to take calcium supplements with food, which helps minimize the gastrointestinal side effects common with calcium. To minimize side effects, avoid taking large doses of calcium all at once. For example, if you're looking for 1,000 mg per day as your total daily dose, then split it into two doses: 500 mg with breakfast and 500 mg with dinner. Formulas that are sold as cap-sules or liquid are generally easier to digest than tablets. Finally, moderation in all things, so don't overdo the calcium, especially if you have kidney disease.

Side effects from calcium supplements include flatulence, gastric disten-sion, constipation, belching, and increased risk for calcium kidney stones. So if you can, get your calcium from your diet instead of from lab-created supplements—your whole body will be happier!

So What Else Can You Do to Have Beautiful Bones?

✳ **Start sweating**—Exercise builds bone mass, especially weight-bearing exercise: weightlifting, jogging, stairclimbing, step aerobics, dancing, and tennis. Plus it makes you leaner and firmer. Pump it up several times a week—and no, chasing kids around the house and vacuuming don't count.

✳ **Take minerals and vitamin D *now*—**It's never too early to start supplementing, and never too late to reverse bone damage.

✳ **Switch your saltshaker—**Get rid of that cheap, white table salt (which is sometimes used for industrial purposes!). This popular seasoning has been chemically stripped of natural minerals and reduced to its simplest form of sodium chloride. I never use it at my house because it is nutritionally void and may cause your body to dump calcium. Instead, use healthier forms like Redmond's Real Salt (www.realsalt.com). Or, for a real treat, look at the amazing gourmet salts at www.seasalt.com (their phone number is 800-353-7258). These specialty salts range in price from $10 to $20 and their gourmet gift sets run about $50, but in my opinion they're well worth it.

✳ **Skip the alcohol—**Drink more water instead, because alcohol harms our osteoblasts (bone builders) and makes it hard to take up calcium and important B vitamins from our meals. In addition, alcohol attacks the liver and pancreas, causing vitamin D production (crucial for bone health) to come to a screeching halt.

Suzy's Secrets from Behind the Counter
Timing Is Everything . . .

Bone-building mineral supplements are best taken at night because calcium is taken up into your bones during the wee hours of the morning. Besides that, taking these supplements later means that you feel fewer gastrointestinal side effects!

Skeleton Builders with Strange Names

I've listed the following skeleton builders in the order that I would take them myself. You can combine them all if you want, adding one supplement to your regimen each week. All of the supplements listed below can be taken along with the Building Blocks listed on page 41.

Lactobacillus Acidophilus, Sporogenes, and Other Probiotics

In my opinion, many disorders start in the gut, and everything we eat is "information" for our body. Probiotics don't build bone, but because they improve the gut lining, they help us absorb bone-building nutrients from our food so that we *can* build stronger bones. So we need to make sure that the GI tract is full of the friendly bacteria to get the most from our foods, vitamins, and mineral supplements. You can get probiotics from eating yogurt, drinking kefir, or taking a probiotics supplement, sold in pharmacies and health-food stores.

Horsetail, a.k.a. Equisetum arvense

Despite the strange name, many cultures have enjoyed horsetail for centuries, using it as a remedy for bladder ailments, gout, and arthritis. Horsetail is actually a plant extract, but it's rich in silica, a mineral that is absolutely critical to bone and cartilage formation. Silica is found all over planet Earth in the form of sand. We need it for lovely skin, beautiful hair, and strong nails as well as for our teeth, tendons, and arteries. Silica helps us use our calcium properly, and I can't resist telling you that seafood, green leafy veggies, and whole grains are rich in silica too.

Horsetail extract is safe in normal doses; you just have to make sure you have the right form of horsetail, *Equisetum arvense,* not its toxic cousin, *Equisetum palustre* (Marsh Horsetail). It's a bit of a drug mugger with potassium, so balance it with lots of the potassium-rich foods I recommend above. *Dosage: 1 gram in capsule or tea form, two or three times daily.*

Ipriflavone

Ipriflavone is a lab-created substance taken from soybeans. Clinical studies show that it is an alternative worth considering in the prevention of osteoporosis in postmenopausal women. It's not viewed as a treatment, although ipriflavone does happen to increase bone thickness. The supplement may possibly lower white blood cells, so don't take it if you're prone to infection or suffering from cancer or any other disease that compromises your immune system. *Dosage: 200 mg three times a day with meals*—and be sure that you are taking *calcium citrate 500 mg twice daily* as well.

Clinical Trials for the Curious

Strontium is a mineral found in grains, just like many other trace minerals, such as zinc, selenium, vanadium, chromium, boron, and so forth. It's gotten a bad rap because the organic, stable form of strontium is sometimes confused with a cancer-causing radioactive form produced by nuclear reactors. What's fascinating about strontium is that it's such a minor component of bone, yet it's a major contributor to bone health. This trace mineral may be twice as effective at building bone than the bisphosphonate drugs Fosamax and Actonel. That's according to two recent large, double-blind, placebo-controlled trials using strontium ranelate, a semi-synthetic version of the mineral available by prescription in European countries and sold under the brand name Protelos. The trials prove strontium plays a major role in skeletal health. In the study, postmenopausal women were given a combination of strontium ranelate along with calcium and vitamin D. Results showed the combo could dramatically build bone mass, reducing the risk for spinal deformities and hip fractures, compared to calcium and vitamin D alone.

In the 2004 study, published in the *New England Journal of Medicine,* strontium ranelate increased bone mass in the spine by 14.4 percent after just a year and a half and reduced the risk of vertebral fracture by 41 percent after three years of use.

Because Protelos is not available in the United States, people who want strontium take the dietary supplement called "strontium citrate," which is sold in health-food stores and online. You'll see it as "strontium" or "strontium citrate" on the label, and versions are made by Solgar, Vital Nutrients, and Pure Encapsulations, among others. One thing here: Protelos is a drug, a patented version of the strontium mineral, whereas strontium citrate is a dietary supplement, so don't expect to find clinical trials backing the supplement. That just doesn't happen too often. But it's clear to me that strontium is beneficial to the bone, in moderate doses. It costs less than $20 a bottle, considerably less than the price of prescribed bone builders such as Fosamax, Boniva, and Actonel.

Warning: Stick to the dosages on the label; more is not better. *Dosages hover around 200–350 mg elemental strontium.* The supplement is best taken in the morning, which allows you to take a little calcium at bedtime. Avoid strontium if you have impaired kidney function. Side effects could include mild stomach upset, though this can be minimized by taking the supplement with some food.

Menaquinone, More Commonly Known as Vitamin K$_2$

K$_2$ is a natural vitamin and a powerful player that helps build bone mass without harm to the liver. It's found in fermented soy products like natto, miso, tempeh, and soy sauce, and also leafy greens. I recently learned from a study that K$_2$ works even better when taken with vitamin D$_3$. You can take K$_2$ as a supplement along with HRT to boost bone mass, or by itself. But do be careful, since K$_2$ also reduces the effects of blood-thinning drugs like warfarin, Plavix, aspirin, and heparin, so your dosage of those meds may need adjustment. You will have to work closely with your physician to adjust your medication dose, and your doctor will probably also want to give you blood tests to make sure your blood is clotting in a healthy way. Vitamin K$_2$ Liquid is available from Thorne Research; *a typical dosage is 15 drops two or three times a day.*

What If You Could Exercise Your Bones Without Sweating?

The first nondrug treatment for osteoporosis is in sight. The Juvent 1,000 is a gentle, vibrating platform that looks a lot like your bathroom scale, and you just stand on it. The gentle vibrations encourage better circulation in your body, improve balance and coordination, and strengthen your muscles. It's currently sold in Europe, Canada, Australia, and online, but the company is hoping to get the FDA's approval by 2009 as a bona fide treatment. Meanwhile, the National Aeronautics and Space Administration plans to install the device on the International Space Station in 2007 to help counter the bone loss that astronauts experience in zero gravity. The cost for this space-age technology (aliens not included) is $2,500 (www.juvent.com).

> *Beware of other brands sold in the U.S. that offer "whole body vibration." The devices made by Power Plate, Turbo-Sonic, and Galileo look similar to Juvent, but the shaking is exponentially more forceful and unconfined. Such technology is designed for athletic training, not for the repair of brittle fragile bones, and it would likely be harmful to people with osteoporosis.*

4

Do You Have the Guts to Throw Away Your Antacids?

So now we need pills to help us eat—has it really come down to that? Why do we rely on so many drugs when eating should be the most natural thing in the world? But yes, many people have to take strong medicine to help them deal with indigestion, heartburn, and reflux. And those who can't afford over-the-counter acid blockers or that "little purple pill" that makes you blue in the face when you put out the "green" for it (a.k.a. Nexium) just put up with these problems or others like constipation, diarrhea, cramps, and gas.

However, the answer to healing your gut once and for all isn't found at your pharmacy—it's in your fridge. So I'm going to teach you how to solve common medical problems by changing what you eat. Don't worry—it will be easier than you think! And in the rare case where you do need acid blockers, I'll tell you how to stay safe on them and replenish the nutrients the drug mugger takes!

Digestion 101—It's Very, *Very* Simple

* Your gut has to break down food into teeny-tiny parts so that all the nutrients, vitamins, and minerals can be absorbed by the rest of the body.

* Your gut has to get rid of useless or dangerous waste from your food.

Yes, it's that simple, yet complex diseases can result when even one small aspect of that process goes wrong. For example, if your gut doesn't have enough "friendly" protective bacteria, what I call "good bugs," then dangerous yeasts, molds, fungi, chemicals, and bacteria can take over, often as the result of your ingesting such medications as antibiotics, birth control pills, and HRT. You're taking the meds your doctor has prescribed—but you're creating new health problems as a result, because your friendly camp of "good bugs" was destroyed. Without healthy flora, you don't absorb nutrients and medications as well either.

For that problem there's a simple solution: Replenish your friendly bacteria with probiotics. Eat a daily serving of kefir or unsweetened yogurt with live active yogurt culture; or buy some probiotics at the pharmacy or health-food store and follow the directions on the bottles. See how easy it is? Look for products that contain lactobacillus acidophilus and bifidobacterium, among others.

So if you want great general health, be careful what you put into your mouth, because food "speaks" to your body. Please, save those chili dogs for a tailgate party! Because when your gut cries out for help, it sounds like this: gas, bloating, diarrhea, constipation, cramps, reflux, or heartburn. And when your gut is more severely weakened, damaged, or torn, it "speaks" in more disturbing ways, including autoimmune disorders, generalized fatigue, anxiety, depression, inflammatory bowel disease, and colon cancer.

Finding Relief from Your Antacids

Like most Americans who suffer from heartburn, you probably don't have the guts to throw away your antacids, and who could blame you? I think every medicine chest should have some sort of antacid, for that rare occasion when that grande bean burrito revisits you at 2 A.M. But if you're taking antacids more than once or twice a month, you almost certainly need to eat differently to prevent the digestive problems from arising in the first place. You also will want to make sure that the valve (sphincter) between your stomach and esophagus stays shut. If that valve is weak and the slightest acid seeps up (refluxes) into your esophagus, you will feel the burn.

Antacids and other gastrointestinal (GI) meds have a number of side effects, not to mention the danger that they'll ease your symptoms without addressing the underlying condition, possibly masking a serious disorder. Let's take a closer look at the conventional options that are currently out there:

Antacids

These sop up the acid in your stomach for quick short-term relief. Terrific—just as long as you restrict them to occasional use. OTC antacids like Mylanta, Riopan, and Maalox usually contain magnesium and aluminum hydroxide.

Some people experience an "acid rebound" effect from these treatments. The antacid works by lowering the acid levels in your stomach, but when the meds leave your system, the acid comes surging back at even higher levels and you get terrific heartburn. Rebound is especially common with antacids that contain calcium carbonate, such as Tums, Rolaids, or Titralac.

If you're going to take antacids, do it while you eat, because that's when the acid is most prevalent in your stomach—it's busy breaking down your food. Antacids will buffer the burn for two to three hours. The most common side effect with aluminum-containing antacids (like Amphojel) is constipation, whereas magnesium-containing antacids such as Milk of Magnesia can cause diarrhea. The possibility of diarrhea increases if either type of antacid includes a "sorbitol" sweetener. I think the best antacids are combinations of aluminum and magnesium or calcium. Two popular brands are Maalox and Mylanta.

Acid Blockers: H2 Blockers and Proton Pump Inhibitors

H2 blockers reduce the amount of acid your stomach makes by sitting at the doorways of your cells and interfering with your own ability to secrete acid. They take more time to kick in (compared to antacids), but once they start, they relieve symptoms for a longer period of time. OTC choices include Zantac (ranitidine), Tagamet HB (cimetidine), and Pepcid AC (famotidine). Their strengths may differ, but their effectiveness is about equal. I'm partial to Pepcid and Zantac because Tagamet has more neurological side effects and interactions with other medications that you may be taking. Pepcid Complete is nice because it combines an H2 blocker and an antacid all in one formula.

Proton pump inhibitors slow down your body's round-the-clock production of acid. However, they won't begin working for about a day, so they're not your thing if you want quick relief. Most of these drugs require a prescription, such as Aciphex (rabeprazole), Nexium (esomeprazole), and Prevacid (lansoprazole). However, Prilosec (omeprazole) is available over-the-counter as Prilosec OTC. Although acid-blocking drugs like this are good at their job, I wish more people and especially more practitioners considered the bigger picture: Why is the acid a problem for this person—and more importantly, is it really the acid that is the problem?

Suzy's Secrets from Behind the Counter
Acid Blockers Are Drug Muggers!

Acid blockers change the environment in your gut by altering the relationship between acid and alkaline, which need to be in balance for good digestion and good health. As a result, acid blockers make it harder for you to maintain healthy levels of folic acid, vitamin B_{12}, vitamin D, and such essential minerals as calcium, iron, and zinc. That's why some people who live on acid blockers end up with painful mouth sores, gum disease, depression, low libido, low thyroid, and anemia. So eat well and replenish with these nutrients every day if you take an acid blocker. I would certainly prefer if you could eliminate these medications once and for all by healing the underlying cause of your troubles, but if you have to take these drugs or were ever on them for more than six months, the following supplements could help you replenish what the drug mugger stole:

* B-complex, *50–100 mg once daily*
* Vitamin B_{12}, *500 mcg daily*
* Calcium citrate, *600 mg daily*
* Vitamin D_3 cholecalciferol, *1,000–2,000 IU daily with food*
* Zinc gluconate lozenges *(10–15 mg), dissolve 1 lozenge once or twice daily*
* Nu-Iron, *150 mg–1 capsule 2 or 3 times a week with food for three months* (back off if you get constipated, and don't be alarmed if it turns your urine or stools dark).

What's Wrong with Acid Blockers?

Okay, this is a controversial topic, and your doctor is likely to tell you something different. But if you'd like to know what your 24-hour pharmacist thinks about this issue, based on almost two decades of experience and research, here it is:

Acid blockers alter your pH, making your stomach less acid and more alkaline than normal. That part's not controversial. But many medical professionals just brush that off as a minor matter, whereas to me, it's major. As we said in

Digestion 101, your gut has to break down food into teeny-tiny parts so that all
the nutrients, vitamins, and minerals can be absorbed by the rest of the body.

Altering your stomach environment and raising your pH (by blocking the
acid) affects your ability to absorb drugs, minerals, and nutrients. It also compromises your ability to digest food normally—both of which could make you
even sicker!

I'm frankly a bit baffled as to why "excess acid" has been identified as a problem in people, especially as they get older. After all, as we age, the level of virtually every other substance in our bodies declines: DHEA, estrogen, testosterone,
thyroid, androstenedione, GABA, serotonin . . . So why would acid go up?

Well, in most cases, it doesn't. Studies confirm that acid levels tend to go
down with the aging process. And some cutting-edge researchers believe that
most people taking acid-blocking drugs actually need *more* acid!

Some people do need to suppress acid, of course, but heartburn is not usually a problem of too much acid—in many cases, it's a problem of what and
how we eat. When stomach acid is measured properly, scientists have found
that the overwhelming majority of acid reflux sufferers have too *little* acid. The
problem is usually related to acid seeping up into the esophagus.

Paradoxical as it seems, knowledgeable physicians have successfully treated
tens of thousands of people who suffer from indigestion, heartburn, and related
conditions with natural, inexpensive hydrochloric acid supplements (betaine
hydrochloride or trimethylglycine) along with enzymes, healing foods, dietary changes, or appropriate prescription meds. The treatment is individually
based, so finding your dream doctor is crucial (see Part V).

Like I said, lots of doctors don't see it this way—but some do, and they may
eventually win over the others. Meanwhile, just remember how many billions
of dollars are spent on antacids and acid blockers each year and maybe be a
little skeptical about why we need so many pills to help us eat. These pills shut
down acid production for temporary relief, but they do nothing to strengthen
a weak valve. They only buffer a burn.

Symptoms of Low Acid—Does This Sound Familiar?

Bear in mind that the following could indicate many other medical conditions.
It's shocking to realize that these symptoms could be due to low acid, yet many
people who suffer with these symptoms are treated for *excessive* acid and given
acid blockers!

* adult acne

* bloating, belching, and flatulence immediately after meals

* chronic yeast infections

* eczema or other skin problems

* hair loss in women

* heartburn

* indigestion, diarrhea, or constipation

* multiple food allergies

* redness or dilated blood vessels in the cheeks and nose

* soreness, burning, or dryness of the mouth

* undigested food in the stools

* weak, peeling, and cracked fingernails

* weight gain

Many of you are probably taking acid blockers to treat these symptoms (which could be a sign of low acid), so you may be making yourself worse in the long run. If you have these symptoms and think you are suffering from low acid, I want you to do some more reading. Don't just go off your acid-blocking drug without your doctor's blessing and another plan of action. It's important to work with a knowledgeable physician, though my experience has taught me that some people will insist on treating themselves because hydrochloric acid supplements are widely available at health-food stores nationwide. So if you insist on self-treating, look for these key words on the label: "betaine," "betaine hydrochloride," or TMG, which is short for "trimethylgycine." Some supplements also contain digestive enzymes along with healthy acids.

Most people who take a high-quality acid supplement experience no side effects and enjoy better digestion. I myself take an acid supplement with every meal. But some people take too much. If you do, or if you take acid when you don't really need it, you'll know in about ten minutes—when you get heartburn! So start at the low end of the dosage and slowly over the course of several weeks work your way up to more—and never exceed dosage guidelines on the label. These supplements are generally taken 15 to 20 minutes before a meal.

Acid supplements aren't for everyone, of course, and they should never be taken at the same time as aspirin, Motrin (ibuprofen), prednisone, or any other anti-inflammatory medicine, except with the blessings and supervision of a skilled physician.

Better Ways to Banish the Burn—No Doctor Required!

✳ Sleep with your bed at a tilt—you can use firm pillows to prop yourself up or invest in one of those fancy adjustable mattresses.

✳ Don't eat within three hours of going to bed.

✳ Don't drink milk at the first sign of heartburn—it could make things worse.

✳ Keep healthy levels of acid in your stomach. There are many brands of acid supplements sold at health-food stores, and Thorne Research makes one called B.P.P.

✳ Keep healthy levels of enzymes in your body (see Chapter 14).

✳ Stop swallowing air as you eat—oxygen in your stomach may cause more burn, especially if you don't produce enough natural acid. If you swallow too much air it will make you burp frequently too. Try not to rush through your meal and don't think about anything that makes you anxious. Make sure your dentures fit properly, and chew your food slowly. It may also help to drink beverages after you've chewed and swallowed your bite. Avoid soda, it's carbonated and makes creates more gas which you have to expel.

✳ Supplement with these gut-detoxifying nutrients:

> SAMe (S-adenosylmethionine)—*200 mg once or twice daily* Look for enteric-coated brands sold at Walgreens, CVS, and health-food stores nationwide.
>
> Vitamin B_{12}—*250–500 mcg daily*
>
> L-glutamine—*1,000–2,000 mg twice daily* (It feeds your small intestine.)
>
> Vitamin B_6—*50 mg daily* (or *20–30 mg* of the vitamin's active form, P5P)

Phosphatidylcholine—*200–400 mg three times a day*

Cod-liver oil—*1 teaspoonful daily* (I like Nordic Naturals': It's enhanced with natural orange essence so it tastes good and it's very pure.)

Better Ways to Manage Belching, Bloating, or Gas

✳ First, dump the dairy. Try cutting down on milk, cheese, and ice cream. If you don't see improvement within two weeks, you can return to your previous dairy intake.

✳ Next, reduce your intake of sweets and carbs, which fuel yeast growth. Yeast contributes to all three of these symptoms.

✳ Then reduce or eliminate "combustible" vegetables and legumes that you know set you off, such as baked beans, green beans, broccoli, potatoes, and turnips.

✳ Try Beano, an over-the-counter food enzyme that stops gas before it starts.

✳ Consider supplementing with enzymes and betaine hydrochloride or TMG, as I explain above.

✳ If the vegetable approach doesn't work, try these inexpensive remedies: Gas-X, CharcoCaps, or Phazyme, all available OTC at your health-food store and many pharmacies. And until these approaches start working, save your marriage—sleep in the other room!

Get to the Bottom of Your Problems!

If you have completed various treatments to no avail; if you take GI meds of any sort routinely; or if traditional stool tests at your lab haven't pointed the way to a successful treatment, I want you to get tested again, this time by a special lab that does better detective work. My two favorites are EnteroLab in Texas (www.enterolab.com) and Genova Diagnostics in North Carolina (www.gdx.net). Both will provide you with awesome home test kits. Only practitioners can use Genova's test, and your own doctor can become one of their practitioners just by faxing them his or her license. You don't have to have a doctor order these specialized tests. EnteroLab.com sells their test kits directly to the public. Test results are easy to understand and can be shared with any doctor or used for self treatment.

Cleanse and Detoxify

If you're really serious about getting and staying healthy, consider Thorne's Medi-Clear or Metagenics's Ultra InflamX to reduce inflammation, improve many uncomfortable GI problems, heal your gut, and basically make you feel better! They contain nutrients and botanicals that work synergistically—better together than alone. I've tried both and been recommending them successfully for years.

Folk Remedy in Your Fridge—The Bitter Taste of Relief

There's an old folk remedy for heartburn that some people swear by: one glass of water with one tablespoon of apple cider vinegar. To make it more palatable, you can add some honey. Or you can include apple cider vinegar in your daily diet as a salad dressing with fresh oil, or in cole slaw. It works because it provides your gut with a form of acid—and recall that many people are acid-deficient.

Symptoms and Possible Solutions

* **Bad breath (halitosis)**—Try a liver detox (cut out alcohol, caffeine, fried foods, preservatives, and high-fat foods for three months) OR go on a candida diet (no sugar or foods containing yeast for three months) and take probiotics.

* **Constipation**—Take probiotics and eat foods rich in fiber (apples, pears, berries, carrots, broccoli, and whole grains).

* **Gas and bloating**—Try enzymes (lipase, amylase, and protease) as well as healthy forms of hydrochloric acid (betaine HCl). Enzyme formulas should generally be avoided in patients with gastritis or ulcers.

* **Hemorrhoids**—Eat fiber-rich foods, drink lots of fresh pure water, and take silica supplements derived from spring horsetail (*equisetum arvense*). I recommend *500 mg three times a day*. I like the Natural Factors brand. Also take Thorne's Diosmin HMC, specifically formulated to help ease hemorrhoids and varicose veins—just follow the directions on the label.

One Man's Meal Is Another Man's Poison

Remember the famous saying? Well, it's true. Why do some people enjoy a cool glass of milk while others wind up with diarrhea, cramps, gas, and allergies? Because some people can't break down milk's protein and instead form antibodies to it. In most people, the sensitivity is due to casein, but there are other protein offenders which become a trigger that sets off discomfort in your body.

Why can some people happily eat whole-wheat bread, breakfast cereals, and pastas, while others develop autoimmune diseases from them? Because some people can't break down wheat, wheat products become a poison to them.

You're born with some sensitivities; others you acquire, especially if you beat up your body with bad foods that create tiny holes in your GI tract, a condition called "leaky gut." Otherwise harmless proteins find their way out of tiny holes in your damaged gut, bum a ride in your bloodstream, and take up residence in various organs, your brain included. To defend you, your brain sets off a full-body alarm, including a cascade of "protective" chemicals that can affect your breathing, circulation, and other bodily functions. Your body is trying to keep you well—but instead, it's making you sick because it's attacking the protein which is now circulating!

For example, Sandy doesn't know she's allergic to casein, even though she visits her doctor frequently with complaints of allergies, bronchitis, fatigue, and asthma. To help her temporarily deal with her symptoms, she takes the best our pharmacy has to offer—strong antibiotics, antihistamines, nasal sprays, and inhalers—which costs her $300 to $400 per month and years of needless suffering. She could spare herself a lot of pain and expense if she'd realize that she's casein-intolerant. For her, rice milk, soy milk, and almond milk would be better choices, and if she wanted an animal-derived milk, then goat milk would be a choice.

Or consider Audrey. She's had multiple sclerosis (MS) for years, as well as headaches, lack of coordination and balance, and deterioration of the nervous system. Gluten—a protein found in wheat, rye, barley, and gluten-contaminated oats (oats processed in factories that process other grains)—is triggering her immune system to send her brain a desperate message: "We are under attack!" So Audrey's body releases a crew of inflammatory chemicals to defend her body from the perceived poison. These powerful chemicals are supposed to destroy toxic invaders. Instead, they are slowly destroying Audrey's own body in this painful autoimmune disease. Other symptoms of gluten sensitivity include abdominal bloating, pain, heartburn, gas, diarrhea, constipation, fatigue, joint pain, osteoporosis, and possibly infertility. The scariest and least-talked about symptoms of gluten intolerance are the neurological changes such as neuropathy, brain fog, headache, memory loss, gait ataxia, and MS-like symptoms.

A small but significant study published in the *Journal of Neurology* found that when ten patients with MS were put on a gluten-free diet, nine of them experienced relief from their symptoms within months. Could Audrey's body relax and begin to heal if she stopped eating gluten?

Of course, there are many other conditions with symptoms similar to Sandy's and Audrey's, so I don't want you jumping to conclusions. But you might at least consider the possibility that you're suffering from food sensitivities and perhaps find a nutritionist or a physician who's open to helping you sort through different hypotheses.

Thyroid Conditions and Gluten Sensitivity

Figures vary, but approximately 1 in 120 to 300 people are gluten-sensitive. I've heard other experts say that number is closer to 30 percent. And if you have irritable bowel syndrome (IBS) or any type of autoimmune thyroid disorder—including Graves' disease, Hashimoto's, and autoimmune thyroiditis—you have an even greater possibility of being gluten-sensitive. That's because when you were just an embryo, your thyroid shared cells with your nervous system and your gut. Now, as an adult, your thyroid gland still shares the same triggers as your gut, so the foods that send off an autoimmune alarm play havoc with your thyroid as well as your digestive system. Accordingly, research shows that people with autoimmune thyroid disease often have gluten-related GI disorders as well, including celiac sprue, a form of gluten sensitivity.

If you think your thyroid or other conditions may be aggravated by gluten, avoid all gluten-containing foods for at least three months—six is even better. If your thyroid condition improves, your doctor may even be able to lower your medication dose. Some people do go through a withdrawal phase in which symptoms actually worsen for a few weeks, but that's rare.

Diseases Associated with Gluten or Casein Sensitivity

 ✳ Autoimmune disorders (lupus, multiple sclerosis, rheumatoid arthritis, Graves' disease, Hashimoto's, celiac sprue, Sjogren's Syndrome)

✳ Psychiatric or neurological disorders such as Parkinson's, dementia, autism, schizophrenia, attention deficit hyperactivity disorder (ADHD), or epilepsy

✳ GI problems (Crohn's disease, irritable bowel syndrome)

✳ Fibromyalgia or chronic fatigue immunodeficiency syndrome (CFIDS)

✳ Diabetes, especially if cow's milk was given too early in infancy

✳ Skin conditions (psoriasis, eczema, scleroderma, itchy or chronic rashes)

✳ Respiratory problems (asthma, bronchitis, sinusitis, earaches)

✳ Osteoporosis

> A good, gut-friendly diet includes lots of fresh fruits and vegetables—preferably organic—as well as nuts, seeds, hormone-free meats and poultry, and fish. Drink plenty of fresh, clean water—and feel free to juice.

Reintroducing Gluten and Casein

The best physicians disagree: Some feel that once you are sensitive, you are sensitive for life (although your sensitivity level may vary over the years). Others say that sensitivities can be overcome simply by eliminating the offending food for a year or two and then slowly reintroducing it. You'll just have to experiment and see what's right for you—or work with a nutritionist, naturopath, or physician whom you trust. Keep in mind that there is a continuum with food intolerance. For example, while most people deal with mild problems with wheat, others develop serious conditions like celiac sprue. People with celiac should eliminate wheat. A simple (anti-tTG) blood test can detect celiac. If you don't test positive, you may still be intolerant to wheat. People experience sensitivity in their own unique ways.

This reminds me of a study published in the *Annals of Rheumatic Diseases,* which discussed three people who were diagnosed with lupus (systemic lupus erythematosus, or SLE). They were treated for years with various strong immune-suppressing drugs and steroids. Then, during the study, they were found to be gluten-sensitive, not afflicted with lupus after all. The scientists

Clinical Trials for the Curious

The condition known as celiac's disease really describes a gluten allergy, and I suspect that many autoimmune disorders are driven by wheat allergies. How can a loaf of bread cause so many problems? Follow the trail of crumbs to the brain of a sensitive person and see how destructive gluten is. In a 2006 study published in the *Journal of Neurology*, researchers tested 215 people with neuropathy—a condition that causes burning, tingling, or "pins-and-needles" sensations most often in the hands or feet, but also in the face and other parts of the body. Gluten sensitivity was found in almost one-third of the patients (29 percent) with neuropathy. Could we conclude that adhering to a strict gluten-free diet would translate to less pain? This particular study did not determine this, but in my opinion, it's worth a try because the condition is maddening for those who are afflicted with it.

In another interesting study published in the *Journal of Neurology, Neurosurgery, and Psychiatry* in 2003, researchers put 43 patients on a gluten-free diet for one year to see if their "gluten ataxia" (loss of coordination) would resolve. After one year, there was significant improvement in the gluten-free group.

---

concluded that a person can have non-intestinal symptoms of gluten allergies, and determining the correct diagnosis is crucial.

If you want to try reintroducing gluten and/or dairy, here's what you do:

＊ Eliminate the offending substances for six months to a year, as long as possible.

＊ After that, bring in gluten-containing foods only (still leaving out the milk and other dairy) and see how you do.

＊ If after a few months you are still feeling well, then bring in the milk and other dairy and see how you do. Within a few weeks, you'll know whether you need to get back on your diet.

You should be able to tell when something triggers your sensitivities because you get those old symptoms—indigestion, headaches, brain fog, fatigue, diarrhea, and all the rest. You may get different symptoms, too, which is why some researchers believe your sensitivity persists for life.

part II

Above the Neck

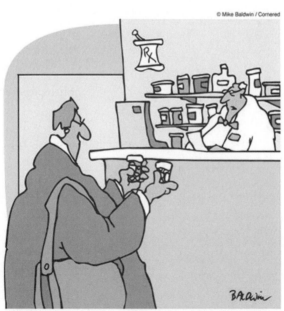

© Mike Baldwin / Cornered

"Take the green pill to feel hunky, the
yellow pill to feel dory."

5

Antidepressants

Do You Need One to Be Happy?

Depression can churn through your life like a hurricane, leaving devastation in your home, your workplace, and, of course, your body, where it all spawned. An estimated 15 million American adults are afflicted with major depression—it's the leading cause of disability in the United States in people ages 15 to 44.

Depression afflicts women far more frequently than men. In fact, many women sink to an emotional low around the age of 30 with no apparent explanation. Here's the good news: The tips I share with you in this chapter can help both recent and long-time sufferers, even the ones who have tried everything. So take heart and read on!

Despair and Depression: The Many Faces of Sadness

For most people, the blues are fleeting and go away on their own within days or weeks. But for millions, depression lingers for months, even years. When you're depressed, you feel empty and numb. Nothing seems to matter and you feel irritable, confused, and unable to concentrate or even to make simple decisions. Insomnia comes with a lot of emotional and physical baggage, including weight problems—either losing a lot or gaining too much. You try to pull yourself together, but feelings of guilt and worthlessness override your efforts. Tears fall for no reason and without warning.

Depression Comes in Many Forms:

✳ **Dysthymia (neurotic depression)**—This is chronic depression with a long history of poor self-esteem and despair. Your mood is generally down but doesn't reach the lower depths.

✳ **Manic-depression (bipolar disorder)**—Your mood swings high and low, from happy and frenzied to sad and hopeless, perhaps with some "normal" periods in between.

✳ **Postpartum depression**—This is the depression and anxiety that occurs after the birth of your baby. Teenagers and women with a history of depression are most often affected because of the rapid drop in hormones that occurs after a baby is born.

✳ **Anxious depression**—When depression combines with anxiety, this is the result, perhaps including some aspects of obsessive-compulsive disorder (OCD), suicidal thoughts, and hypochondriac fears of illness.

✳ **Agitated depression**—In this case, depression is hallmarked by agitation and may also include insomnia, panic attacks, and a general sense of dread or doom.

SSRIs: Not So Sexy

One of the most popular types of antidepressants is the Selective Serotonin Reuptake Inhibitor, or SSRI for short. Blockbuster SSRIs—Paxil, Prozac, Zoloft, Celexa, and Lexapro—can do wonders for your mood, but they also take the punch out of your pajamas. They can squash sex drive, delay orgasm, create impotence, lead to painful erections, promote pain on climax, cause premature ejaculation, and lead to penile "anesthesia." I don't know anybody who's in a good mood when their sex life is ruined, so consider switching to a medication that is less sexually disruptive (Buspirone or Effexor, or one of the older tricyclics) or ask your doctor for a prescription of cyproheptadine and amantadine, two drugs that barge in and counteract sexual side effects for some people.

You can also try a natural over-the-counter antidote—ginkgo biloba. Yes, that's the same herb that's used for memory loss. It works by restoring blood flow to the genitalia, which SSRIs tend to block. Try *60–120 mg, three or four times a day for as long as you're taking SSRIs.*

Drugs Don't Work Forever

Prescription antidepressants may work well for you at first—but over time, they often lose their effectiveness. Generally, prescribed antidepressants such as SSRIs (the most popular) help your brain retain the hormones that boost your mood—but they don't make any more of these important chemicals. So for a while, your brain is fooled into thinking that hormone levels are higher and your mood improves, but after a few months or a year, the effect wears off—and you're still suffering from your original shortage of brain chemicals. In fact, you may feel even worse after you stop your meds: Deceived by the temporary drug-induced good mood, your brain has become far less efficient in using tiny amounts of hormone, so now you've got a small supply of hormones *and* you're using them less efficiently.

The answer? Nutritional supplements and "Good Mood Foods." That way, when your meds lose effectiveness, your brain is in better—not worse—shape than before. Don't underestimate the impact of food. More serotonin is produced by your gut than by your brain, so eating healthy, living foods really can improve your mood.

Foods to Fight the Blues: Good Mood Foods

Eat small, regular meals and snacks to keep your stomach full and your blood sugar levels steady. Make sure your diet is rich in the following foods:

* whole grains and legumes

* nuts and seeds, especially walnuts, almonds, and flaxseed

* lots of fresh fruits and vegetables, especially green leafy ones like kale, chard, and turnip greens

* lots of low- or nonfat dairy: skim or 1% milk, reduced-fat cheese, nonfat yogurt

✳ high-quality, low-fat protein: turkey, fish, organic chicken, cage-free omega-rich eggs, tofu—in small amounts if you've been diagnosed with "agitated" depression (in which you frequently feel angry and upset); in high amounts if you've been diagnosed with "sluggish" depression (in which you frequently feel sluggish and tired)

✳ Also, cut back on sugar, refined carbs, alcohol, caffeine, and processed foods. They may taste good momentarily, but their initial high is often followed by a depressing "crash," plus they alter your body's ability to produce happy brain chemicals.

Step Away from the Chocolate!

Ice cream, chocolate, truffles, and cookies—these delicious treats can literally medicate you. Evidence proves that sweets make your brain release endorphins—chemicals that make you feel more blissful, less achy, and less cranky. And that's not all. About an hour after indulging in such melt-in-your-mouth luxuries, the mood-boosting hormone serotonin joins the party.

Alas, this sweet effect works temporarily, but it only makes your condition worse in the long run. Sugar highs are usually followed by the sugar blues, as your blood sugar crashes and you feel worse than before. Sugar contributes to weight gain, which can promote depression, for both physical and psychological reasons. As if that weren't enough, sugar feeds candida, an otherwise natural yeast that grows out of control in the presence of excessive sugar and starches. Candida overgrowth can also cause depression, among other things—so pass on the desserts until your mood improves.

Downer Drugs

If you haven't felt like yourself lately, and if you can't identify a specific loss, stress, or anxiety, check inside your medicine cabinet. More than 1,200 drugs can cause or worsen "depression." In an August 2006 study published in the *Archives of General Psychiatry,* researchers examined nearly 5,500 adults and children ages 6 to 18. They concluded that those treated with antidepressants were about 1.5 times more likely to attempt suicide, and 15 times more likely to die of the attempt, than those not treated with an antidepressant.

The FDA now requires that antidepressants be packaged with literature warning that these drugs have been associated with suicide and thoughts about death, especially in children and teens. Stop in at any pharmacy and ask for a free "patient package insert"—the little paper that has all that fine print and unadvertised side effects on it. Here are a few of the major downer drugs—so ask your pharmacist if you suspect that a medication you're taking may be bringing you down:

THESE MAY CAUSE DEPRESSION	WHAT THEY'RE FOR
Accutane (Isotretinoin)	Acne
Acid blockers (Pepcid, Zantac, Axid)	GERD and ulcers
Alprazolam	Anxiety
Ambien	Insomnia
Anabolic steroids	Muscle growth
Beta-blockers, oral and eye drops	Reduce blood pressure
Birth control pills/patches	Oral contraceptive
Butalbital	Headache
Chemotherapy	Cancer
Digoxin	Heart
Hormone replacement drugs	Menopausal symptoms
Prednisone	Anti-inflammatory
Quinolone (Cipro, Levaquin)	Antibiotics
Valium	Sleep and anxiety

If you're taking a downer drug that is causing you to feel suicidal or agitated, DO NOT suddenly stop taking it without consulting your physician. You might end up with withdrawal effects such as dizziness, unusual dreams, nausea, vomiting, anxiety, tremors, and possibly seizures. Ask your doctor or pharmacist about tapering off slowly and switching to something safer. Once your medicine is completely out of your system, you should no longer have these intense feelings.

Adrenal Burnout—Does Your Engine Need an Overhaul?

Your adrenal glands are your "stress motor," and when you are coping with too much stress—a busy schedule, a demanding family, chronic illness—that motor can get worn out. This helps explain why some formerly happy-go-lucky women come down with depression in the prime of life: Their adrenal glands just can't take the pace. Red flags of adrenal burnout include fatigue, achiness, low blood sugar, low blood pressure (you may feel dizzy when you stand up), and of course depression. Recent studies indicate that reduced serotonin, which is targeted by most antidepressants (SSRIs), may not be as much a causative factor in depression as the long-term presence of elevated stress hormones like cortisol. For more on adrenal fatigue, see Chapter 1.

So what do you do if your depressed mood is from adrenal burnout?

✳ Avoid irritating people and situations. Try not to obligate yourself to certain people if they drain your energy.

✳ Learn to do something you've always dreamed of doing. Fulfilling yourself by learning to play the guitar, or bead, or speak another language can be satisfying and may take your mind off heavier subjects.

✳ Don't sweat the small stuff. So what if the lawn man shows up an hour late, or your friend backs out on dinner? Beating others up for minor indiscretions like this (to their face or in private) only makes you look bad—and feel bad. Take the higher road and understand that people are going through their own life situations. You don't need any more of those unhappy chemicals floating around, so redirect your energy to something nice.

✳ Eat better. Skip the sugary sweets and the temporary pick-me-ups like caffeine.

✳ Take up yoga or Pilates. Exercise boosts happy hormones, plus toning up will make you feel sexy again.

✳ Do something nice for someone else. I know you feel bad and want instant gratification to make yourself feel better, but it's true that giving to others makes you feel really good. Just watch someone glow about a random act of kindness that you shared. It will make your day better!

✱ Nourish your adrenals. Of course, you can consider prescription medication—hydrocortisone tablets are a synthetic form of cortisol available by prescription only. But there are lots of over-the-counter natural herbs or vitamins that feed the adrenal glands and give you noticeable relief within weeks. Consider the supplements that I recommend for adrenal burnout in Chapter 1: licorice extract, Panax ginseng, DHEA supplements, Rhodiola, and pantethine, plus Eleuthero.

Are You Being Thwarted by Your Thyroid?

Thyroid burnout can cause depression too, and it often goes hand in hand with adrenal fatigue. Are you tired all the time? Frequently cold? Are you constipated, gaining weight, moody, and suffering from low sex drive? Poor thyroid function will reduce your levels of T3 hormone (triiodthyronine), a powerful "happy brain" chemical.

To find out if you're low in thyroid hormone, check out Chapter 1, where I outline some instructions on how to home-test your thyroid function by taking your temperature and then explain exactly how to improve your thyroid health with over-the-counter products from your health-food store: iodine; zinc; copper; selenium; tyrosine; vitamins C, E, and B_{12}; and Ashwagandha extract.

Suzy's Secrets from Behind the Counter

Keep an Eye on the Estrogen

Every prescription drug that contains estrogen (even birth control pills) has the ability to cause depression because these drugs rob your brain of nutrients needed for good mood. So if you're taking estrogen in any form, please eat the "Good Mood Foods" listed in this chapter and consider the supplements I recommend under "Hormonal Havoc" below.

Hormonal Havoc: The Estrogen-Progestin Paradox

Ladies, we need both our estrogen and our progesterone to feel happy and emotionally stable. Both their absolute levels and the balance between them can vary widely—and this variability can cause depression and other psychological symptoms, including insomnia, irritability, anxiety, and tearfulness.

Doctors often prescribe artificial estrogen and progestin drugs as hormone replacement therapy (HRT) to help menopausal women relieve hot flashes, protect bones against breakage, and improve mood and emotional stability. This might seem to make sense, but there's a catch: These are synthetic, lab-created hormones, so our bodies don't recognize them or process them correctly. As a result, our hormone levels rise—but the meds also drive out essential nutrients and vitamins. Over the long term, this can cause depression.

For example, our precious B_6 is "drug-mugged" by HRT. We need B_6 to convert tyrosine into its active mood-boosting relatives dopamine and norepinephrine, which give us energy and make us feel more cheerful and optimistic. B_6 is also used to convert 5-HTP to serotonin—one of our most important "happy" hormones, and one that also makes us feel better about ourselves. So you can see how HRT might act indirectly to bring some women down.

Unfortunately, most doctors are unaware of the way birth control pills and HRT deplete our nutrients—but now *you* know, so ask your doctor about taking the following supplements for as long as you take your medication. These are intended to help ease depression related to the drug-mugging effects of hormones, but may help anyone with the blues.

   ✳ **Vitamin C**—*200–500 mg of buffered C daily*

   ✳ **Vitamin B₂ (riboflavin)**—*50 mg every morning* or *30 mg activated "R5P" daily.* (Your urine may turn bright yellow, but don't worry—it's harmless!)

   ✳ **Vitamin B₆**—*25–50 mg every morning* or *10–20 mg activated "P5P" daily*—but back off if you get bad dreams

   ✳ **Vitamin B₁₂ (cyanocobalamin or methylcobolamin)**—about *500 mcg daily* or have your doctor give you an *injection of 1,000 mcg once or twice a month*

   ✳ **Vitamin B₉ (folic acid)**—*800 mcg*

   ✳ **Tyrosine**—*100–500 mg once or twice daily, morning and afternoon.* Avoid if you have anxiety or heart problems.

✳ **Magnesium chelate or glycinate**—*200–300 mg once or twice a day.* These forms should not cause diarrhea; however, if you develop diarrhea or any stomach discomfort, back off on the dose.

✳ **Iodine**—Iodoral is a good brand, *12.5 mg in the morning.*

This regimen is much easier to follow if you can find a quality brand of B-complex to take each morning along with tyrosine, magnesium, iodine, and C. B-complex vitamins usually contain many Bs, so you'll also be consuming other B vitamins than those listed above, such as pantethine, niacin, and thiamine. Taking extra Bs is even better for your adrenal and hormonal health. Check out Chapter 13 on Hormone Replacement for more information, and see Part V for a complete list of drugs that wipe out magnesium and vitamin C.

Suzy's Secrets from Behind the Counter
Replenish Your Riboflavin

If you're prone to menacing migraines, try taking about *400 daily mg* of riboflavin. If you're taking birth control pills and get migraines or any other type of debilitating headache around your period, it's possible that the pill is wiping out this vital nutrient. One study in 2000 showed that this mighty B nutrient could help prevent migraines as well as prescribed beta-blockers such as metoprolol. Another study compared high-dose riboflavin (400 mg daily) to placebo sugar pills. Eight people, primarily women ages 18 to 65 years, were selected for the study. The women all met the International Headache Society's diagnostic criteria for migraines with or without aura. The double-blinded study took place at six centers in Belgium and Luxembourg, and participants kept detailed records of their headaches, including frequency, duration, pain levels, nausea/vomiting, and even adverse side effects that they may have experienced. Those patients who took the riboflavin showed, on average, two fewer migraines per month compared to those taking the placebo. Also, the duration of attacks was shorter, and they experienced three fewer days of misery, pain, nausea, and vomiting!

This study is important to share with you because riboflavin is very inexpensive, and it has far fewer side effects than migraine drugs, which can affect the heart.

Add Vigor with Vitamins

Depression can occur when your brain runs out of one or more nutrients or enzymes necessary to crank out the "happy brain" chemicals: norepinephrine, dopamine, serotonin, GABA, and epinephrine.

One commonly depleted nutrient is folic acid (a.k.a. folate). In fact, a deficiency of this B vitamin could result from the use of drug muggers such as estrogen-containing drugs, aspirin, ibuprofen, naproxen, metformin, and seizure medicines. (For a more comprehensive list of drugs that mug your folic acid, refer to Part V.) So if you think you are losing your mind, it could be true—and, happily, reversible! Psychiatric symptoms of folate deficiency include low appetite, forgetfulness, depression, insomnia, crankiness, fatigue, and anxiety.

Now, in order for you to use folic acid, your body has to convert it into a biologically active form, known as 5-methyltetrahydrofolate, or 5-MTHF. For most people, this is easy, but some "Folate Misbehavers" can't perform this simple chemical conversion, so they frequently show signs of folate deficiency. Some 20 to 30 percent of the population suffers from this problem, making them far more likely to develop depression, as well as catastrophic illnesses such as heart disease, dementia, diabetes, Alzheimer's, Parkinson's, breast cancer, and cervical cancer.

A simple blood test of your "homocysteine" levels may lend some insight. If it's high, you could be a Folate Misbehaver. In that case, just take "body-ready" folate so your body doesn't have to convert it. Thorne Research's 5-MTHF and Metagenics's FolaPro are two brands of "body-ready" folate, a type of folate that is activated for you. You'll also want to take an additional *500 mcg of* B_{12} *per day as well as 50 mg of a B-complex*—the extra Bs will support the whole process. Even if you're not a Folate Misbehaver, supplementing with B vitamins can still have dramatic effects on your physical and mental health.

Pay Attention . . .

Folate Misbehavers may develop concentration problems, or even Attention Deficit Hyperactivity Disorder (ADHD). When people with ADHD supplement with activated folic acid 5-MTHF that seems to help. You'll be happy to know that the vitamin doesn't interact with any ADHD medicine. So if you or your child is suffering from ADHD, talk to your doctor or psychiatrist about 5-MTHF or folic acid supplements, which are sold over the counter.

Each of the following supplements is a consideration if you want to stabilize your mood or improve depression. These are in no particular order, and it's okay to combine a few if they feel right for you.

Ten Supplements That Can Add Zest to Your Life

1. **L-tyrosine:** a natural building block for some important mood regulators: dopamine, norepinephrine, and epinephrine. Too little tyrosine can lead to depression, low blood pressure, and low body temperature—and you also need this amino acid for healthy adrenal, thyroid, and pituitary gland function. Try *500–1,000 mg twice a day (upon rising and at 3 P.M.).* Don't take it too late in the day because it acts a little bit like caffeine. In fact, if you're trying to kick the caffeine habit, L-tyrosine can help suppress latte urges.

People who take MAO inhibition antidepressants or appetite suppressants or people with high blood pressure should not take tyrosine.

2. **5-HTP:** short for 5-hydroxytryptophan, which turns into serotonin, one of your happy brain chemicals. Your body makes 5-HTP from its precursor, tryptophan, which is found naturally in turkey, dairy, nuts, eggs, and seeds. Taking a supplement of 5-HTP can ease depression, anxiety, panic attacks, and insomnia within a week or two because the 5-HTP turns into serotonin. 5-HTP is also a natural appetite suppressant and can help curb a voracious sweet tooth! Some studies show it works as well as—or even better than—SSRI antidepressants, such as Prozac, Zoloft, Paxil, and Celexa. Get capsules; try *25–100 mg at bedtime* because it usually causes drowsiness. If you're one of those people who get more "energetic" after taking this, then swallow your capsules earlier in the day. Taking it *with a little* B$_6$ helps produce more of your major mood booster, serotonin.

This supplement can increase the side effects of some prescribed antidepressants, which also create more serotonin in the brain. So if you're taking antidepressants, DO NOT take 5-HTP without your doctor's approval and supervision. Too much serotonin is dangerous.

Doctors generally suggest slowly weaning the medication down while bringing in the 5-HTP.

3. **Rhodiola rosea:** a centuries-old root that's been used by Russian athletes and cosmonauts to increase energy. After all, it comes from Siberia, where people have long had to cope with stressful conditions! Rhodiola is an "adaptogen," which means that it only affects chemicals in your body that are out of balance; it ignores the ones that are in healthy ranges. Effects can be dramatic within weeks, and anyone suffering from depression will benefit because Rhodiola helps normalize serotonin, dopamine, and other neurotransmitters that are crucial to your mood, energy levels, and ability to cope with stress. I call it nature's Valium because it relaxes you and makes you feel like you can conquer any problem—we should all be so lucky! Don't worry, there's no risk whatsoever of addiction. And since Rhodiola can help with manly problems such as erectile dysfunction, premature ejaculation, and prostate problems, you can recommend it to your partner, too. *Try one 50 mg capsule twice a day.*

Make sure you get Siberian Rhodiola rosea root extract and not some cheap knockoff made by fly-by-night manufacturers riding on the coattails of legitimate companies.

4. **St.-John's-wort (*Hypericum perforatum*):** an herb that's been used for centuries to boost mood, stabilize emotions, and relieve neuralgia by increasing levels of several key substances involved in mood. St.-John's-wort helps ease mild to moderate depression when taken for three to four consecutive weeks. Optimal effects can be seen within two months. It comes in many different forms—capsule, tea, and extract, any of these are fine, but make sure you get a standardized extract of 0.3 percent Hypericin. *A typical dosage is 300 mg two or three times daily.*

You shouldn't take St.-John's-wort if you're on HIV medication, chemotherapy, cyclosporine, MAO inhibitors, tramadol, dextromethorphan (found in cough syrups), or other antidepressants. Do NOT suddenly stop taking any prescription medication in order to take St.-John's-wort.

5. **Magnesium:** has dramatic effects on your body. Diets high in sugar, carbs, and processed foods tend to flush out magnesium. Magnesium can relieve anxiety and agitation, and some studies suggest that it can help reverse suicidal depression. You also need this essential mineral to balance your calcium levels and stabilize your mood and heart function. *200–400 mg per day* should be fine; get your doctor's approval to take more than that. Magnesium chelate and glycinate are terrific forms of this nutrient and are sold widely at health-food stores.

6. **Vitamin D:** This nutrient is particularly helpful to people who become depressed each winter in a condition known as Seasonal Affective Disorder (SAD). Our bodies make vitamin D from sunlight, and recent studies show that increasing numbers of people are deficient in D because they shy away from the sun or live in areas with fewer daylight hours. Not enough D causes our mood to suffer, so *try 1,000–3,000 IU per day taken with food* during the winter season when daylight hours have dwindled. Cod-liver oil is the best source of this nutrient; I like Nordic Naturals' Arctic Cod-Liver Oil because of the flavor (www.nordicnaturals.com). (For more on drugs that wipe out vitamin D, see Part V.)

Don't take too much D. Unlike other vitamins, which are excreted quickly, D stays in the body. And too much D can cause weakness, bone pain, kidney stones, and heart problems.

7. **Vitamin C:** Lots of drugs erode our stores of vitamin C, which we need for balanced brain chemistry and many other things. Vitamin C converts amino acids into neurotransmitters that boost mood; for example, it helps convert 5-HTP to serotonin, a crucial brain chemical to keep us balanced and positive. Some studies support C's use in people with bipolar disorder, too. *Try 500 mg three or four times a day* of a buffered C. (See Part V for drugs that deplete vitamin C.)

Vitamin C is best taken in small, frequent doses during the day, rather than one very large dose, which can upset copper balance in the body. I like the buffered kind—it's easier on your stomach.

8. **Essential Fatty Acids (EFAs):** EFAs support good health for your heart, your immune system, your gut, and, of course, your brain. We can't make EFAs, so we have to get them from an external source, such as fish oils, krill oil, flaxseed, borage oil, or black currant oil. If we don't eat enough foods that are rich in EFAs, particularly cold-water seafood, we can develop all sorts of brain problems, including depression. Some people are concerned about the recent mercury-contamination scares. This is why I recommend high-quality supplementation. If you are a vegan, supplement with flaxseed: Just sprinkle it on everything. But if you don't mind an animal product, or if you eat a typical American diet laden with fast food, you'll be better off with omega-3 fish oils, *1,000 mg taken three times a day with meals.* Make sure your bottle contains both DHA and EPA. And get a high-quality brand so you don't burp up fish during the day.

9. **SAMe:** Short for S-adenosylmethionine, SAMe (pronounced "Sammy") is an amino acid that boosts mood and reduces arthritis pain at the same time. SAMe helps neurotransmitters latch onto their receptor sites in the brain and has been used successfully in Europe for many years. Interestingly, the nutrient also helps reverse liver damage even in people with a history of alcohol abuse. *Try 200–400 mg one to four times daily on an empty stomach;* get an enteric-coated brand.

> *People who take psychoactive drugs or antidepressants, or who have bipolar disorder, should avoid SAMe.*

10. **Phenylalanine:** This essential amino acid comes in two forms. The "L" form occurs naturally in food, and the "D" form is the lab-created version. Most supplements are a mixture of the two and are designated as DLPA, which gets converted into two powerful mood boosters, tyrosine and phenylethylamine. These substances also improve memory, reduce pain, and suppress appetite. *Dosage is 200–250 mg once or twice daily.*

Breathe Deeply—It Could Boost Your Mood

Try a whiff of such pure essential oils as jasmine, grapefruit, bergamot, cinnamon, mandarin, or peppermint. These brain pick-me-ups work quickly and safely to lift your mood. Buy an essential oil diffuser with the right blend of essential oils to make your home smell like an exotic garden.

Sweat Your Way to a Sweet Life

It's harder to launch an exercise program—and to stick with it—than it is to exercise itself. But studies have repeatedly shown that sweating can make you happy. It works because exercise releases "feel-good" chemicals all over your body; plus it distracts you from the endless chatter in your brain. *Try 15–30 minutes a day, three times a week.* You can play with dumbbells, ride a bike, walk the dog, or my favorite, turn on some music and just dance!

6

Frazzled, Frustrated, and Freaked Out

Coping with Anxiety and Stress

Are you feeling frazzled, frustrated, and freaked out? Has that state of mind become more familiar to you than anything vaguely approaching serenity or calm? I think everyone experiences fear or worry, technically termed "anxiety," with such symptoms as shakiness, jumpiness, irritability, hot flashes, dizziness, chest pain, muscle tension, weakness, or diarrhea. Some degree of anxiety is natural—but if the angst is starting to affect your decision-making abilities, memory, or nighttime rest, then it may be time to take some action.

For many people, out-of-control anxiety is the result of chemical imbalances. You can address this condition in a wide variety of ways, and yes, the tranquilizers your doctor prescribes may indeed be one of them. But before you go that route, just give the ideas in this chapter a try—no doctor required! You may be pleasantly surprised. And remember, you don't need a formal diagnosis to know you're frazzled—after all, you're the world's leading authority on how you feel.

One of the first ideas you should try is replacing frazzle and frustration with two other "f" words: *forgiveness* and "being in the *flow.*" I am constantly amazed at how much those two concepts help to calm me down, and you may be delighted with how they work for you, too. Letting go of anger and resentment really cuts back on the frazzle factor in one's life. I've found it especially helpful to listen to Eckhart Tolle's wonderful CDs, *The Power of Now, Stillness Speaks,* and *A New Earth*: He's so calming and sensible. So put him in your medicine cabinet next to those tranquilizers and supplements. Seriously, play his CDs when it's quiet at night, or as you drift off to sleep. He has a slow, relaxing voice, so do not operate machinery or drive a motor vehicle while listening to Eckhart!

What's Freaking You Out?

Let's begin with a tour of the various anxiety disorders. Do you see yourself in one or more of these descriptions? Don't stress—it'll be our little secret!

* **Generalized anxiety disorder**—Anxiety is normal—but constant anxiety is not. If you feel fretful or worried all the time, if your anxiety rarely has a logical explanation, or if your anxiety regularly interferes with what should be pleasant occasions, especially times when you might otherwise be resting or relaxing, you may have generalized anxiety disorder. Prescription tranquilizers are the conventional treatment for this condition—but like I said, read on, because in a few pages, I've got some natural OTC suggestions you can consider too.

* **Social anxiety disorder**—This is where you freak out at the idea of having to go to a party, speak in front of a few coworkers, or spend time in other social situations. The terror in your mind is so deeply entrenched that you get cold, clammy hands; tremors; dry mouth; shortness of breath; or break out into a cold sweat; or you simply isolate yourself. This is a seriously debilitating condition, and it's different from just being shy. The drugs Effexor and Paxil are promoted for this; however, in a few pages, I'll share some natural options that may help as well.

* **Panic attacks**—Triggered by random events, your "fight or flight" button gets clicked and suddenly, frightening symptoms make you feel as though you're going crazy or even dying. Pounding in your chest, shortness of breath, dizziness, sweating, and a choking sensation may last for up to an hour. About 5 percent of the population experiences

such an attack once in their lifetime, but some people are prone to more frequent incidents. Panic attacks may be estrogen-driven, so women suffering from PMS or estrogen dominance are especially vulnerable. Episodes have also been associated with deficiencies of certain minerals such as zinc or magnesium.

✳ **Obsessive compulsive disorder (OCD)**—The brain gets stuck—as if with a mental cramp—on one particular fear, thought, or urge. Fear of dirt, germs, or bodily secretions are common obsessions for some people, who then compulsively wash their hands or sweep their immaculately clean houses. Some people with OCD hoard useless stuff or develop elaborate rituals. If you spend a lot of time stressing over senseless urges or thoughts, or if you feel that your life is dominated by rituals you can't control—counting, cleaning, or keeping your possessions arranged in a strict order—you might have OCD. Luvox and SSRI antidepressants such as Zoloft, Prozac, Paxil, and Celexa are generally prescribed. I have also heard that DHA fish oils, St.-John's-wort, and passion flower herb may help. Work with a holistic physician, herbalist, or naturopath to find your correct dosage as you explore these and other alternatives.

✳ **Posttraumatic stress disorder (PTSD)**—The stress most often starts in childhood, but it could also result from a physical or emotional crisis experienced as an adult, like the survival of a traumatic event like 9/11 or Hurricane Katrina. Sometimes, a vivid flashback occurs out of the blue as the person with PTSD re-experiences memories of sexual abuse, combat stress, or other traumatic events. Sedatives, tranquilizers, and some antidepressants may help temporarily, but psychological counseling and hypnosis offer long-lasting results.

"You Are Getting Sleepy, Very Sleepy . . ."

A well-trained therapist with a relaxing voice can help you unwind and move past traumatic childhood memories that get trapped inside your head, causing current anxieties, phobias, or panic attacks. One of the most famous hypnotherapists is psychiatrist Brian Weiss, MD, author of such bestsellers as *Many*

Lives, Many Masters (Simon & Schuster 1988) and *Through Time Into Healing* (Simon & Schuster 1992).

Dr. Weiss's conventional practice was turned upside down when he began helping a client named Catherine who suffered from depression, anxiety, and recurrent nightmares. He had been using hypnosis because a fear of choking kept Catherine from swallowing the medication he wanted to prescribe, and indeed, under hypnosis, Catherine successfully recalled several childhood memories that contributed to her anxieties. But one day when Dr. Weiss asked her to go back to the time from which her symptoms arose, she began to recount an experience of death by drowning—four thousand years ago. This past-life experience was the key to her present-day trauma, and when she had processed that ancient memory, she was able to overcome her fears.

Even if you don't believe in past lives, hypnosis has a great track record of helping people to quit smoking, stop compulsive eating, and overcome PTSD—plus it won't damage your liver and kidneys like drugs can. A natural antidote to anxiety, hypnosis can help you regain calm in otherwise stressful situations. It's truly powerful stuff!

I asked Dr. Weiss about finding a good hypnotherapist, and he suggested that people who require psychotherapy along with hypnosis should "choose a qualified, licensed mental health professional with experience in hypnotherapeutic techniques and certification from an excellent training organization." These would include the American Council of Hypnotist Examiners, the American Board of Hypnotherapy, or the National Guild of Hypnotists (see Resources).

Drugs Can Play Tricks with Your Mind!

You might very well be the most rational, patient person in the world, but if you take one of the meds listed below, your alter ego may emerge. That's right; drugs can actually change levels of key neurotransmitters in your brain, causing you to feel anxious, spacey, or irritable. According to the pharmacist's gold-standard resource, *Clinical Pharmacology*, the following drugs have the potential to spark personality changes, even delirium or psychosis—where you have trouble staying in touch with reality. Simply put, you feel like you're out of your mind! Look in your medicine cabinet. Do you take any of the following drugs?

Meds That May Mess with Your Mind

* H2 acid blockers used for GERD and heartburn like ranitidine, cimetidine

* Antihistamines containing diphenhydramine or hydroxyzine, used for allergies, itching

* Cough/cold remedies that contain phenylephrine or pseudoephedrine

* Chantix, the anti-smoking pill, which, in 2008, was linked to psychiatric problems, including suicide

* Antibiotics used for infection, particularly fluoroquinolones such as Cipro or Levaquin

* Erectile dysfunction drugs, such as Viagra

* Corticosteroids used for inflammation and autoimmune disorders, such as prednisone, dexamethasone

* Provigil, the drug used for narcolepsy

* Stimulants used for ADHD such as methylphenidate, dextroamphetamine

* Antiviral drugs used for herpes-type infection such as acyclovir and valacyclovir

* Appetite suppressants such as phentermine or diethylpropion

DO NOT stop taking any prescription medication without consulting your physician. Some drugs have to be weaned off slowly to prevent harmful withdrawal effects. Ask your doctor or pharmacist about alternative options, and then get your doctor's permission to discontinue.

Suzy's Secrets from Behind the Counter
Fight That Fog!

Medicines can cause brain fog and memory loss—especially drugs used to treat allergies and colds, high blood pressure, high cholesterol, heart rhythm abnormalities, glaucoma, menopause, depression, anxiety and pain, and inflammation. But now there's a terrific option that I think could help you reverse brain fog, prevent Alzheimer's, and ease the symptoms of Parkinson's disease, multiple sclerosis, and Lou Gehrig's disease. The nutritional supplement BrainSustain, formulated by the famed neurologist and author Dr. David Perlmutter, could sweep those cobwebs away.

This unique product promotes brain health by facilitating energy production and communication among brain cells as well as protecting you from dangerous free radicals. The product's key ingredients, which include ginkgo biloba, acetyl-L-carnitine, CoQ10, phosphatidylserine, NAC (N-acetylcysteine), and vitamin D, have been extensively studied at some of the world's most respected medical institutions. You can find out more about this fabulous supplement at www.brainsustain.com.

Mood-Creating Chemicals

Your brain functions courtesy of a group of chemicals known as neurotransmitters, which transmit messages from one nerve cell to the next. Some of the most common are serotonin, norepinephrine, GABA, dopamine, and epinephrine (adrenaline), and their circulating levels dramatically affect your mood, personality, and responses to stress. For example, low levels of dopamine may be associated with Parkinson's disease or Attention Deficit Hyperactivity Disorder (ADHD), while high levels can induce agitated depression, in which you frequently feel angry, agitated, and upset. Likewise, too much norepinephrine can make you feel aggressive and panicky. Low serotonin is tied to depression, whereas too much serotonin can lead you to feel manic and hyper, creating agitation, tremors, and insomnia.

As you can see, healthy levels of neurotransmitters keep you thinking clearly and responding to situations with appropriate emotions. You need the right vitamins and minerals to create these brain chemicals and help them work properly. For instance, run out of B_6 and you can't make serotonin, which in turn leads you to feel withdrawn, depressed, and overcome with sugar cravings. So if you're overcome with anxiety, it's not necessarily an emotional problem—you may be struggling with easy-to-fix nutritional imbalances. Please note that many conditions share common symptoms, and it's important to have the proper diagnosis from a physician rather than trying to piece one together yourself. This is especially important before attempting self-treatment with natural remedies that alter your neurotransmitters.

Of course, you don't have to be a complete slave to your brain chemicals. No matter what's going on in your body chemistry, you can make some choices about how you handle stress—whether you keep reliving every frustrating incident that happens to you, for example, or learn somehow to let them go; whether you overschedule yourself or make time for de-stressing; even whether you devote some time to learning how to meditate, use creative visualization, or listen to a relaxation tape. Mind, body, and spirit—all work together to create a sense of health and well-being.

Massage Me Before I Have a Meltdown

One of the quickest ways to reduce stress is to get a massage. This is not just an emotional reality but also a physical one: Massages reduce cortisol—a major stress hormone that contributes to disease.

The physical action of the hands upon your skin and muscles enhances blood flow and circulation, releasing stagnant lymph and allowing it to carry away with it waste products and pain chemicals. The lymph and increased blood flow allow more oxygen to nourish your cells, too. Besides all this, an hour of massage may be the only time you get to take a deep breath all month! It might seem unbelievable, but I've found hundreds of research studies to support massage therapy for dozens of conditions, including arthritis, autism, depression, aggression, headache, anorexia nervosa, ADHD, and even spinal cord injuries. For example, one study found that immediately following massage therapy, subjects' depressed mood, anxiety, and stress hormone levels were measurably reduced. Following ten days of massage therapy, people's pain and insomnia also showed improvement.

I'm sure I'm not the only person who believes in a nice relaxing rubdown, because a study back in 1997 found that visits to chiropractors and massage therapists combined represented 50 percent of all visits made to complementary and alternative practitioners. In Austria, a patient's massage is often covered by insurance, and 87 percent of patients with back pain receive massage.

Studies support massage as a way to reduce muscle tightness, relax the mind, calm anxiety, and lessen the sensation of pain. One study in the *Scandinavian Journal of Rheumatology* found that massage eased rheumatoid arthritis pain.

So go to a health club, reputable salon, or chiropractic clinic and find a massage therapist who can loosen you up with soothing hands or—the latest craze—hot stones! It's terrific! If undressing freaks you out, don't worry; you only have to remove clothing to the level that you are comfortable with. And for a real treat, find a licensed massage therapist who comes to your home. At your house, you can relax with a cup of herbal tea, heat your "cover-up" towel in the dryer, light a candle and a stick of incense, and put on some quiet music for a deeply relaxing massage that taps into all five senses. Talk about a melt-down—mmmm!

Choices That Can Make You Anxious

Sometimes the way we live our lives and the boundaries that we set for ourselves and our families make us anxious. It's completely within your control, and within your rights, to make choices that are healthier for yourself. Give yourself permission to relax. Consider the following lifestyle changes that can have a dramatic impact on your frazzle factor. I promise that making even one of these changes will help you feel less anxious.

* Stop overcommitting yourself to every cook-off, party, wedding, and social event in your city.

* Set reasonable goals. This is important for you—and those whom you call to bail you out.

* Learn to expect those "unexpected" setbacks, delays, and obstacles.

* Remember that it's okay for you to say "no." It's a real word, and it comes with the power to restore your energy.

Foods That Can Make You Anxious

* **Caffeine**—If you're prone to nervousness, insomnia, or panic attacks, lay off the caffeine. Studies have shown that as little as 200 mg of caffeine—the amount in about 2 cups of coffee—can cause anxiety or trigger a panic attack in some people. True, if you have brain fog, caffeine *can* temporarily clear it, but it's short-term and there are better ways, so read on.

✳ **Artificial sweeteners**—I say pass on the pretty little packets, because the effect of these pretend sweeteners can creep up on you. While these sweeteners are FDA-approved, in my opinion, they're dangerous to people who are anxiety-prone, because they behave as excitotoxins—literally, they excite nerve cells to death. Some clinical research has associated artificial sweeteners with migraines, seizures, depression, fatigue, hearing loss, tinnitus, and memory loss, not to mention anxiety and panic attacks. I'm particularly concerned about children because their developing brains may be affected by chemicals currently deemed "safe" by the FDA. My recommendation is to use only the sweeteners produced by Mother Nature, which are therefore easily recognized, processed, and eliminated from your body.

✳ *Natural cane sugar or brown sugar*—not the bleached and processed white sugar that is probably in your cabinet.

✳ *Stevia*—this calorie-free natural dietary supplement is derived from a naturally sweet plant native to South American forests. It is heat-stable, so you can cook with it and use it in any food or beverage. It's great for diabetics, people with insulin resistance, and those who are counting carbs because it's low on the glycemic index. Stevia looks just like any other artificial sweetener—white and powdery—and you can get it in most health-food stores, including the big chains like Whole Foods, which sells little packets if you want to carry them with you. It's fascinating to me that the FDA has gone to such great lengths to keep people in the dark about what I think is a natural and safe sugar substitute—at one point they instituted a "search and seizure" campaign! Apparently there is big money in the artificial sweetener business, and stevia interferes with that. Today, stevia is grown all over the world, including China, Germany, Malaysia, Israel, and South Korea.

✳ *Agave nectar*—another natural sweetener 75 times sweeter than sugar that you can pour into any food or beverage. It's just sap extracted from the agave plant, and just like stevia, it's low on the glycemic index. Generally, ⅓ cup of agave syrup is equal to 1 cup of sugar, but you may have to experiment. Try Melissa's Organic Low-Glycemic Agave Nectar at www.melissas.com. Agave nectar looks just like honey, but it's safe for diabetics because it won't spike blood sugar levels.

✳ *Vegetable glycerine*—It's a clear, thick liquid with a natural, moderately sweet taste. It's almost all fatty esters made from coconut or palm oil with a little water. Because it doesn't affect your blood sugar levels, it's safe for people with candida, diabetes, and hypoglycemia.

✳ *Evaporated cane sugar*—Rich in molasses, vitamins, and minerals, cane juice is evaporated and then crystallized. The result is a delicious sugar that will enhance all of your favorite recipes and will easily be recognized by your body. It can be replaced one-for-one with refined white sugar.

✳ *Honey*

✳ *Maple syrup*

✳ *Brown rice syrup*

✳ *Molasses*

✳ **MSG**—Monosodium glutamate—another excitotoxin—is found in many canned foods because MSG suppresses canned foods' tinny taste. MSG and other food additives may contribute to neurological conditions, such as depression, neuropathic pain, anxiety, schizophrenia, Parkinson's, Lou Gehrig's, epilepsy, migraines, and bipolar syndrome. My advice would be to cut back on MSG and its other aliases: "glutamate textured protein," "hydrolyzed protein," "calcium caseinate yeast food," "sodium caseinate autolyzed yeast," and "gelatin yeast nutrient."

✳ **Alcohol**—Many people who suffer with anxiety turn to alcohol to calm them down—but honestly it's not the greatest choice. Sure, a glass of wine can soothe away the day's troubles, but you have to be careful because too much alcohol is harmful to the body. Not only can it destroy brain cells, liver cells, and the stomach lining, but it's also habit-forming and in some people can actually spark agitation and panic attacks.

> Birth control pills are drug muggers, wiping out vitamin B_6, which can lead to irritability and mood swings. Consider B_6—also called "pyridoxine"—as part of your good mood regimen and take about *50mg each day*, or *20mg P5P*, its active form.

Feed Your Brain: The Ten-Ingredient Rule

Have you ever realized that "stressed" spelled backward is "d-e-s-s-e-r-t-s"? But reaching for feel-good foods like ice cream won't solve your problems—in fact, all that sugar, fat, and caffeine (like candy bars and soda pop) will actually rev up your brain and boost your stress levels. My advice? Make a clean sweep of your kitchen and toss out hidden candy bars, processed TV dinners, and unhealthy oils, like the corn and canola oil found in potato chips and French fries. Substitute fresh for canned foods and drink lots of water—either filtered or bottled.

Next, read the labels on every item you buy, and if you see lots of big, giant words in the ingredient list, leave the item on the shelf. Don't eat anything that has more than say, ten ingredients, because processed foods contain all sorts of man-made chemicals that attack your brain, whereas healthy foods contain natural substances that feed your brain what it needs. In fact, eat as many one-ingredient foods as you can, preferring a slice of apple (ingredients: apple) to a slice of apple pie (ingredients: a lot more than an apple!).

Of course, gooey brownies are allowed sometimes. But for most of your meals, I have in mind bright, colorful foods rich in nutrients that will support your neurotransmitters. M&Ms don't count.

Eat Like a Rabbit

You could literally walk through your produce department with a blindfold and pick randomly, pretty much knowing whatever you grab will be good for you—after all, they're all single-ingredient foods! My personal favorites include:

※ **Asparagus**—because it is very alkalinizing (when we're stressed, we're acidic)

※ **Avocado**—because it's a great source of glutathione, which helps our livers break down toxic substances that can cause anxiety

※ **Blueberries**—because they're chock-full of antioxidants that protect your brain and eyes from cancer, plus they're low in sugar

＊ **Citrus Fruits**—oranges, if I had to pick—because they're high in vitamin C, which vacuums up waste from your brain, plus helps your body make neurotransmitters

Worrywarts Like to Meditate

Next time you see someone worrying, ask them, "Are you meditating?" Of course, they'll shout "No!" at which point you could say, "But worrying is just negative meditation!" Most worriers engage in negative meditations all day long unless they actively choose what to think about.

You can retrain your brain to focus on positive thoughts if you try. Here's how. Pretend that every single thought in your head is broadcast aloud . . . that helps you instantly refocus on a positive, peaceful, or complimentary concept rather than a negative, aggressive one. Try this approach for forty-eight hours nonstop and you will begin to automatically find more good in your day than bad, which at the end of the day produces far less stress.

From Worrier to Warrior in Ten Easy Minutes

Want a simple recipe for reducing stress? Just sit still and quiet all the mental chatter—for only ten minutes.

Now, if just the thought of taking that much time out of your busy day stresses you out, take a baby step and buy an inspiring CD by Wayne Dyer or Marianne Williamson. Try playing it in your car or on your MP3 player. You might also try playing some calming instrumental CDs in your home, especially if children are around—it induces a calm mood much better than TV.

If you're a warrior woman who is determined to relax even if it kills you, meditation is for you. Honestly, it's not that hard—it's just like thinking, except you concentrate on only one thing, such as how it feels when your child hugs you, or the beauty of a flower. Candles and incense (perhaps some of the Nag Champa incenses sold in metaphysical bookshops and mall kiosks) can help set a peaceful mood. Just sit and be mindful of your breath and of any sensation you feel in your body. When negative thoughts enter your brain—and they will—let them float away and redirect your thoughts to something pleasant. You might also try repeating a word or phrase like "I am love," or "All is well" and then imagining your body lying in warm sand on a beach or sitting right inside a rainbow.

The National Institutes of Health reports that meditating regularly can reduce cortisol, blood pressure, and stress hormones, and therefore lessen anxiety. In a fascinating 2005 study printed in the *Proceedings of the National Academy of Sciences*, Tibetan monks proved that meditation makes you happy. The Dalai Lama dispatched eight of his most accomplished Buddhist practitioners to the United States so their brains could be scanned with electroencephalograph (EEG) testing and magnetic resonance imaging (MRI) as they meditated. The goal was to see how their images differ from yours and mine. The art of deep meditation is centuries old, and the eight monks each had logged anywhere from 10,000 to 50,000 hours of practice. A control group of ten students with no meditation practice also took part in the study. Each group was asked to focus on unconditional compassion or, as the Dalai Lama's teaching puts it, the "unrestricted readiness and availability to help living beings." Researchers chose that focus because it's easier to think of feelings rather than to try to recall and focus on memories, images, or objects. Both groups experienced positive changes in their MRI and EEG results; however, the monks showed powerful spikes of gamma brain waves, an extremely heightened state of awareness. The monks also had very bright areas of activity in the left pre-frontal cortex, the part of the brain that elicits happiness and positive emotions.

So take ten minutes to meditate, or at least give yourself a sixty-second brain vacation several times a day. Just close your eyes and take five good deep breaths, relaxing your shoulders and your forehead. You may be surprised at how refreshed you'll feel!

Destress with Software

HeartMath software programs are technologically cool ways to help you get into the right emotional state. Their computer program called Freeze-Framer helps you transform stress into positive energy. The Freeze-Framer system includes computer software and a little finger sensor that you wear on one finger while sitting at your computer. You then begin to relax and feel positive emotions, and as your heart rhythms smooth out, a dreary black-and-white image of, say, a jungle forest, brightens up right before your eyes. Maintain this calm, clear, and balanced mood, and you can make the computer image teem with waterfalls, animals, and flowers. The longer you hold this positive state, the more spectacular the scenery! Their latest gadget is the personal pocket stress-reliever called emWave, a handheld biofeedback device that works the same way. (For information, contact 800-450-9111 or visit www.emwave.com.) Cost: $200–$400.

Mood-Altering Weeds and Other Brain-Saving Nutrients

You can calm yourself with any of the nutrients listed below, which are sold in health-food stores and pharmacies nationwide—no doctor required! However, do ask your doctor and pharmacist whether these products will interact with any medications you're taking. And don't just stop taking your current antianxiety meds—talk to your doctor about how you might taper off.

I've listed the following supplements in the order that I'd begin taking them. It's possible to take all of these together—just get your doctor's blessings and bring a new supplement in every week, not all at once.

1. **Trancor:** Made by Metagenics, this is the perfect calming combination for anxious worrywarts who just can't help themselves. It contains a blend of vitamin B_6, magnesium, taurine, NAC (N-acetylcysteine), and green tea extract, and works to increase GABA and suppress glutamate in the brain. In English, this means that you will feel aaaah, so nice and relaxed! I love this product and recommend it particularly if you have irritability or anxiety related to PMS—but don't take it if you're on antiseizure drugs like Tegretol (carbamazepine) or Neurontin (gabapentin). Metagenics products such as Trancor are available through health-care professionals only, so you won't find this one in health-food stores, although you can buy all the ingredients separately at pharmacies and health-food stores. If you want Trancor, search their website at www.metagenics.com to find a practitioner near you. *Dosage: 1 capsule four times daily.*

2. **Omega-3 fatty acids:** a.k.a. fish oils, which contain EPA and DHA. You can take these with the Trancor, no problem. These substances—especially the DHA—penetrate the brain tissue and help all your neurotransmitters communicate with one another for better

brain function and mood. Also, fish oils lower inflammatory chemicals, which leads eventually to higher serotonin levels, leaving you feeling calm and good about yourself. Omega-3s help prevent or ease ADHD, high cholesterol, heart disease, arthritis, Alzheimer's, depression, and autoimmune disorders. Sardines don't sound so bad right about now, huh? *Try 1,000–2,000 mg twice a day with a meal.*

3. **Magnesium:** You won't need this if you take Trancor, but in case you buy these nutrients one at a time, you should know that even the slightest deficiency of magnesium can cause nervousness, high blood pressure, depression, migraines, and PMS. Soda pop and white-flour foods are void of magnesium, so maybe your anxiety is tied—at least in part—to what's on your plate? Eat whole grains, green leafy vegetables, wheat bran, chocolate (yeah!), legumes, seaweed, nuts, and pumpkin seeds. Or take magnesium chelate or glycinate: *100 mg three or four times a day.* Because magnesium enhances serotonin, divide up your doses so that you get a steady dose of "feel-good" chemicals throughout the day. For added punch, *take a B-complex or some B$_6$ once daily.* And if you're having a particularly upsetting moment, try taking about *50– 100 mg* of magnesium right then and there. Magnesium works very quickly to calm you, and it also relaxes your large muscles so it's good for cramps as well.

4. **Chamomile tea:** Sip to your heart's content, because the chamo- mile is a natural sedative. I like blends that contain other soothing herbs like passionflower, lemon balm, valerian, or orange blossom. Of the many yummy brands available, one of my favorites is Chamomile Lemon Tea by The Republic of Tea. It is sweet and blended with various fragrant herbs.

5. **L-Theanine:** Meditation in your teacup, L-theanine is what's nat- urally found in green tea. Theanine is the term used to describe an amino acid that acts in your brain called "gamma-ethylamino-L- glutamic acid." Now you know why we just refer to it as theanine! You may be confused at this point because it's true that most teas contain caffeine, so how can green tea be so calming? The credit goes to thean-

ine, which begins to relax you in just 30 to 40 minutes. According to a study published in 2001 in *Alternative and Complementary Therapies*, theanine lulls your brain into producing alpha brain waves, which are also produced when you meditate. It also sparks the production of GABA, a relaxing brain chemical that is highest when you sleep. GABA is the same chemical that floods your brain after you pop a sleeping pill such as Valium, Ambien, Sonata, Lunesta, or Restoril.

The sense of well-being from green tea could last for hours. Just make sure to read labels carefully, and don't confuse L-theanine with L-threonine. *Dosage: 100–200 mg of L-theanine at the first sign of stress, and every four to six hours if needed.* Or drink three to four cups of green tea per day, any flavor!

6. **Lavender:** Lavender can be found in bath gels, eye pillows, lotions, teas, and aromatherapy oils. The scent is very soothing and purifies both body and spirit. It can also ease depression, agitation, and insomnia. For some people, its effects are immediate.

Buy some pure essential lavender oil and dab 5 to 10 drops on a tissue that you keep in your purse (in a zip-top bag if you want). Whenever you're stuck in traffic or feeling stressed, take a whiff for instant calm. I promise you—this really works! Or put some lavender oil drops right into a hot bath by candlelight. Hey, why not? Don't you need a little relaxing "me-time," too?

7

Headaches Can Be Cured If You Know the Cause

Your brain is like the motherboard of your computer, so if it's not functioning properly, your whole system malfunctions. It's very frustrating to have a strong physical body, yet you are unable to enjoy life because your head feels like it's going to explode.

If you have chronic headaches, the pain is intensified with emotional anguish when well-meaning friends or relatives look at you like you're crazy, or whisper that you look so well and "maybe it's all in your head." Yeah, it is! Just because you can't whip out an MRI showing a bona fide ice pick in your brain doesn't make your pain any less authentic. I understand you, and I also suspect that even simple things like reading this chapter could feel like a chore, but stick with me because in five minutes, you'll learn tips and tricks to help you feel better than you have in years.

A Word to the Wise

By and large, most people with headaches will never have to face a diagnosis like a brain tumor, meningitis, or intracranial hematoma, but just to be on the safe side, why not rule out all the scary stuff first? Please comply with your doctor when he asks for labs, tests, or scans. Don't ignore head pain that is accompanied by numbness or blurred vision, or that occurs with coughing, sneezing, or bending over. These symptoms and any sudden-onset headache that worsens over 24 hours are a warning sign to get help.

Get Control of the Pain

Headaches are much easier to fix if you know what kind you are experiencing. It's safe to say that most people have experienced a tension headache at one time or another. You know, the kind you get from fatigue, eyestrain, tension in your neck, anger, or worrying too much. You can take control with some quick and simple remedies below; here is my list of Headache Halters.

Headache Halters

1. Take hot showers; the warmth relaxes tension and pressure in the head.

2. Apply a very hot compress to the area of pain for two minutes, then follow it for two minutes with a cold compress. The change in temperature creates a "pumping" action and could help relieve pain, drain your sinuses, or distract you enough to break the pain cycle.

3. Take minerals, in particular magnesium and calcium. Take about 200 mg of magnesium chelate or glycinate every morning, and about 400–500 mg of calcium citrate at bedtime. These minerals are usually deficient in people with migraines, as well as people with anxiety, another condition that could go hand in hand with constant headaches.

4. OTC analgesics like acetaminophen (Tylenol), ibuprofen (Motrin or Advil), or naproxen (Aleve) can be used occasionally; they reduce inflammation and pain. Serrapeptose is a natural anti-inflammatory that could be used instead of these drugs.

5. Get a massage. The therapist's job is to feel your pain and make it go away! Besides, studies show that massage reduces pain by releasing endorphins.

6. Try chiropractic care. Gentle chiropractic care may help some people whose headaches stem from a misaligned vertebra in the neck.

7. Apply pressure on the web of skin between your index finger and thumb for a few minutes—this area is an acupressure point.

8. Avoid Migraine Maker foods because they can trigger headaches (see page 103).

Headaches Come in All Shapes and Sizes

Sinus Headache

Sometimes the nasal membranes get so inflamed that mucus and air can't flow freely between the sinus cavities and the nose, creating excess pressure behind the eyes, across the forehead, and even down into the teeth. People who are prone to sinusitis often have allergies too; you'll want to boost your immune system. (Read Chapter 18 for more on this.) Try the Headache Halters previously mentioned as well as the following tricks, which can be done together:

1. Eliminate dairy. It causes a high incidence of congestion in people who are allergic.

2. Run a humidifier. Breathing moist air loosens congestion.

3. Try OTC decongestants like Sudafed (pseudoephedrine) or medicated nasal sprays, but only for three days or less.

4. Irrigate your sinuses to cleanse them of mucus, pollen, and bacteria. There are many brands of nasal irrigation devices; they range in price from $15 to $100. Brand names include Nasaline, SinuPulse Elite, and HydroPulse.

5. Purchase magnolia flower herb—also known as Xin Yi Hua—which can help clear blocked sinuses, relieving congestion and unstuffing your nose. It's available as a tea or oral supplement.

6. Ask your doctor for a prescription for a steroid such as Flonase or Nasonex. These are squirted into the nose and can reduce inflammation

after a few days. If used long term, you will have to replenish what these drug muggers steal, so supplement with calcium, vitamins C and D, potassium, and folic acid; a good multivitamin should be able to replenish what the drug mugger stole.

Suzy's Secret from Behind the Counter

Breathe Easy with Botanicals

This is a great trick if you have a cough or cold, and also if you are prone to sinus headaches. To a pot of boiling water, add two or three drops each of eucalyptus and tea tree essential oils. Then leaning over the pot at a safe distance so as not to burn yourself, carefully cover your head with a towel and breathe in the moist air.

PMS Headache

A PMS headache is often labeled as a migraine, which we will talk about in depth shortly. This headache occurs either when you start your period or a few days before and is usually accompanied with other premenstrual symptoms such as emotional sensitivity, food cravings, and anxiety. You can try my Headache Halters, especially the minerals and the OTC pain relievers, which should be started one week before your period is due. Also, consider these tips and tricks, which can be done together:

1. Take 5-HTP, an OTC dietary supplement that helps your body create serotonin. *Dosage: 50–100 mg each night.*

2. Eliminate xenobiotics as much as you can; these are substances that behave like estrogen, only they're hormone disrupters and can trigger headaches. You'll find them in some shampoos, plastic containers, paint, and pesticides. Read Chapter 25 for a complete list of these harmful estrogenic substances.

3. Try a supplement called I3C (Indole 3 Carbonal), which is extracted from cruciferous veggies such as broccoli, cauliflower, and Brussels sprouts. *Dosage: 100–200 mg once daily.*

Cluster Headache

This headache wakes you up around 1 A.M. and feels like someone just stabbed you in the eye! It is one-sided and may also be accompanied by tearing and nasal congestion. Men get this nine times more frequently than women, and cluster headaches affect about 1 million people in the United States. Unlike a migraine, the pain usually subsides within a few minutes, but the attacks come in clusters, four or five times a night. Please refer to the upcoming section on food triggers because tyramine-containing foods should be avoided. Here are other valuable tips and tricks; you can do all of these together if needed:

1. **Oxygen:** Could abort a cluster headache within minutes; your physician will order a small tank for your home. Inhale the oxygen as soon as the attack wakes you.

2. **Melatonin:** People with cluster headaches are often deficient in the "sleep" hormone, so take about 3–6 mg every night, 30 minutes before going to bed.

3. **Pyridoxine or B$_6$:** Take 50 mg daily, or 20 mg daily of its active form, P5P. Back off if you start to get bad dreams. B$_6$ is also helpful in preventing migraines.

4. **Taurine:** Helps boost melatonin in your body and protect your heart and nervous system. Take 200–500 mg twice daily every day.

Sex Headache

Like a cruel twist of fate, this headache can happen during sex, and sometimes at the point of orgasm. The pain is bilateral and feels like you just got clubbed in the head, lasting for about an hour. It occurs mainly in men and has been called an "exertional" headache because it can be induced by exercise, too. If your man is prone to these, he ought to stop when he feels the headache coming on. But if that's not doable:

1. Slow down the pace of your sexual activity (or exercise); it's the *rapid* rise in blood pressure that causes it.

Tonight, Honey, I Have a Headache

We usually think that headaches are the excuse to get out of sex, but did you know that a romp in the sack could stop a migraine in its tracks? All those endorphins have a euphoric effect, acting like morphine in the body, and as levels of tension go down, so does the headache pain. The more powerful the orgasm, the greater the release of endorphins, and therefore the more headache relief you can expect.

2. Change positions. (The idea is to avoid crooks in the neck or excessive blood pressure in the head.)

3. OTC pain relievers such as ibuprofen or naproxen (one dose) taken an hour before activity may help; prescription indomethacin is also a choice.

Migraines

With most "typical" migraines, there is usually a warning—called an "aura"—before the pain. The aura has been described as a flash of colored lights, or a halo around objects; sometimes it is a moment of dizziness, nausea/vomiting, or double vision. Then the pain sets in and ruins a few hours, or even days. Doctors try to classify migraines as "typical" or "atypical." But this is hard to do because symptoms vary so much from person to person, and from migraine to migraine. For example, an atypical migraine may include the aura, but no pain (known as a "silent" migraine), or it may include facial nerve pain, or it may occur bilaterally, instead of on just one side. Don't worry about what kind of migraine you have; the care and treatment is the same because it's the nervous system that sets off the whole cascade of misery.

Some aggravating factors that trigger migraines include stress, certain smells, bright lights, hormonal changes, insomnia, and foods. You can try any of my Headache Halters, especially the minerals, as well as these tips and tricks:

1. **Butterbur (*Petasites hybridus*):** This is an herbal extract that reduces the frequency of migraines by improving blood flow in the brain; unfortunately, it could take up to two months to work. Butterbur

may also relieve painful urinary spasms, allergies, and asthma, plus the remedy is safe for kids. Be careful when choosing products; some inferior brands contain pyrrolizidine alkaloids, or PAs, which are toxic to the liver. Purified butterbur that is PA-free is sold under the proprietary name of "Petadolex." Adults should take 50 mg of Petadolex three times daily for a month, then reduce to twice daily for four more months. Children 6 to 10 years old can try 50 mg once daily, while older kids and teens can try 50 mg twice daily. When you're symptom free, try to taper off. Side effects include belching and nausea.

2. **Riboflavin:** One of the B vitamins; take about 200–400 mg once or twice daily. It may impart a harmless bright yellow color to your urine. Foods rich in this nutrient include peas, lentils, nuts, dairy products, broccoli, and asparagus.

3. **Feverfew** *(Tanacetum parthenium)*: This herb is related to the sunflower. It helps reduce the frequency of migraines, increases levels of serotonin, and reduces inflammation. Quality is imperative. Feverfew may thin the blood, so do not combine it with prescribed blood thinners. Gaia Herbs has a liquid herbal extract of feverfew; take 30–40 drops in a little water, three times daily. Whole plant extracts seem to work better than standardized extracts.

4. **Digestive acids:** People who are low on digestive acids seem to be more prone to migraines and headaches. This is not for everyone, however; if you take acid supplements when you don't need them, you will seriously feel the burn. But if you need these healthy acids, they are sold at health-food stores as "betaine hydrochloride" or "trimethylglycine," and you take one at each meal. An easy trick to see if acid supplements could help you is to drink a homemade acidic cocktail of two teaspoons apple cider vinegar in a cup of water. Honey is fine if it helps you get it down. Drink this at the first sign of a headache. If it aborts your headache, that's a clue that digestive acids will help you. (There's more on digestive acids in Chapter 4.)

Migraine Makers

This could sound weird, but food "speaks" to your body by causing it to release various hormones and neurotransmitters during digestion, some of which cause headaches.

Many people report food as a trigger for their pain, and so I've put together this list of foods that I call migraine makers.

Tyramine

Tyramine causes an increase of norepinephrine, which increases blood pressure and can cause a headache. You'll find tyramine in lots of things, such as chocolate, blue cheese, brie, Gorgonzola and other aged cheeses, beans, and red wine; it's also in cultured dairy products such as yogurt, sour cream, buttermilk, and some sauces and condiments, especially those that contain vinegar. This includes salad dressing, ketchup, olives, pickles, marinades, sauerkraut, and soy sauce. By the way, people who take MAO inhibitor drugs should avoid tyramine-containing foods because the combination could be lethal.

Sodium Nitrate or Nitrite

These are preservatives added to keep foods fresh, but these chemicals open up tiny blood vessels, increasing blood flow and thereby leading to pressure and pain. They're found in most meats because they give the meat a fresh pink color, protect against Clostridium botulinum, and impart a "cured" taste. Avoid bologna, pastrami, pepperoni, corned beef, smoked fish, bacon, sausage, and hot dogs.

Monosodium Glutamate (MSG)

MSG is a flavor enhancer that's often found in canned foods and Chinese food. It's the hardest of all the food triggers to avoid. See Chapter 6 to learn much more about this migraine maker, which is sold under the trade name Accent, among others. An estimated 20,000 tons of this stuff is used annually, and it's often found in soups, diet foods, bouillon cubes, peanut butter, nuts, salad dressing, frozen pizza, doughnuts, hot fresh baked bread, and fast food.

Alcohol

Maybe skip that Appletini because alcoholic beverages, including beer, wine, champagne, and liqueurs, expand your blood vessels, and some contain tyramine, which we talked about earlier. Plus, you could wind up with a hangover headache—like you need anything else to deal with.

Vitamins and Herbs

Some people take niacin to reduce their cholesterol, but it can cause a headache because it increases blood circulation. Ginkgo biloba and vinpocetine are two other migraine makers which people use to improve their memory.

Nightshade Vegetables

It's hard to pinpoint if these foods are a problem because headaches (and arthritic flare-ups) could take up to two days to become evident. Tobacco products are on the list of foods to avoid as well as tomatoes, potatoes, eggplant, cherries, peppers (sweet peppers and chili peppers, but not black pepper), tomatillos, and cape gooseberries.

Artificial Sweeteners

If you try only one thing, try going off artificial sweeteners for even one month as a trial. I can't tell you how many people have thanked me for relieving their headaches with this trick. There is much more about this in Chapter 7.

Caffeine

Caffeine is found in soda, coffee, tea and (in small amounts) in dark chocolate and cocoa. It actually goes both ways, meaning it can relieve a headache for some people, but in others, it can cause one. If you find that it helps you, indulge in a latte and make it a double shot or try the OTC med called Excedrin Migraine.

Fruits

It's usually dried fruits, such as figs, raisins, and dates, that are the problem, because they contain preservatives—usually sulfites—that trigger headaches. Fresh citrus fruits, including papayas, avocados, raspberries, kiwifruit, and pineapple, could also be a problem, but I'm not sure if it's the pesticides they contain that trigger your pain, or the fruit itself. Why not try organic fruits first and see if you still have a problem? If so, give them up altogether.

Head-Banging Drugs

It may come as a shock, but some meds cause headaches. Look in your medicine cabinet, and if you find any of the following medications, ask your doctor for an alternative. Don't just suddenly stop taking them, however, since this could be harmful.

* nitroglycerin (for heart disease)

* blood pressure meds

* medication used to improve circulation

* proton pump inhibitor drugs (acid blockers) that treat ulcers

* seizure meds

* oral contraceptives (the Pill) and hormone replacement therapy

A Minute About Medication

It started in the 1990s when Imitrex injections were introduced. Triptans would prove to be a godsend for headache sufferers. They work in various ways, partly by increasing serotonin, the same happy brain chemical that saves us from depression. Triptans also latch onto brain cells, squeezing off tiny cranial blood vessels which cause pain. If taken at the first sign of a migraine, these drugs can stop an attack in its tracks, though they do nothing for prevention.

Over the years, the triptan family has grown to include some popular meds such as Zomig (zolmitriptan), Amerge (naratriptan), Maxalt (rizatriptan), Axert (almotriptan), Frova (frovatriptan), and Relpax (eletriptan).

Botox Makes Headlines

In 1999, the pretty poison used to remove wrinkles was shown to reduce the frequency and severity of headaches, especially tough migraines. This benefit was discovered quite by accident when patients who received the shots in their foreheads also noticed that their headaches disappeared for months at a time. Today, specially trained doctors use a special type of botulinum toxin called Myobloc, which they inject in appropriate locations on the head, face, and neck to help relieve headache pain.

Each type of triptan has a personality of its own, so if one doesn't work for you, it's okay to try another. Nasal sprays and dissolving tablets are available in some brands, which are a real plus if you tend to vomit with your headache.

Triptans come with a book full of warnings because they affect blood pressure and heart rate. They should be avoided by people with high blood pressure, diabetes, or a family history of heart disease, stroke, or coronary artery disease. While allergic reactions do occur, the most frequently reported side effects include wooziness, chest pressure, flushing, drowsiness, and odd sensations such as tingling or warmth. A rebound headache may occur when your medicine wears off, prompting you to take another dose. This could be dangerous (unless otherwise prescribed) because overuse of migraine medication keeps the cycle of rebound headaches going on.

Suzy's Secrets from Behind the Counter

Count On the Power of Peppermint

Peppermint, in both the herbal and essential oil forms, is a powerful headache remedy. Sniff the aroma of pure peppermint essential oil as soon as you feel a headache coming on, or put a drop on your temples and the back of your neck. Peppermint relieves pain, relaxes tight muscles, and is known to bring rapid relief. You'll find peppermint as an herbal tea as well, and since it helps with tummy upset and nausea, it is a definite plus if your headaches make you feel sick to your stomach.

When You Just Can't Put Your Finger on It

Some people get headaches that move around and change intensity or spark facial pain. When the headaches act weird, it's very hard for a doctor to put his finger on it. These problems could arise after whiplash, a sports injury, a fall or other trauma causing inflamed muscles or tendons, a herniated disk, or even a nerve root irritation in a tooth. A compassionate pain specialist, dentist, neurologist, or anesthesiologist can help you with any of these:

✳ **Temporomandibular joint syndrome (TMJ)**—This tiny jaw joint lies near your ear, but it can cause unbearable pain that radiates to your eye, cheekbone, temple, teeth, and jaw. A TMJ dentist can shave down your teeth, and fit you with a bite guard if your teeth are misaligned. Pain relievers should be prescribed to help you laugh and eat again.

✳ **Post-herpetic neuralgia (PHN)**—If you've recently had shingles, you could be left with this painful syndrome. The burning neuralgias are disabling. Lyrica is a prescription medication that may work for you. There are supplements that might prove helpful, too: alpha lipoic acid, *200 mg three times daily*, and B$_{12}$ (methylcobalamin), *1,000 mcg daily*.

✳ **Ernest syndrome**—In this syndrome, the facial pain and headache begin around the ear and radiate from the temple to the jaw. It's the result of damage to the stylomandibular joint, which can happen after head trauma, dental work, a car accident, or a surgery that required anesthesia. To learn more, visit www.ernestclinic.com.

✳ **Temporal tendonitis**—This is a migraine mimic and includes temple headaches with pain radiating over the ear to the back of the head. You might also experience sensations of a swollen cheek, toothache, ear pain, and the feeling your eyeballs may pop!

✳ **Trigeminal neuralgia (TN)**—Imagine that someone plugged the nerves in your face into an electrical socket. The lancinating pain can occur from shaving, brushing your teeth, or even a slight breeze. The attacks come in episodes and then disappear; fear of the next attack dominates your life. Anti-seizure meds (such as gabapentin or Trileptal) may help, and procedures called "gamma knife" and MVD sometimes help. For more information and support, visit www.tna-support.org.

✳ **Atypical facial pain (AFP)**—To understand this disorder, imagine living with nonstop TN. If you have AFP, try an integrative approach

Why Bread Might Be Bad for You

Gluten, the protein in wheat, barley, and rye, can create inflammatory chemicals in the body and damage the coating around your nerves (called myelin). It's impossible to get real, lasting relief from any sort of pain if your nerves are raw and exposed. With gluten sensitivity, you will have a problem absorbing nutrients from food and supplements. Some scientists today suspect that many neurological complications are tied to gluten sensitivity, and there are even a number of cases mentioned in the medical literature where people with celiac disease—severe gluten sensitivity—were able to reduce their facial pain by eliminating gluten. There are tips on going gluten-free at my website, www.DearPharmacist.com, or at www.celiac.com.

for the pain that includes using prescription medications, herbs, essential fatty acids, and nerve blocks, which can be administered by an anesthesiologist. Some people call this disorder "the suicide disease" because it is so excruciating and nonstop.

Suzy's Secrets from Behind the Counter
Think Chili for Pain Relief

If you're suffering from facial pain caused by Trigeminal Neuralgia, Atypical Facial Pain, or Post-Herpetic Neuralgia, think chili—in the form of hot chili pepper cream. Wait until your facial pain has subsided a bit and then gently rub the cream, whose active ingredient is capsaicin, into your face. It doesn't erase pain on contact, so don't be disappointed. Begin by applying it twice a day (but never during an attack or you will prolong the pain) and work your way up to using it up to four times a day. At first, capsaicin causes a burning sensation, but it wears off with continued use. Capsaicin reduces "substance P," a chemical found in nerve endings that tell your brain there's pain. After a few weeks, you will numb your nerve endings, so your brain never gets the message that there's pain. The creams are sold at pharmacies for under $10. Wash your hands carefully after each application, so you don't get the pepper cream in your eyes.

8

Snoring and Other Things That Go "Boom" in the Night

Does your guy sound like an English bulldog with a sinus infection? Or maybe he's more like an engine that's misfiring—rat-a-tat-a-tat. By and large, it's the men who snore—twice as many as women—and ladies, you know this can be *really* annoying. Your guy will tell you it's no problem, except for the poking, kicking, and jabbing he gets from you to shut up! Of course, women snore, too, and even more so after menopause because progesterone levels drop and this hormone is needed to stabilize the musculature of your airway.

But snoring is more than an annoyance. Some snorers get morning headaches and daytime fatigue, while their bedmate suffers with daytime drowsiness and irritability. Snorers also are at higher risk for diabetes, high blood pressure, stroke, and heart disease.

According to the National Sleep Foundation, snoring is the primary cause of sleep disruption for approximately 90 million Americans—37 million suffer from it on a regular basis. So if you or your mate snores occasionally, don't worry—it may just be related to minor sinus congestion, a cold, or allergies. It might even be the result of sleeping on your back, especially if you're carrying a few extra pounds. But if either of you makes regular night music, read on.

Hardly the Sound of Music

When you inhale during sleep, air comes in through your nose or mouth, then passes across the back of the roof of your mouth toward your lungs. On its way, the air whizzes by your tonsils, adenoids, and uvula—that little tag of tissue hanging off the roof of your mouth. If any part of this passageway is blocked or restricted, air travel is hindered, your throat dries out, and your airway tissues vibrate, causing that snoring sound. (So maybe you could stick a harmonica in your bedmate's mouth and be serenaded back to sleep?)

The most common reason for snoring is being overweight: That extra weight coats your mouth, tonsils, and throat with extra tissue, restricting the airway—and producing those golden growls. So shedding excess fat can reduce snoring dramatically. In fact, it's possible that half of all snorers could cure themselves just by slimming down. A hint that you've reached "snoring weight" is a shirt collar size greater than 17 inches for a man and 16 inches for a woman. I know dieting isn't fun. But believe me, it beats the alternatives—see more of the graphic details below.

> Alas, earplugs probably won't solve the problem of a snoring bedmate: The average snore registers somewhere between 60 and 90 decibels, while your average earplug shuts out only about 30 decibels of noise, leaving a lot of sound to exasperate you.

Snoring—especially the really loud, gasping kind—might come from many problems, but one of them is age, most likely because our throat muscles and tissues begin to sag and vibrate. Most of the time, snoring doesn't signify anything serious, but heavy snoring might actually indicate a serious disorder: Obstructive Sleep Apnea (OSA), in which you literally stop breathing for seconds or even a minute at a time. Then, when you finally do inhale, you sound as if you're choking or gasping. This cycle—quiet, choking, and snoring—goes on all night long, for 30 to 300 times a night! It is a biological cry for help, because you are literally suffocating.

An estimated 18 million people suffer from apnea—twice as many men as women—with the added long-term effects of irritability, depression, sexual dysfunction, memory loss, increased pain in the body, and daytime drowsiness. Snoring may seem funny sometimes, but apnea is nothing to giggle about: Some 38,000 people die from apnea-related complications each year. In fact, a 1990 study reported in the journal *Chest* found an increased number of strokes in patients who had obstructive sleep apnea, so it's truly not a laughing matter.

High blood pressure and heart disease are also associated with sleep apnea, though researchers aren't sure which causes which. One thing's for sure: People with sleep apnea wake up feeling exhausted—a hallmark sign. So if you think you have OSA, see a specialist as soon as possible. Medications won't work for apnea—you really just need more oxygen in your lungs—so check out the re-sources and devices listed at the end of this chapter.

Other causes of snoring include:

* chronic or seasonal allergies

* chest cold or sinus infection—anything that can block the nasal passages

* deviated septum

* enlarged or swollen tonsils

* hypothyroidism, a condition that also causes alterations in muscle tone (For more on hypothyroidism, see Chapter 1.)

Kids Snore, Too

About 10 percent of all children are habitual snorers. Around age 6 or 7, children's tonsils and adenoids grow faster than the rest of their bodies. At night, this tissue relaxes and may obstruct the airway during sleep.

Most childhood snoring is nothing to worry about—your child will likely grow out of it—but some 2 or 3 percent do suffer from OSA. If your child isn't sleeping soundly, his or her learning could be impaired during the day, so be firm with your doctor, who might overlook the possibility of OSA or chalk up sleep-deprivation symptoms to behavioral problems.

Ten Tips for Nighttime Noisemakers

1. Don't drink alcohol before bed: It causes your muscles to relax and your tongue to flail into the back of your mouth. This causes more flapping of the airway and more noise.

2. Sleep on your side. That way, your tongue doesn't fall back into your throat and your airway stays open—especially helpful if you're a "mouth" snorer. An old trick is to sew a pocket to the backside of your pajamas and stick a tennis ball in there. If you flip onto your back while you're asleep, you'll get an instant reminder to roll onto your side.

3. Try a bedtime concoction: one cup of warm water laced with 1 tablespoon each of honey and cider vinegar. This old folk remedy will lubricate your throat and maybe even turn down the decibels.

4. Don't kink your neck forward with overstuffed pillows—it restricts your airway.

5. Elevate the head of your bed 4 to 6 inches.

6. Run a humidifier. Dry air can cause nasal congestion and clogging of the airway, which worsens snoring. Ionizers that clean the air are also great.

7. Avoid milk (even soy milk) before bed. There are two strikes against dairy:
   Thick drinks like milk create more mucus in the throat and trigger more episodes of snoring. Ice cream, cheese, and other dairy products could do the same.
   Milk can be a major allergen for some—and allergies contribute to snoring.

8. Avoid antihistamines if possible: They tend to relax your throat muscles, which can cause snoring. They also dry out your throat—and the drier it is, the noisier you are.

9. Quit smoking. Smoking encourages your body to produce more mucus, a factor in snoring. Besides, why compromise your lung capacity any more? There are many great nicotine-withdrawal products available over-the-counter to help you kick the habit.

10. Put a little pillow beneath the small of your back. This support for your abdomen will help expand your lungs and open your airway.

Approach Pills and Sprays with Caution

When the sound of slumber becomes shocking to you or your bedmate, you may resort to trying to solve the problem by taking sleeping pills or giving them to your partner, but beware! Most sleeping pills worsen snoring because they relax you too much, causing your throat and tongue muscles to slacken. This is not good: You want those muscles to remain firm. Can you guess why? I'll give you a hint. *People who are awake don't snore.* Their mouth and neck muscles remain firm, allowing air to flow freely in and out, without obstruction.

As for supplements and sprays, proceed with care: Some are worthy indeed, but some are useless, not to mention expensive. The Federal Trade Commission (FTC) has become much more involved in investigating these products, and as a result of their scrutiny, the market changes constantly.

Suzy's Secrets from Behind the Counter

Exercise Your Snore Muscles!

One super way to cut back on snoring is to strengthen and tone your neck, throat, and tongue muscles. As we've seen, many snorers have lost that tone from a variety of factors, including age—but you can tighten up those muscles without even breaking a sweat. Just complete this simple exercise routine at least once a day—you can even do these exercises right before bed:

1. Hold a pencil between your teeth for up to five minutes. Grip it firmly but not painfully.

2. Press your finger gently against your chin for up to three minutes.

3. Push your tongue against your lower row of teeth for about five minutes.

Sleep Clinics: New Help for the Night's Most Wicked Nuisance

Sleep clinics are popping up everywhere, serving as keen reminders for us to get the rest that is crucial to optimal health—and to our very survival.

﹡ Plug in your address and zip code to find a sleep center near you at www.sleepcenters.org.

﹡ For general information on sleep and disorders, try www.sleep foundation.org.

﹡ For support group information and other great resources, visit the American Sleep Apnea Association (ASAA) at www.sleepapnea.org.

Spiffy Stuff to Help You Sleep

I recommend all of the following products—they're natural, noninvasive, and often effective. They don't work for everybody, though, so you may need to experiment to see what works for you.

﹡ **PillowPositive**—This patented cervical pillow has been dubbed the "sleep apnea" pillow because it's helped people with mild cases of this disorder—so don't expect results if you've got a moderate or severe condition. The pillow extends your head and neck into the same position they're in if you were undergoing CPR, allowing you to lie back and get more airflow into your passages. Its removable inserts make it somewhat adjustable, enhancing your comfort. Manufactured by LifeSleep Systems. Cost: $120.

A lot of other companies make this type of pillow, which is amazingly comfortable, especially if it's made of memory foam—the type of foam that supports alignment of your neck, shoulders, and spine. It reduces both snoring and muscle tension. You can tell if your pillow is made of memory foam if it holds the imprint when you stick your hand into the foam. These support pillows last for many years, so even though they may seem expensive, you really get your money's worth out of them.

✳ **Helps Stop Snoring**—This product—available as gargle or spray—contains fifteen essential oils, including peppermint, lemon balm, fennel, sage, citronella, and lavender. It was developed in the UK to induce better sleep, calm inflammation, and lubricate your throat and passageways. Some people swear by-products like these, although critics argue that the essential oils might seep into your lungs as you sleep, possibly causing pneumonia. Fortunately, this is extremely rare and there are many satisfied users of sprays—in fact, the product's website boasts about a double-blind clinical British study which found that 4 out of 5 sufferers got relief. The findings were published in a 2004 issue of *Phytotherapy Research,* an international journal that publishes research articles. You can buy "Helps Stop Snoring" spray in most pharmacies in the UK and on the Internet. Cost: $10.

✳ **Snore Stop**—You can buy this product at any pharmacy as a throat spray, a chewable tablet, or an "extinguisher"—another type of throat spray. Snore Stop is a combination of all-natural homeopathic ingredients that shrink swelling of the soft tissues of the throat while eliminating built-up mucus in your nasal passages. Cost: $20.

✳ **Marjoram oil**—This essential oil has been touted as a remedy for snoring. It's typically sold in a jar, and the oil saturates a type of sponge. Leave the jar open on a nightstand or dresser, allowing the oil to gradually fill your bedroom with a pleasant scent.

✳ **Breathe Right**—These drug-free nasal strips are sold over-the-counter in every pharmacy. They're adhesive strips that resemble a thin Band-Aid; they gently pull on both sides of your nose, helping it to flare and opening your nasal passages. They're great for the kind of snoring that's caused by a cold or congestion. The same company makes a Breathe Right throat spray that claims to be effective for up to 85 percent of snorers. Cost: less than $15 for a pack of strips or for the spray.

✳ **Silent Snore by Dr. Frank**—This product—found at most pharmacies—contains a naturally occurring substance, MSM (methylsulfonylmethane), which might be able to curb the snore-producing vibrations at the back of your throat. One study of thirty participants showed a 90 percent success rate. Just give yourself one or two minty sprays each night to the back of your throat, then swallow—and don't drink or eat afterward. Cost: $10.

＊ **Anti Snor Therapeutic Ring**—Talk about jewelry with a purpose: While you sleep, you wear this pretty, sterling-silver ring on your left pinkie finger, where it puts the squeeze on some of the Chinese acupressure points associated with sleep. The gentle pressure may relieve your snoring within a few days, or you can take advantage of the company's money-back guarantee within thirty days. Choose from one of four sizes at www.antisnor.net. Cost: $50.

＊ **Noiselezz**—This relatively new antisnoring device consists of a soft plastic appliance that looks like a dental guard and prevents your lower jaw from falling backward, keeping your tongue from vibrating against the soft tissues at the back of your throat. You don't usually need a fitting as this appliance fits most mouths—but I'd advise consulting with your dentist before wearing one, since people with temporomandibular joint (TMJ) syndrome may find that it increases their pain. Noiselezz fits over your dentures, too, assuming your dentures are also fitted properly. Buy it through a dentist who's familiar with it, or online at www. nosnorezone.com. Cost: $65–$70.

＊ **Sleep Right**—The only no-boil night guard that adjusts and protects against teeth grinding. It is sold at many Target stores and online at www.sleepright.com or 888-792-0865.

＊ **SomnoGuard**—This is another fitted soft appliance that looks like a clear plastic impression for your teeth. It works best for people who are "closed-mouth" sleepers. Actually, it's pretty similar to Noiselezz. It's best to have your dentist custom-fit you so he or she can check for TMJ at the same time. However, fitting instructions come in a CD-ROM with the product. More information is available at www.nosnorezone. com. Cost: $65–$70.

＊ **Snore Free**—A plastic ring with two magnets attached at each end, this device was developed by a former NASA scientist. Just attach it to your nose and let the magnets naturally stimulate your sensory nerves to open your nasal passages. (It looks a bit like a ring dangling from the bottom of your nose, hooked into each nostril.) You can expect results within two weeks, and the product claims to be 80 percent effective. It's available from a British company that is located at www.healthymagnets.co.uk. Cost: $20.

✳ **CPAP (Continuous Positive Airway Pressure)**—This is not the sexiest-looking device, but at least it's worn in the dark! The older devices are just face masks that push air into your mouth and prevent the collapse of the upper airway passages during your sleep—a common problem for people with sleep apnea. The CPAP won't cure snoring, but it does stop—or at least minimize—snoring as long as it's worn. Since the product is a face mask, it tends to bother people with claustrophobia. Newer designs are sleek and more comfortable because they fit under the nostrils and don't cover the eyes. The device must be prescribed for you by a specialized sleep doctor from a sleep clinic after an overnight sleep study. You might resemble a Klingon—but at least you won't sound like one! The smallest and lightest CPAP that I could find on the market is called the GoodKnight420G, which retails for about $300 and is made by Puritan-Bennett. Your insurance plan may cover a CPAP machine, if you have OSA. You can find more product information at www.cpap.com, or call 800-356-5221. Talk with a sleep specialist to see if this device is right for you.

Procedures of Last Resort

Treatment of snoring is not generally a condition that health insurance companies or Medicare will cover, because they consider it cosmetic, unless you're diagnosed with Obstructive Sleep Apnea or some other qualifying disorder. If you feel you need one of these "last-resort" procedures, try to find a helpful doctor who will either bill your procedures as "office visits" or write you a "medical necessity" letter.

✳ **Pillar® Procedure**—During this brief outpatient procedure, three tiny inserts (18 mm long) are placed in your soft palate, stiffening and adding structural support to reduce or eliminate the flutter that causes snoring and/or the collapse that causes OSA. This FDA-cleared treatment does not require general anesthesia, and most patients see noticeable improvement within a few weeks, though the full effects may take three months. In a one-year study, Pillar Procedure reduced obstructive sleep apnea in 81 percent of patients. The procedure isn't routinely covered by most health insurance plans, but some offices will work with you. You can find a doctor in your area who performs the procedure at www.pillarprocedure.com. Cost: $1,500–$2,500.

✳ **UPPP (Uvulopalatopharyngoplasty)**—You'll need anesthesia for this one. A surgeon will remove the back of your soft palate and uvula, along with any excess tissue in the throat, such as tonsils and adenoids. This is an older procedure than the laser- and radio-powered ones, with the risk of removing too much of your palate, possibly causing a hoarse voice and the embarrassing sight of liquids backing up into your nose or even spewing out of it. That may make interesting dinner conversation for your 4-year-old, but otherwise, it is very embarrassing and quite uncomfortable. Still, some people need this procedure, which is successful about 30 to 50 percent of the time. If you have OSA, your insurance may cover this procedure. Cost: $5,000–$7,000.

✳ **LAUP or Laser-Assisted Uvulopalatoplasty**—Similar to UPPP, this approach is less invasive and more comfortable. It's an outpatient procedure that uses local anesthesia, and you'll need three to five of them to improve a sagging, floppy palate. LAUP relies on lasers, not to remove your tissue but to slowly scar and tighten it, allowing easier airflow. Some doctors have revised this standard LAUP treatment into a one-step treatment where tissue is actually removed. Either way, you'll probably have no bleeding, but you may be stuck with a sore throat that lasts for about a week, relievable by pain meds like acetaminophen or hydrocodone. It doesn't seem to be incredibly effective if you have sleep apnea, although it's a very popular treatment option. You may be able to arrange for reimbursement from your insurance company. Cost: $1,500–$3,000.

✳ **Somnoplasty**—This outpatient procedure is similar to LAUP but uses radio frequency energy instead of lasers to shrink and tighten the soft tissues in your upper airway. It is sometimes abbreviated as "RPM," which stands for Radiofrequency Palatal Myoplasty. Reshaping these upper airway tissues stops the palate vibration and prevents subsequent snoring. For each of three treatments, you'll have to spend about an hour in your doctor's office, although you'll only be exposed to radio waves during ten to fifteen minutes of that time. After each treatment, you should be able to return immediately to your normal activities. There are several varieties of Somnoplasty, so make sure that the one you're having is covered by your insurance policy. Cost: $1,000–$2,500.

✳ **Genioglossus advancement**—In this surgical procedure, your tongue is moved forward, preventing it from falling backward and vibrating. The doctor makes a small slice in your tongue, then tugs forward some bone attached to the tongue and fastens it to its new position with a screw. This procedure is often done along with Maxillomandibular Advancement (MMA), which basically breaks your jawbone in a few places and then shifts it forward. MMA is also used cosmetically, to correct a receding chin, and is usually performed by maxillofacial surgeons. Insurance plans usually cover this if you have a diagnosis of OSA or something other than "snoring." Cost: about $8,000–$10,000.

9

A Nation of Insomniacs

Do You Really Need a Pill to
Get a Good Night's Sleep?

I f you used to sleep like a brick, but now wish you had one to knock yourself out—you have insomnia. According to the National Institutes of
Health, more than 70 million people in the United States deal with sleep
troubles, but fortunately we have Starbucks to get us through the day! I call it
my "brains in a cup."

All kidding aside, too many insomniacs are relying on stimulants to make
up for lost sleep. Sleep patterns do alter as we age, but the average adult needs
seven to nine hours of rest in order to feel human the next day. Without that,
you may become tired, accident-prone, frazzled, frustrated, and freaked out.
So here's some "bedtime reading" to help you sleep.

Has TV Made You Think You're an Insomniac?

Ignore those sleep-med commercials you see on TV. Drug companies spend
billions of dollars to convince you that a good night's sleep is easy to achieve.
Sure, at the price of $5 a pill! The newest short-acting agent that can put you to
sleep will go by the brand name Indiplon if it ever gets a thumbs up from the
FDA. It seems that—try as they might—the makers are having problems getting FDA approval and marketing bucks so they can't get a chunk of the change
that is currently shared by Lunesta, Sonata, and Ambien. By the way, Ambien

lost its patent in 2005, so a generic is out. Guess what, the makers are now promoting the new and improved version, Ambien *CR* instead. Cha-ching!

You may need to consider sleep meds—but only after you've exhausted all other potential remedies. Many deceptive ads paint prescription meds as "non-narcotic" to imply safety, suggesting that you can't get addicted to them. But even non-narcotic drugs can cause physical dependence and addiction, meaning that you come to rely on them in order to fall asleep, and you need higher and higher doses as time goes by.

What's really scary is that you may not even realize you're addicted to a prescription sleep aid until you try to stop taking it—and face withdrawal symptoms. The only sure way to avoid addiction is to restrict your use to once or twice a week. If you rely on prescription sleep aids more than three times a week for two weeks in a row, read on, because my information could help you get a good, deep sleep *every* night—medication-free.

Is Your Bedroom a Place of Bedlam?

You might not even have insomnia—it might just be your lifestyle. For me, the desire to watch all those TiVo'd reality shows interferes with my sleep. You may be facing other distractions. So turn off Leno and Letterman and make a concerted effort to get rid of computers, hidden chocolates, TVs, and snoring husbands. (Check out Chapter 8 for more tips on that last one!) And if your teenagers are staying up too late, take the cell phone, computer, TV, and iPod out of the room: All that texting, IMing, and "MySpacing" will keep them up at night!

Which Kind of Insomniac Are You?

Some people opt for a sleep study, or "polysomnography," to answer this question. If you check into a sleep clinic, you won't exactly be sleeping at the Ritz, but you will benefit from special doctors observing you and designing your treatment. Or, if you want to try self-diagnosing, use the following descriptions. Remember, you may be a combination type.

✳ **The Creepy Crawler**—You fall asleep just fine. But then you wake up at an unreasonable hour, maybe 3 or 4 A.M., and no matter how hard you try, you can't fall back to sleep. You consider vacuuming or putting away the dishes, but at that hour, family members will wake up and retaliate by duct-taping you to the bedpost. You resort to creeping around the house or surfing the Internet instead. (The technical term for this problem is Sleep Latency Insomnia.)

✳ **Antenna Head**—You climb into bed at a reasonable hour (say, 10 P.M.) and lie there as your brain becomes an antenna for every thought on the planet. Your head goes into "rewind" mode as you think about what you should've done, what you might have said, and what you still need to do. Around 1 or 2 A.M., when you are fully maddened, you might doze off. (The medical term for this condition is Sleep Onset Insomnia.)

✳ **The Bed Bugger**—You might fall asleep just fine and even stay in bed for eight hours, but the night is long and your sleep is fitful. You may have bad dreams or night sweats, or just toss and turn. Sheets usually wind up tangled around your legs or on the floor. Someone with an aerial view would think that you had a case of the bedbugs. (The doctors call this Poor Sleep Quality.)

By the way, if you're a Bed Bugger's spouse, you've probably noticed that Bed Buggers tend to thrash so much that they either wind up throwing your sheets to the floor or entangling you both like a mummy. So if your man is a Bed Bugger, buy one fitted sheet for your mattress and then two flat twin top sheets, one for each of you. I've tried this one, and it really works!

Is Your Medication Giving You Bad Dreams?

Certain drugs are skilled at crossing through a very thin layer of cells surrounding your brain, the so-called blood-brain barrier. Then, when the medication gets to your brain cells, it does odd things, like trigger the release of mood-altering neurotransmitters, hormones that can spark hallucinations, rage, uninhibited behavior, vivid abnormal dreams, and nightmares. So if you're sleeping poorly and you're taking one of the following meds or something similar, ask your doctor about an alternative. This is not a complete list.

＊ **Breathing medications**—AccuNeb, Ventolin or Proventil (albuterol), Volmax

＊ **Blood pressure medications**—Aldomet (methyldopa), atenolol, nadolol, bisoprolol, carteolol, Carvedilol, Coreg, Corgard, Inderal (propranolol), Lopressor HCT, Zebeta, Ziac

＊ **Acid-blocking drugs**

＊ **Appetite suppressants**

＊ **Alzheimer's drugs**—Aricept (donepezil)

＊ **Sleeping pills**—Ambien (zolpidem), Sonata (zaleplon), Ativan (lorazepam), Klonopin (clonazepam), clorazepate, Dalmane (flurazepam), Halcion (triazolam), ProSom (estazolam), Serax (oxazepam), Valium (diazepam), and Restoril (temazepam). It's ironic that sleeping pills make this list!

> Scientists studied fifty insomniacs and found that the people who visualized a relaxing scene, such as a waterfall, fell asleep twenty minutes faster than those left to their own devices. But here's the kicker: Those who counted sheep took the longest to drop off!

＊ **Antidepressants**—Zoloft, Prozac, Celexa, Lexapro Cymbalta, Wellbutrin, BuSpar (buspirone)

＊ **Antibiotics**—Cipro (ciprofloxacin), Biaxin, Levaquin (levofloxacin), Trovan, Tequin

＊ **Parkinson's drug**—Levodopa

＊ **Phenobarbital**

＊ **Eye drops for glaucoma**—Timoptic, Timoptic XE (timolol), Ocupress

Hormonal Havoc

Estrogen dominance—described more fully in Chapters 11–13—produces a wide variety of symptoms, including insomnia. Progesterone has a calming, antianxiety effect on the body. Taming the estrogen is the key, though, because it allows the "voice" of your progesterone and testosterone to be heard. So if you think you're suffering from estrogen dominance, ask your doctor to evaluate you. Also consider my Hormone Helpers in Chapter 11, to tame your estrogen. You may sleep better within a few weeks, even if you've suffered for years.

> *DO NOT take progesterone or any hormonal supplements carelessly, even if they're "natural." They could seriously disturb your menstrual cycle—and your health—if you don't follow the instructions in Part V, or on your product label.*

Restless Legs Syndrome (RLS): No Rest for the Weary

It might be the most annoying thing you've ever felt—an irresistible urge to move your legs while resting or trying to sleep. You may also feel an itchy, tugging, or otherwise weird sensation in your thighs or calves, as though a bunch of bugs were crawling all over you. Sometimes, with no warning, your leg or arm jerks out of control, though the symptoms may subside when you stand up and walk around.

You're not going bonkers. You've probably got restless legs syndrome (RLS), an under-diagnosed disorder that also causes insomnia. Many elderly people develop this condition, as well as those afflicted with fibromyalgia or Chronic Fatigue Syndrome. RLS is maddening, and it's often left untreated—or else it's treated with the kind of potent drugs used for Parkinson's, chronic pain, or epilepsy. Requip was the first drug approved for the treatment of RLS—in 2005—and it's still very popular. Mirapex is another medication in the same class and was approved by the FDA in November 2006. Commercials for the drug are rather interesting, and if you're not paying attention to the TV, you might miss the part where the announcer says, "...tell your doctor if you experience increased urges to gamble or have sex." The first time I heard that, I had to play it back with my DVR because I couldn't believe my ears. And as a pharmacist, my first thought was, "Woo hoo, Mirapex is gonna put Viagra out of business!"

So back to these urges... now I don't know about you, but if I get an urge to gamble, or have sex, it's not my physician that I think to call! How would the conversation go, anyway? "Hey, doc, I'm feeling a little frisky and I'm headed to Vegas to play blackjack, could you fax a refill prescription to Caesar's Palace before these urges subside?"

Mirapex and Requip were originally approved for the treatment of Parkinson's disease. They affect muscle control and tremors by boosting levels of a brain chemical called dopamine. But when you increase dopamine—your passion hormone—you also increase urges of all sorts (!), which explains the interesting side-effect profile. Narcolepsy is also a possible reaction to this medication, but don't worry, when you eventually wake back up, your legs won't hurt.

So at this point, you're probably wondering if I agree with the use of these types of medication. I think that if you've tried all of the recommendations below and you want to try medication, go ahead. Just be sure to discuss your discomfort with your physician first to make sure that your RLS doesn't indicate kidney disease or blood sugar abnormalities. If these meds work for you, and you tolerate them well, take them with my blessings.

What Can You Do Right Now?

✳ Reduce or eliminate caffeine.

✳ Older antihistamines and over-the-counter sleep aids (containing diphenhydramine) might make your condition worse. Try Claritin (loratadine) or Alavert instead.

✳ Take some nutritional supplements. Start with the lowest doses and if they don't help, work your way up:

> ✳ *Folic acid*—I like the "body-ready" forms sold as Thorne's 5-MTHF or Metagenics's FolaPro. Take *1 tablet daily (about 800 mcg)*. If you have trouble finding these special activated forms of folic acid, take a higher dose of the regular kind that is sold over-the-counter at pharmacies nationwide—*about 800 mcg twice daily*. More if your doctor permits.

> ✳ *Calcium-magnesium citrate or chelate*—Find a combination of about *600 mg calcium and 200 mg magnesium*, and then follow the directions on the bottle. (Solaray makes a good one.) Magnesium is fantastic for eliminating cramps and, most importantly, for inducing sleep. In a study of more than 200 patients,

magnesium chloride was found to induce the kind of sleep that is restful and uninterrupted. Unlike most prescription drugs, magnesium supplementation did not cause morning fatigue or daytime anxiety in participants, and, sorry to tell you, it caused no wild urges to gamble and have sex!

* *Iron—150 mg of Nu-Iron (iron polysaccharide complex) each day for one month, taken with food.*

    Note: Iron may impart a harmless black or greenish discoloration to your urine or feces, but don't worry—that's normal. Also, don't take iron for more than three months (unless directed to do so by your physician) because too much of the mineral over time, or excessive doses, can tilt your ratio of copper to zinc out of balance. Finally, a 2002 study found that red grape juice and prune juice could seriously squash the amount of iron you absorb from your supplement, so don't take your iron with either of those fruit drinks.

* *L-carnitine—500–1,000 mg twice daily with food.* The nutrient is imperative for muscle health.

* If you take blood pressure pills, tricyclic antidepressants, medicine for diabetes, or statin cholesterol drugs, you may need only a supplement of **Coenzyme Q10** (*100 mg*) and B-complex (*50 mg*), both each morning. Yes, it could be that simple!

* You might reduce cramping by upping your **potassium** with a daily 8-ounce serving of Gatorade or a similar electrolyte drink. Also, potassium-rich foods (figs, bran, apricots, raisins, squash, beans, baked potato with skin, watermelon, or spinach) are helpful.

A good resource for more information is the Restless Legs Syndrome Foundation: www.rls.org.

Are Pills in Your Medicine Chest Keeping You Awake?

Some one thousand drugs can interfere with sleep, causing you to feel wired, hyper, "buzzed," or otherwise arousing your brain waves. If your medication is on the following list, it may be causing insomnia, so ask your doctor for an alternative:

* **Antidepressants**—Wellbutrin, Zoloft, Prozac, Paxil, Lexapro, Celexa

* **Cough/cold remedies** containing the decongestant pseudoephedrine or phenylephrine. These are frequently (but not always) labeled as "non-drowsy."

* **Estrogen-containing drugs**—birth control or hormone replacement pills, patches, injections, and creams

* **Evista** (raloxifene)

* **Guarana**—found in natural weight-loss products and energy drinks and bars

* **Statin cholesterol drugs**—Lipitor, Zocor (See Chapter 2 for complete list.)

* **Drugs for Attention Deficit Hyperactivity Disorder (ADHD)**—Ritalin (methylphenidate), Adderall (amphetamine salts), and Dexedrine (dextroamphetamine)

* **Most diet pills**—both prescription and OTC

* **Steroids for inflammation**—prednisone, methylprednisolone, Orapred

* **Breathing medicines**—albuterol, salmeterol, theophylline, Advair, Xopenex, Atrovent, and Rhinocort—and these include inhalers as well as tablets, syrups, and pills

* **Thyroid medication,** especially if your dose is too high, or if you mistakenly take it at night. To avoid sleep problems, all thyroid supplements and meds should be taken upon arising.

Vitamins and Minerals: Your Secret Sleep Allies

Calcium has a calming effect on the body, while **magnesium** relaxes your muscles. So they're both good for all kinds of insomnia, not just RLS. When purchasing either calcium or magnesium, buy the "calcium citrate" or "magnesium chelate" or "glycinate" forms, since they're easier on the tummy and better absorbed into your bloodstream. You can get a combination formula, or buy these supplements separately; either way, go for doses of *500–1,000 mg* calcium and *200–300 mg* magnesium. And of course, get your doctor's approval before self-medicating, since these minerals do affect the heart—usually in a good way, but your doctor still needs to be aware of what you're doing.

Vitamin B$_{12}$, technically known as cyanocobalamin, is also crucial to your health and sleep. Signs of a B$_{12}$ deficiency—which is pretty common—include fatigue, weakness, constipation, low appetite, numbness and tingling in the hands or feet, depression, confusion, memory loss, and sores on your tongue or outer corners of your mouth. If you run low on B$_{12}$, you can't make melatonin, your sleep hormone, so you could get insomnia, or worse, an upside-down cycle where you sleep all day and stay up all night. (For more on melatonin, see below.)

You can take B$_{12}$ in a relatively inexpensive pill form—I often recommend bigger doses than conventional standards because it's hard to get B$_{12}$ out of your gut and into your bloodstream. Or most doctors will happily write you a prescription for injectable B$_{12}$, which you'll get as one simple shot in their office, or you can even inject yourself at home. If you choose oral supplements, take *500–1,000 mcg daily*. Taking B$_{12}$ in combination with "intrinsic factor" can really boost absorption. Just look for these at your health-food store. With either pills or injections, you'll spend less than $20 for a six-month supply.

Everything You Always Wanted to Know About Sleep Aids—But Were Too Tired to Ask

If you take any prescription or over-the-counter sleep aids, these medications will seriously slooooow you down. Makes sense: Sedatives are intended to provoke sleep, so naturally, they'll slow your breathing, heart rate, digestion, and even your thought processes. So follow these suggestions to keep yourself safe at any speed:

  ✳ Before taking prescription meds, try the less potent over-the-counter remedies—but make sure your doctor and pharmacist approve.

* As with any medication, start with the lowest dose.

* Never stop a sleep med abruptly—taper off, ideally with a doctor's help. Weaning off prescribed sleepers could take months.

* Never ingest alcohol within twelve hours of taking a sleep aid—you could slow your heart rate and respiration to a deadly level.

* If your insomnia is part of a bigger problem, such as depression or pulmonary disease, treat both conditions at the same time for the best results.

Are Sleeping Pills Ruining Your Sleep?

I know this sounds crazy, but it's true: Sleep drugs can actually *interfere* with your sleep! That's true for pretty much anyone who takes them for more than a few weeks, because they don't allow your brain to follow its natural sleep cycle, which is supposed to alternate between rapid eye movement (REM) and non-rapid eye movement (NREM) in nightly cycles that usually last about ninety minutes. Most sleep medications alter or even obliterate a particular stage of sleep—usually REM sleep—which means you're not resting well, even though you feel like Silly Putty. Sleepers also might increase NREM sleep, decrease slow-wave sleep, decrease "density" of REM sleep, and interfere with your cycle in other ways. Long story short, you fall asleep, but your body is not really getting the benefits that a full cycle is supposed to provide—and sleep deprivation is the result. So you wake up feeling unrefreshed, and you're tired and groggy all day long. Even more alarming, many prescription and OTC sleep aids cause a paradoxical reaction in about 10 percent of people who take them, triggering nightmares, talkativeness, mania, tremors, hyperactivity, and anxiety. As your 24-hour pharmacist, I need to warn you about overdoing it. Taking more than the recommended dose of your sleeper may cause breathing problems—it can slow down your respiration.

You'll Sleep Better Without a Nightcap!

Alcohol interferes with normal sleep patterns. A little may put you to sleep, but drink too much and you'll wake up in the middle of the night from the havoc alcohol plays with your REM sleep, inhibiting deep sleep—not to mention that it sparks more bathroom trips. If you're not sleeping well, go alcohol-free for two weeks and I bet you'll start feeling more rested overall.

Sleepytime Plants

Herbal extracts have been used medicinally for centuries all over the world. In the U.S., plant extracts come in all shapes and sizes: capsules, teas, tinctures, and ointments, among others. Now, I'm all for natural aids, but you should remember that any substance, even a natural one, can give you an allergic reaction—so stop taking these herbal products if you notice any adverse effects. I recommend you get your doctor's blessings if you have any psychiatric condition or take sedating medications like painkillers, muscle relaxers, sleeping pills, and certain antidepressants.

Often, herbal products combine two or more sleep-inducing herbs, so look for teas, tinctures, powders, or pills that contain any of the following:

* **Chamomile (*Matricaria recutita*)**—great for Antenna Heads and Creepy Crawlers. Chamomile belongs to the ragweed family, so stay away from it if you are allergic to ragweed.

* **Lemon balm (*Melissa officinalis*)**—indicated for Creepy Crawlers and Bed Buggers. People with thyroid conditions may find that this herb makes their conditions worse. Avoid using it excessively; limit its use to only a few days at a time each month.

* **Passionflower (*Passiflora incarnata*)**—good for Creepy Crawlers, Antenna Heads, and Bed Buggers. Also great for easing muscle twitches—it may even have some benefit for people with epilepsy. Start with low doses because this one's powerful and you may wind up with morning fatigue. Also, do not confuse this type with a relative called "blue passionflower"—it is NOT the same thing.

* **Valerian root (*Valeriana officinalis*)**—suggested for Antenna Heads and Bed Buggers. It shortens the time needed to drop off to sleep, without creating any morning hangover effect. It's particularly helpful for people with elevated blood pressure due to stress and worry

because it relaxes the tiny muscles of the artery walls. It's a myth that valerian root is related to the drug Valium. Start with very low doses because you may be sensitive to it. In certain people, valerian can paradoxically cause insomnia and even heart palpitations.

✻ **Lavender (*Lavandula angustifolia*)**—ideal for Antenna Heads. Interestingly, when applied to the skin as a lotion or oil, lavender seems to soothe burns and ease bug bites. For sleep, try inhaling the aromatic scent of lavender, or drink a pure herbal tea.

The Melatonin Miracle

Melatonin is a hormone that is secreted from the pineal gland, which serves as our "master clock." It fluctuates according to our circadian rhythm, telling us when to sleep, how long to sleep, and when to wake up. Our melatonin levels decline as we age, which is one reason we start losing sleep. Melatonin declines if we are stressed, too. We can boost our melatonin levels with a dietary supplement that's sold in pharmacies and health-food stores. Don't expect results the first night, but if you stick with it, you'll probably see results in about three weeks. Do make sure you're taking a B-complex each morning, because the melatonin won't be as effective without it. The B will energize you, so take that in the morning; the melatonin relaxes you, so take that at night about an hour before bedtime.

My recommendation is to start with a *1 mg* dose of melatonin nightly and if that doesn't help after three weeks, work your way up—add *1 mg* every three weeks—until you've reached the maximum dose of *3 mg*. This is quite a large dose by some experts' estimates, and it's not safe for everyone. For that reason, and because melatonin is a hormone that has far-reaching effects in your body, it's best to take a saliva test to determine hormone levels. Just call one of the labs that I list in my Resource section. With a test, you can custom-fit a dose of melatonin that is perfect for you. Some people get noticeable improvement within four weeks, but if you don't, you could do one of three things:

1. Switch brands to find one that is more effective for you.

2. Bring in another sleep supplement to augment the melatonin— for example, passionflower.

3. Wean off it altogether because something other than low melatonin may be causing your insomnia.

You won't hear me say this often, but take a synthetic version of melatonin.
The "natural" kind is usually derived from cows and seems to trigger allergic
reactions more frequently in people than the lab-created versions that are not
animal-derived.

Melatonin has other effects in the body beyond its use as a sleep aid. Scientists say that melatonin may:

* minimize or ease jet lag

* cut cravings for cigarettes, hypnotics, and tranquilizers (benzodiazepines)

* prevent cluster headaches

* ease autoimmune disorders, especially multiple sclerosis

* protect against skin cancer and other tumors that could cause breast,
prostate, and lung cancer

* ease tinnitus, a.k.a., an incessant ringing in your ears

It's rare for people to notice any side effects from melatonin, but it has been
tied to asthmatic attacks, so if you suffer with asthma, especially nocturnal
asthma, stay away from it altogether.

For all others, I should tell you that some experts suggest taking this hormone only twice a week, rather than every single night.

A 2003 study in the *Journal of Allergy and Clinical Immunology* found
that people who suffered with lung problems, bronchospasms, or asthmathic
attacks had higher levels of melatonin.

Magic Mushrooms

For centuries, Chinese and Japanese herbalists have revered the Reishi mushroom for its ability to improve liver and cardiac function as well as to enhance
sleep. No, these mushrooms are no relation to the hallucinogenic kind from

the 1960s and 1970s! In fact, there are references to this medicinal mushroom as far back as 100 BCE. Give them a month or two before your deep sleep improves. There are many good brands that have "Reishi" on the label. I've tried JHS Natural Products' formula called Reishi Gano 161, available at www.jhsnp.com. Cost: $20–$30. Great for Creepy Crawlers, Antenna Heads, and Bed Buggers.

5-HTP: The Natural Relaxant

A precursor to serotonin—a hormone that lifts depression, elevates mood, and promotes good sleep—5-HTP occurs in your body naturally, but you can also take it as a supplement. You get a double benefit from 5-HTP, because in the body, it goes on to make both serotonin *and* melatonin. Serotonin helps improve mood, and melatonin regulates sleep. Start with *50 mg* taken around dinner, and after a week increase to *100 or 150 mg* if necessary. Some people feel stimulated by 5-HTP; if you're one of those, take it earlier in the day or try something else. Don't take it with prescribed antidepressant drugs. Great for Creepy Crawlers and Antenna Heads.

Suzy's Secrets from Behind the Counter

Timing Is Everything

If you're having trouble sleeping, it could just be a matter of *when* you're taking your meds for other ailments. So before you reach for the sleepers, please ask your pharmacist to review all your medications. There's a simple rule in pharmacy: *Take energizing meds in the morning and relaxing ones at night.* Thyroid hormone, newer SSRI antidepressants, nasal decongestants, and appetite suppressants should be taken in the morning because they create energy or cause restlessness. Also, diuretics or "water" pills used for blood pressure are morning medicines because they inspire bathroom trips. Likewise, pain pills, muscle relaxers, antipsychotic meds, Alzheimer's drugs, and blood pressure pills should be taken at night because these can make you feel drowsy or dizzy.

To fall asleep, breathe deeply. Try to make your hands and feet warm up and get tingly. The blood flow into your extremities and away from your brain will help relax you.

If You Really Need Sleep Meds . . .

Some of you will implement every suggestion I offered and still not sleep. My friend Marita has tried *everything* and says she can't afford to go sleepless any longer because her nightly sprees on QVC are costing her too much! So for her—and you—medication may be the answer. The nice thing about sleeping medications (both prescription and over-the-counter) is that they begin working the very night you take them.

It's impossible for me to list every single agent here, but I'll share some popular ones that are currently on the market, in case you're already taking something that isn't working well enough. For any sleep med, keep a "sleep diary" to track how well you're responding. Jot down any changes, for example: "had enough energy to clean today, woke up refreshed, had more patience at my job." Also, take note of anything peculiar, such as "got dizzy and bumped into two walls, had a bad dream, threw up breakfast, couldn't remember my boss's name . . ." With a diary, you'll know within a few days whether or not you want to continue that drug.

Over-the-Counter Sleep Aids

Over-the-counter (OTC) sleep aids are sold everywhere, in many different brands, but usually with one of two ingredients, either diphenhydramine or doxylamine. Both of these are a type of antihistamine, similar to the kind found in cold or allergy meds. These medications are not addictive, but they do tend to interfere with deep sleep because of the way they monkey with your REM and NREM cycles. They are relatively safe unless you have angina, heart rhythm problems, glaucoma, enlarged prostate, difficulty urinating, or breathing problems. Typical side effects are morning fatigue, poor coordination, blurred vision, dry mouth, and daytime drowsiness. Some popular brand names are Sleepinall, Sominex, Nytol, Simply Sleep, and Unisom. Sometimes, these medications are combined with pain relievers like acetaminophen and marketed as Tylenol PM. Another pain reliever/sleep aid combination is Excedrin PM. The "PM" in a product's name is a dead giveaway that it has some sort of sleep aid in it.

Prescription Sleep Aids

✳ **Antidepressants**—The FDA may not have approved these medications for insomnia, but they are routinely prescribed because they are sedating. Two examples are trazodone (Desyrel) and amitriptyline (Elavil).

✳ **Benzodiazepines**—These hypnotics dampen the nervous system and cause the brain to release a hormone called GABA. These drugs may cause next-day hangover and daytime drowsiness, and they're addictive. They take about thirty minutes to an hour to cause drowsiness, and their effects are long-lasting. Ah, you think this is good. Well, maybe so, maybe not. Long-lasting drugs are more likely to cause morning hangover. These drugs affect sleep patterns and may interfere with REM sleep. Some popular ones are temazepam (Restoril), estazolam (ProSom), clonazepam (Klonopin), triazolam (Halcion), oxazepam (Serax), flurazepam (Dalmane), lorazepam (Ativan), and alprazolam (Xanax).

✳ **"Z" drugs**—These drugs get their name from the Z in their chemical designation. They're promoted as being better than older benzodiazepines, but I think their efficacy and addictive potential are about the same. It really depends on what study you read and, dare I say it, on who funded the study! Their advantage over benzodiazepines is that they work very quickly, within five or ten minutes, so take them and immediately hit the sack. They mimic your sleep cycle much better than benzodiazepines. Z drugs don't linger in the body, so you're less likely to have a morning hangover, but then you also might not get a full night's sleep. Examples of popular medications in this group include zaleplon (Sonata), zolpidem (Ambien), eszopiclone (Lunesta), and cyclopyrrolone (Indiplon).

✳ **Melatonin agonists**—This is a new kind of sleeping pill, a prescription med that mimics the actions of our natural sleep hormone, melatonin, but with a far more potent effect. It works according to our circadian rhythm, helping people to fall

Avoid sleeping pills or sedatives when you fly: They slow down the blood flow in your legs. Given that you're cramped up in a tiny space, you've got the perfect recipe for a blood clot. Sure, it's unlikely, but it is possible, especially if you are elderly or have circulation problems. I say, save the sleepers for when you land and tuck yourself into your hotel room.

asleep faster and stay asleep longer. The first and currently only drug in this class is ramelteon (Rozerem). For full disclosure, I served as a clinical consultant for the manufacturer back in 2006. This type of drug may be safer for certain people who require medication: As of 2006, clinical trials had shown no evidence of physical addiction or next-day hangover, since this med hones in on the brain's "master clock" rather than showering your entire brain with GABA like other popular sleep aids do. Because melatonin rather than GABA is produced (as with other sleep aids), deep sleep occurs with little or no next-day hangover. Cost: $85–$100 for a month's supply.

part III

Below the Waist

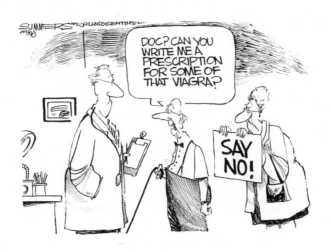

10

When He Wants Viagra and You Want a Valium

When I started working on this chapter, I gathered a group of ten lady friends of assorted ages and took a survey. "What's your biggest sexual issue?" I asked them.

My boldest friend laughed. "I'm tired all the time and he just wants to have sex," she said candidly. "What fool created that pill?"

After the giggles, this sentiment was echoed by other women in the group. They all seemed to feel that they were stuck in neutral while their man was all revved up, thanks to the power of the almighty "blue diamond" pill—Viagra.

As far as I'm concerned, a person's low sex drive might just be a preference. Or maybe it's a natural part of aging. It's certainly not a disease as the drug-makers imply. Do we really need to pharmaceutically enhance sex drives for 60- or 70-year-old men at the expense of their hearts and vision? And what will it take for the rest of us to keep up with them?

The "Diseasing" of Sex

Guess what? There's a new "disease" coming soon, which you'll hear about as soon as the FDA approves a drug to treat it. It's called Hypoactive Sexual Desire Disorder—HSDD for short—and it apparently strikes women like Bree from *Desperate Housewives* who suffer from "decreased or absent sexual fanta-sies and desire for sex." In fact, the drugmakers have already gotten approval for the sex patch containing testosterone, called "Intrinsa," in Europe. It got the nix in the United States because there weren't enough long-term tests to show safety. But no worries, Libigel is almost available. That's a testosterone gel that women apply to their arms; it provides a steady hormone supply and boosts bedroom fantasies and fun. What's next? How about a sex pill called "VaVaVaVoom," which pharmacists will store right next to Viagra?

Now, don't get me wrong. I love sex and I am sure that there are millions of issues regarding arousal, orgasm, and overall sexual satisfaction that do need attention. However, I can't help but notice the tremendous financial opportu-nities that result from turning "low sex drive" into a disease, giving it a diagno-sis code for billing insurance, and then charging exorbitant prices for medications to relieve you. What if I told you that some of those sexual "blahs" might be caused by a whole range of conditions, and might not require these new drugs, which offer no information on their long-term safety or adverse ef-fects. Let's take a look at some culprits in the bedroom . . .

Sexual Culprit #1: Stress

Women who feel burnt out from life are generally not interested in sex, even if they love their partners deeply. When your adrenal glands are pushed to their limit from a hectic, busy, stressful life, your body stops producing its sex hor-mones and starts producing "stress" hormones like adrenaline and cortisol.

I have one friend in her early fifties—normally a lively, sexually open person—who came to me in fear because, she said, she'd suddenly "dried up." She wanted to know if she needed some kind of medication—maybe hormone replacement therapy (HRT). I knew she was a night owl and a workaholic who rarely slept more than four hours a night, so I told her, "You don't need HRT. You just need some R&R, a relaxing CD, and a little TLC!" She took a vaca-tion and on the fourth night called me to say, "Everything is back to normal!" And no side effects, either!

Well, it makes sense, doesn't it? Once you start to nourish your adrenal glands, your body starts making sex hormones again. My friend was lucky, because often, adrenal burnout and the resulting low sex drive can take months to repair. So if you're feeling sexually numb, check out Chapter 1 and start nourishing your adrenals. You'll feel better in a whole bunch of ways—outside the bedroom too.

Sexual Culprit #2: Imbalanced Hormones

Here's another statement that seems almost too obvious: Your sexual vitality, stamina, and arousal are directly affected by the level of sex hormones in your body. So if the delicate balance between estrogen, testosterone, and progesterone is disrupted, you pay a price in the bedroom. Other signs that your hormones are out of whack include hair loss, vaginal dryness, insomnia, fatigue, no muscle strength, and mood swings. So *please,* if you want a long-term fix, don't turn to all those over-the-counter sex pills—correct the hormonal imbalances instead. And guys, using Viagra, Cialis, and Levitra to boost your sex drive is the equivalent of trying to jump-start your car every two miles. I'm saying fix your battery with hormones!

Many physicians don't treat hormone imbalance; they just prescribe a quick-fix pill. It's important to find an endocrinologist, gynecologist, or other type of physician who offers hormonal testing, usually with saliva or urine. (Learn how to find such a doctor in Part V.)

You also need a clever lab. One that I've come across is ZRT Laboratory: I like them because you can test at home and send the results back to them. Not only do they evaluate your hormone levels, they also review your medication profile to see which drugs may be dampening your sex drive. (For more on labs and testing, see Resources.)

Once a hormonal imbalance has been identified, your doctor can help you restore balance, either with over-the-counter supplements, prescription medications, or customized bioidentical hormones.

DHEA: The Fountain of Youth?

One of the key sex hormones is testosterone, the male sex hormone—but believe it or not, this substance is crucial for sex drive in women, too. So if you're feeling blah in the bedroom, you may want to boost your testosterone levels, which can easily be done by upping your levels of a testosterone precursor known as DHEA.

DHEA is naturally produced in our adrenal glands, gonads (ovaries and testes), and brain. Because DHEA goes on to make several other hormones in the body, even a subtle deficiency can cause dramatic health consequences. Likewise, disease, chronic stress, and the aging process all tend to lower our DHEA levels, which is why some experts think that boosting your DHEA levels can make you feel younger and more vibrant.

DHEA is one of my favorite over-the-counter supplements—I agree with those who consider it the fountain of youth! I'm in a bit of a quandary, though, because I can't safely suggest it to all of you. Because DHEA is the precursor to many other hormones in the body, some of which are known to drive the growth of cancer, it simply isn't right for everyone. And if you're not absolutely sure that you're deficient in DHEA, you definitely don't want to randomly supplement yourself with it.

There are other potential problems with DHEA. Even though DHEA is a precursor to testosterone, it's also a precursor to estrogen—and my hormone experts tell me that in men DHEA is more likely to create that female hormone rather than the macho testosterone that they're really looking for. Bodybuilding men, please read that sentence again! According to some studies, DHEA also works for fewer than half the women who try it, and a lot of controversy exists about the possibility of its excessive use increasing the risk of estrogen-driven cancer.

Here are some safety tips if you take DHEA: Please consider taking the supplement Indole-3-Carbinol (I3C) along with it (*about 200 mg twice daily*). The I3C will help drive any extra DHEA-engendered estrogen into healthier forms. Consider chrysin, Metabolic Maintenance's DIM Complex, or Dr. Chi's Myomin—any of these control the amount of estrogen produced from supplemental DHEA.

Having given you all these warnings and safety tips, I still want you to consider DHEA, because if you're one of those people who need it, DHEA can give you back your life by boosting your energy levels, mood, and sex drive. DHEA can also help you fight infection, squash free radicals, strengthen bones, improve memory, and increase your sensitivity to insulin (a good thing if you have insulin resistance, which is also related to weight gain). So get your DHEA levels tested and, of course, ask your doctor whether this supplement is okay for you.

Luckily, it's easy to get a DHEA test: Just order a saliva test from ZRT Laboratory, John Lee's website, or Genova Diagnostics (see Resources for information). I usually recommend using a DHEA skin cream rather than oral supplements because creams bypass the liver and go right into your bloodstream, where they work more efficiently. I have to tell you, though, the best researchers in the world are debating that point, too. Wouldn't it be nice if all the scientists just agreed? While we're waiting for that happy day, Life Extension and Life-Flo are two of the many good brands of DHEA cream which are sold online and in some health-food stores. Oral supplements like tablets, capsules, and sublingual sprays are easier to find at pharmacies and health-food stores. Now, one note of caution: DHEA can be made from wild yam extract in a lab. Some nutritional companies market wild yam extract as a "natural DHEA," but I think this is inaccurate because the body can't convert wild yam into DHEA; it can only be synthesized into DHEA under strict laboratory conditions.

Drugs Can Dampen Your Sex Drive

Low sex drive is a side effect of certain medications, including:

* almost all blood pressure pills

* pain relievers containing butalbital

* acamprosate (Campral), used to cut alcohol cravings

* statin cholesterol drugs

* almost all antidepressants

* acid blockers (ranitidine, cimetidine)

* seizure medications (gabapentin, phenytoin)

* finasteride (Proscar)

* antipsychotic drugs (Risperdal, Zyprexa)

> *If you think one of these drug muggers is robbing you of your sex drive, please talk to a doctor. Do NOT stop taking your meds without a doctor's approval. Some drugs need to be tapered off gradually, so stopping suddenly could make you really sick!*

Viagra Excites Investors, Makes Profits Rise

No other drug has come close to the dizzying heights reached by Viagra (sildenafil)—doctors wrote a whopping 367,857 prescriptions for Pfizer's love pill during its first month out. This impotence drug and other copycats like Levitra (vardenafil) and Cialis (tadalafil) relax blood vessels in the penis, causing more blood flow to the area. Voilà, an erection! A natural amino acid called L-arginine (sold over the counter) is also capable of improving blood flow to the penis.

But here's what you *really* need to know: Impotence drugs and L-arginine improve erectile function, but they won't spur desire or lust. If your guy starts to have an erection, these meds may make him harder—but if nothing's going on down there, none of these drugs will get a fire started, if you know what I mean. That's why I'm so concerned with addressing sexual problems at the root—adrenal burnout, hormonal imbalance, relationship issues, and your overall life situation. Also, Viagra and similar sex pills cannot be taken with nitrate drugs traditionally used for chest pain and angina, because it could result in a dangerous drop in blood pressure. These drugs have interactions with other medications too.

So if you and your mate are not making magic, maybe buy a copy of *The Joy of Sex*, take a massage class together, or put aside a night for an exchange of fantasies—each of you gets one "special request." Don't expect either your relationship issues or your sexual concerns to be resolved by that little blue pill—because although the meds can improve an erection, they can't create one. Love, passion, and your very own sex hormones are the best aphrodisiacs on the planet. Get *them* in balance, and I promise you'll have more punch in your pajamas!

Suzy's Secrets from Behind the Counter

Have Super Sex with Super X!

Super X is nature's Viagra—a plant-based combination of Eastern herbs that gives you big results. It is sold without a prescription, and you take it only when you want it. Its combination of Panax ginseng, Tongkat Ali, and Cistanche deserticola may help spark erection, increase stamina, and delay premature ejaculation. Super X may also cause insomnia—but if you're having fun, who cares? Find Dr. Chi's formula at www.chi-health.com. *Dosage: 2–3 capsules one hour before sex.*

Andropause: Putting the "Men" in Menopause

Andropause is literally menopause for men: It's the term used to describe declining levels of testosterone in middle-aged men, usually after the age of 50. As we've seen, we need testosterone to spark desire. So here are some questions that your guy can ponder to find out whether andropause is drowning that spark.

1. Does he have less strength and endurance?

2. Has he lost the urge to ravish you?

3. Has he lost height and gained weight?

4. Is he cranky or depressed?

Honestly, it wouldn't shock me if every man saw himself in the description, whether his testosterone levels are dropping or not. So please, don't think of either andropause or menopause as a disease. A person's hormone levels are supposed to decline as you get older! But you can support them and keep them in balance if you know what to do—and you can continue to enjoy a satisfying sex life.

In fact, a healthy man whose adrenals are properly nourished can expect a relatively slow hormonal decline, so that by age 70, a guy could brag that he still has about 60 percent of his peak testosterone levels. The problem in andropause is that when testosterone declines, it sometimes upsets a man's estrogen-testosterone imbalance, creating a condition known as "estrogen dominance." Older men with malfunctioning enzymes and men of any age who eat too much hormone-laden meat, fish, and dairy may be more prone to that imbalance. Men who can't activate their B vitamins, particularly folic acid, and men who are exposed to phthalate chemicals or dioxins at work or in a war are also at greater risk for estrogen-testosterone imbalances. There is a lot of information regarding this on Dr. John Lee's website, www.johnleemd.com.

A less-talked-about reason for estrogen dominance (in both men and women) is belly fat. That's because fat cells produce estrogen. Too much estrogen and your guy can sprout voluptuous breasts to go with that rotund belly.

He could get an enlarged prostate too. (To find out what happens to *you* during estrogen dominance, see Chapters 11–13.)

In both men and women, testosterone turns into estrogen with the help of an enzyme called aromatase. So for both sexes, blocking that pathway with an aromatase blocker helps prevent some estrogen from being formed, improving the testosterone-estrogen balance. When the balance is just right, sexual appetite returns. Doctors usually prescribe aromatase inhibitors for women only, mainly for the treatment of breast cancer. However, I know of two over-the-counter supplements that act like botanical aromatase inhibitors: chrysin, derived from the passionflower, and Myomin, a formula made by Dr. Chi. You can also block aromatase by eating soy foods and colorful vegetables. Amazing, huh?

Estrogen—A Guy's Worst Enemy

Many experts, including Dr. Jonathan Wright and the late Dr. John R. Lee, believe that estrogen excess—too much estrogen for a man in relation to his other hormones—contributes to, and maybe even causes, enlarged prostate (BPH) and prostate cancer in men. Their hypothesis flies in the face of more conventional theories that prostate cancer is driven by the conversion of testosterone into dihydrotestosterone (DHT). In fact, that conventional wisdom is why conventional medicine has developed a drug, Proscar (finasteride), to slow down that conversion.

Proscar is the current gold standard for treating men with BPH. But is this drug saving lives, or is it actually putting our men at higher risk for prostate cancer? Well, that depends on what study you read and, of course, who funded it. When I did my own review for Proscar, the top-selling prostate drug in my pharmacy, I found that results were decidedly mixed.

For example, a study published in *British Journal of Cancer* in 1998 considered fifty-two men with BPH who took Proscar over a five-year period. The double-blind, placebo-controlled study reported that men slashed their PSA in half (PSA is a traditional marker for prostate cancer), so the study appeared favorable for the medication. But at the same time, the men in the study experienced a significantly higher risk of developing prostate cancer. Their PSA went down—but their risk of cancer increased.

So I wonder: If testosterone is indeed the driving factor for prostate enlargement, cancer, and impotence, why don't 18-year-olds suffer from these conditions? High as their testosterone levels are, they should have the highest rates of prostate cancer and impotence in the population—yet their prostates are healthy and most of them are virtual studs in bed: not a single problem with arousal or erection.

My conclusion? The problem isn't entirely testosterone—it's also estrogen and the overall balance of a man's hormones. Many studies concur, showing that men with the highest levels of testosterone tend to have the lowest rates of prostate enlargement, while men with the highest levels of estrogen are most likely to have enlarged prostates. In 1996, a study was published in the medical journal *Prostate* proving the role of estrogen as a culprit in prostate problems.

It makes sense because as men age, their ratio of estrogen to testosterone increases, so finding a way to suppress the amount of estrogen, DHT, and another hormone called "sex hormone binding globulin," or SHBG, is critical. Saw palmetto can protect against prostate enlargement caused by DHT, but it can't squash the elevated levels of that extra estrogen and SHBG. You need nettle root to achieve that, and shortly, I'll explain how it works. In Chapter 11, you'll also learn more about my "Hormone Helpers," which can help your man feel better.

As a pharmacist who knows how to balance the risks and benefits of medications, I think your man's goal should be to bring down his estrogen burden as much as possible, which will do all sorts of lovely things: raise his testosterone; rev up his sex life; improve his stamina, strength, and hair growth; and lower his risk of heart disease. Yay! So talk to your physician about ways to lower your guy's estrogen burden, and perhaps also consider some of the "Hormone Helpers" I suggest in Chapter 11.

Suzy's Secrets from Behind the Counter
Find That Fish!

If your guy is concerned about his prostate, suggest that he up his intake of fresh cold-water fish or maybe take *2,000 mg* of fish oil twice daily. The prestigious British medical journal *The Lancet* reports that omega-3 fatty acids—found mainly in fish and flaxseeds—halt the growth of prostate cancer cells.

Impotence and Estrogen

If your guy struggles with impotence and you think it might be caused by excess estrogen, ask him to . . .

✳ lose weight—fat produces estrogen.

✳ exercise—thirty minutes a day of moderate exercise, such as a brisk walk, five times a week.

✳ eliminate alcohol and prescription painkillers (but wean off them slowly!).

✳ get a "glucose tolerance–insulin resistance test" from his physician: More often than not, a man with excess estrogen also has insulin resistance, a common precursor to diabetes and a factor in weight gain. If your man has insulin issues, he will need a diet high in healthy proteins and low in processed carbs.

✳ eat organic fruits and veggies—the more colorful, the better. Organic is important because pesticides often mimic the effects of estrogen in our bodies.

✳ avoid hormone-laden meats, dairy, and poultry; he should go organic instead and eat only grass-fed beef.

✳ avoid touching or inhaling garden pesticides, herbicides, and ant killer—they contain xenoestrogens, chemicals that act like estrogen in the body.

✳ try to minimize contact with dry-cleaned clothes, since dry-cleaning chemicals also imitate estrogen.

✳ try the following nutrients, which will help reduce his estrogen load and improve prostate health:

    ✳ chrysin: *500 mg three times daily*

    ✳ Indole-3-Carbinol (I3C) or diindolylmethane (DIM): *200 mg twice daily* of either

* calcium d-glucarate: *500 mg (one or two capsules) three times daily*

* lycopene: *10 mg twice daily*

* beta-sitosterol *50–60 mg twice daily*

* get enough sleep—anywhere from seven to ten hours a night, depending on his needs. None of the suggestions will do much for someone who's constantly in "frazzle" mode!

Stinging Nettle May Surprise Men with Prostatitis and BPH

In about two dozen studies, stinging nettle *(Urtica dioica)* has shown itself to be a major player in relieving symptoms of BPH and prostatitis (the inflammation of the prostate gland). It works in various ways, including reducing inflammatory chemicals in the body as well as controlling the conversion of testosterone to DHT. Stinging nettle reduces levels of estrogen and, in a fairly amazing act of genius, latches onto SHBG and keeps it from attaching to (and annoying) the prostate. In one study, a nettle root extract was shown to inhibit the growth of prostate cells by 30 percent in just five days. This is fantastic news for the millions of men who suffer with prostate problems.

How do herbs such as nettle root or saw palmetto compare to Proscar (finasteride), our prescription gold standard? In fact, very well. In 2000, a randomized double-blind study published in the *British Journal of Urology* analyzed more than 500 patients. The group was divided and some were given a combination of saw palmetto and stinging nettle, while others were given Proscar.

As expected, urine flow increased and urgency decreased in both groups. Other BPH symptoms also decreased in both groups, but fewer side effects were reported in the herb-treated group.

The Wonderful World of Dr. Chi

I met Dr. Tsu-Tsair Chi, a naturopath and author of *Dr. Chi's Method of Fingernail and Tongue Analysis* (Chi's Enterprise, Inc., 2002), at a national health expo and went on to try some of his powerful Eastern-based herbal formulas—

Studies show that men who are overweight are 30 percent more likely to be impotent than their lean counterparts because fat cells make estrogen. Kill two birds with one stone: Have sex and lose weight—sex burns more than 80 calories an hour!

always with good results. If your guy wants to enhance his sex drive and reverse the uncomfortable symptoms of enlarged prostate, he might try Prosta Chi—*three capsules twice daily after a meal*. It will reduce prostate levels of DHT, improve sexual function, and boost hair growth. It could also improve urinary flow, which means less urgency. And both of you should consider Myomin, which acts as a natural aromatase inhibitor to reduce your estrogen load: *three capsules twice daily after a meal*. They can be taken alone or combined with any of the supplements I've already listed. Find Dr. Chi's products at www.chi-health.com, or call 714-777-1542.

Other Products to Raise Men's Spirits—No Doctor Required!

At some point, you just get annoyed with all the ads, mailings, and unsolicited e-mails for sex pills that will help your man "gain 3 inches" or promote "wild sex all night long!" Most companies are fly-by-night frauds with bogus clinical trials selling useless or dangerous products. So here's the low-down on what's good and what's not in the men's department:

Good:

✱ **PropeL (propionyl-L-carnitine, acetyl-L-carnitine, and alpha lipoic acid)**—This supplement may improve male sexual function even better than testosterone, and it could lift depression and fatigue in some men—and without notable side effects. You can take PropeL with any of the other supplements listed below. *Dosage: for men, three capsules morning and evening; for women, two capsules morning and evening.* Find it at a natural-food store, go to www.life-enhancement.com, or call 800-543-3873.

✱ **Saw palmetto (*Serenoa repens*)**—A terrific herb for men with enlarged prostate and symptoms such as weak stream, night urges to urinate, and that sense that you haven't "finished" peeing. I like Life Extension's brand, called Super Saw Palmetto/Stinging Nettle Root Formula with Beta Sitosterol. Another good one is Thorne's Basic Pygeum Herbal, which contains saw palmetto along with other prostate-friendly nutrients. And, of course, there are many other quality brands at Whole Foods, Wild Oats, Mother Earth, GNC, and Vitamin Shoppe. Dosage: *160 mg twice a day* (standardized extract of at least 85 percent fatty acids).

✳ **Korean (Panax) ginseng**—This herb relaxes muscles in the penis just like those prescribed sex pills do, plus it nourishes the adrenal glands. It's great for guys under tremendous pressure who have "lost that lovin' feelin'." Ginseng has a very safe track record with centuries of use, it's been backed scientifically, and it's cheap. It can thin the blood, which is considered a benefit, but don't take it if you have surgery scheduled or if you also take anticoagulant drugs like Coumadin (warfarin), Plavix, or aspirin. You can *try 500–1,000 mg three times a day;* yes, *throughout* the day, rather than just before sex, like prescribed sex pills.

✳ **L-arginine**—This sexually enhancing amino acid is available by itself or in various sex formulas like VasoRect, sold nationwide. It dilates the vessels leading to the heart, improving blood flow to the heart and the penis all at once. Get your doctor's approval first; it works much like Viagra does, but it's an amino acid, very natural. *Take 750–1,000 mg twice daily.* I like a sustained-release version to create more consistency; try CVS's Life Fitness Arginine TR.

> *If you have herpes types of viruses, like genital herpes or shingles, you need to balance your L-arginine with 1,000 mg L-lysine or you might trigger an outbreak.*

✳ **Ginkgo biloba**—Centuries old and well studied, this herb can punch up sex drive and improve memory. It's the antidote to those nasty sexual side effects from antidepressants like Zoloft, Paxil, Lexapro, Prozac, and Wellbutrin, which can produce delayed orgasm, premature ejaculation, painful erections, impotence, pain on climax, or penile anesthesia. It also improves production of nitric oxide, and it, too, thins the blood, so your guy shouldn't take it if he's on anticoagu-lants. *Dosage: 40–80 mg twice daily*, of a product standardized to 24 percent ginkgo heterosides.

Not So Good:

    ❋ **Maca root (*Lepidium meyenii*)**—Related to turnips and cabbage, this root is rich in calcium, phosphorus, iron, and natural fiber. I'm not convinced it will turn your guy into an all-night lover, but a tiny study did find that it increased sperm count. It's certainly safe to try—look for "pure maca root" and have your guy *take 500–1000 mg in the morning.*

    ❋ **Yohimbe**—It's produced from the bark of an evergreen tree and found in practically every OTC sex formula. There's no hard evidence that it really works, and some reports say the only thing it raises is your blood pressure. I don't recommend it, but it seems to be popular with men. Approach with caution.

    ❋ **Horny goat weed**—Makes me laugh just saying it! Farmers noticed their goats getting aroused on the weed, so shall we assume it does the same for our guys? Some claim it beats fatigue and lifts your guy's spirits to boot—but, ladies, there just isn't as much literature on this supple-ment as there is on other, better-studied sex supplements.

The Nose Knows Who's Hot to Trot

Our sense of smell can tell us who's hot and who's not. Sniffing out the pheromones—the unique scent that we each produce—can subconsciously drive you wild. Zinc enhances our sense of smell (and taste), reduces anxiety, and nourishes our adrenal glands. So a guy can't do any better than zinc when it comes to putting lead back in the pencil! And ladies, you may find that in-creased zinc increases your zing as well. I would prefer that you get it from your diet—just eat more clams, oysters, shellfish, turkey, alfalfa sprouts, wheat germ, and seeds, including pumpkin, sesame, sunflower, and poppy. If you prefer to supplement, try zinc gluconate lozenges, sold at any pharmacy or health-food store. *Dissolve one lozenge 2 or 3 times daily.*

For Longer-Lasting Pleasure . . . ?

If your man is quick to the finish line, he can try numbing creams that contain the anesthetic benzocaine. Maintain, Mandelay, and StayHard are a few reliable brand names. Apply them under the condom. Or for Mr. Natural, a man can also retrain himself by recognizing the "point of no return" and repeatedly backing off before orgasm. He can practice doing this on his own, then try out his new "distance training" on you.

For serious problems with premature ejaculation, a doctor might prescribe an SSRI antidepressant such as Prozac, Zoloft, or Paxil—but these drugs do have many side effects, including, often, a decrease in overall sex drive.

Yes, Yes, Yes . . . There Are Products for Women, Too!

I don't recommend sex pills for women—I prefer that you balance your hormones instead—but topical gels and creams are a different story. In fact, I call some of these products "sex in a tube"! Each brand contains a different blend, and some even contain L-arginine to increase blood flow to your nether regions: Women either love that or hate it because of the added sensitivity. A lot of sex gels also contain menthol or peppermint extract to make you feel even more tingly and help you get to the Big O even faster.

Apply any one of these creams to your clitoris or vaginal area just before sex, and within minutes, you'll feel the zing. You may have to keep experimenting, though, because some of these products work wonderfully for Betty while irritating the heck out of Babs. Check out your local pharmacy, or try these pleasure enhancers:

* **Vigorelle**—A botanical product that contains ginkgo biloba, peppermint leaf, and damiana leaf: $60 for about 30–40 applications; check out www.vigorelle.com.

* **Zestra**—Increases arousal and blood flow to vaginal area without relying on L-arginine or menthol, which may irritate some women; instead, Zestra relies on natural botanical oils. Sold in most chain pharmacies: $20–25 for 9 to 12 uses.

✳ **Emerita's Response Cream**—Contains menthol, niacin, and rosemary to really get things flowing. Sold at many health-food stores: $20 for 25 uses.

Suzy's Secrets from Behind the Counter
More Tingle to the Touch

For a quick and inexpensive sexual pick-me-up, take a shower with peppermint soap, bath gel, or shampoo—it works in a pinch to make you tingly down there and heighten your sensitivity—woo-hoo!

Kegels and "Myself"

Kegel exercises strengthen the muscles in your pelvic floor to help you reach climax more easily. No one can see you doing them, and you don't even break a sweat. Just squeeze your vaginal muscles and hold to a count of three seconds, then release. Repeat this ten times—and then do it three times a day. Work up to squeezing longer.

A small biofeedback machine called Myself, previously available by prescription only, is now being sold over-the-counter. Myself is a training device that teaches women to build endurance and strength in their pelvic floor muscles. In a small clinical trial, the product showed significant benefit, allowing about 50 percent of the women who used it to enjoy fewer symptoms of various types of incontinence. It's sold online at www.deschutesmed.com and in many chain pharmacies. Cost: $100.

For Oy! to Joy

Painful intercourse is often caused by vaginal dryness, a common complaint for menopausal women. The inability to "lube up" could also be the effects of tricyclic antidepressants, antihistamines, smoking, airline travel, or stress. A quick fix is a lubricant, which you can buy over-the-counter—some even warm up when you touch them!

Some women lubricate by inserting an entire vitamin E capsule (400 IU) up into the vagina. This might work, or you can buy a vaginal suppository of vitamin E; I like Wise Woman's brand. *Insert one nightly for two weeks; then after that, twice a week.*

Consuming pure omega-3 fish oil (*1,000 mg twice daily*) will also build up your vaginal mucus. Some studies show that ginseng taken orally can thicken vaginal mucosa, and it's great for your adrenal glands too, so try *400 mg* of Panax ginseng every morning—and be patient. It may take a few weeks before you see results.

Your doctor should consider hormonal creams or bioidentical hormone replacement, such as natural progesterone, which eases endometriosis, another very common cause of painful sex. Women who experience vaginal pain or atrophy could also find relief from DHEA cream. When applied to the skin of the inner thighs, it seems to relieve some of the pain, though it takes a few weeks. To find out more, please check out my discussion of hormones and other feminine difficulties in the upcoming chapters.

11

The Condom Broke

Birth Control Before, During, and the Morning After

It's happened to most women. The mood is set, the music's playing, the passion's about to get totally out of control and then—WHOA!! The sinking realization sets in that the condom broke, or slipped off, and now you are panicked!

Your passionate romp might also go sour from other bedroom bombshells, like realizing that you forgot to take your pill or apply your birth control patch. Or what if your diaphragm got dislodged, or you miscalculated your "safe" day? One of my friends got pregnant—for the fourth time!—because her guy "didn't pull out in time."

So how do you cope with—or, ideally, prevent—this panic scenario? You've got lots of choices, and in this chapter, I'll talk you through the best—and the worst.

Birth Control BEFORE the Main Event

✳ **Abstinence**—Maybe there is no main event? Not having any type of sex is called abstinence, and it's 100 percent effective against pregnancy. Even though it's the "best" way to avoid pregnancy, I don't suggest it for adults—it tends to make one cranky!

✳ **Ovulation method, a.k.a., the rhythm method**—You can identify the most fertile days of each month based on specific bodily signals and then avoid sex during those days. I like the Billings Ovulation Method: Visit www.billings-ovulation-method.org for details. Ladies, be warned: Statistics on their website boast a 99 percent efficacy rate, but I've asked two women who tried a version of this method, and they both got pregnant within ninety days!

✳ **"The Pill" and other hormonal contraceptives**—Oral contraceptives are about 92 percent effective in preventing pregnancy with typical use, and you've got your choice of some fifty brands and generic equivalents—or you can go for the equally effective skin patches, vaginal rings, or quarterly injections. They all work via synthetic female hormones, and they're incredibly popular: Approximately 80 percent of women aged 15–44 have taken the pill, according to the latest estimates from the Centers for Disease Control (CDC). True, hormonal contraceptives are convenient, effective, and for many women, easy. But you may be shocked to learn about some of the drawbacks:

Shocker # 1: You could get pregnant if you switch packs and take your pills incorrectly!

Most birth control pills come in a convenient dial pack that contains 28 pills. There are two types of pills: combination and mini-pills.

Combination pills get their name from their combination of estrogen and progestin (a synthetic female hormone). These are currently the most popular form of oral contraception; the top-selling brands include Alesse, Aviane, Demulen, Estrostep, Loestrin, Lo/Ovral, Mircette, Nordette, Ortho-Cept, Ortho-Novum, Ortho Tri-Cyclen, Tri-Levlen, Triphasil, Yasmin, and Zovia. Other combination contraceptives include the Ortho Evra skin patch; the injection known as Lunelle; and that insertable, transparent, flexible little ring called NuvaRing that you insert inside you like a tampon each month.

Mini-pills are made up of progestin only—no estrogen. Some popular brands include Micronor, Nor-QD, and Ovrette. (A progestin-only shot,

Depo-Provera, is also available—instead of taking a daily pill, the doctor gives you a shot once every three months and you're covered.)

Typically, with combination pills, the last seven in a pack are generally fillers—sugar pills or sometimes iron supplements. Basically, they're just there to help you keep count and to remind you to take your pill every day—so you could toss out those last seven pills and still not get pregnant.

But here's the deal: For some reason I've never been able to figure out, mini-pills' packaging looks exactly the same as that of a combination pill. That means your mini-pill pack contains 28 tablets, just like your combo-pill pack—but with one crucial difference: *All 28 pills are active.*

If you're having trouble tolerating "the pill" and its side effects, your doctor may switch you from combos to minis or vice versa. But if you're used to throwing out those last seven pills in your combination pack and your doctor switches you to the mini-pill, you might forget and throw out *those* last seven pills—and guess what might happen then? You could find yourself an unintentional mom-to-be.

My advice is to just get in the habit of taking every single one of your pills. That way, if you ever switch packs, you'll still be right on track.

Shocker #2: You could get sick and tired from your birth control pills!

Both independent studies and manufacturer pamphlets agree: You're risking as many as one hundred side effects if you're taking any meds that contain hormones—contraceptives, hormone replacement therapy (HRT), or any other hormonal treatments. Many women tolerate the pill (and HRT) just fine, but as your 24-hour pharmacist, I want to share some side effects with you. Most common are abdominal pain, anxiety, breast tenderness, nausea, vomiting, yeast infections, gingivitis, depression, migraines, gallbladder disease, stroke, hepatitis, pancreatitis, low sex drive, fluid retention, and weight gain.

Estrogen-containing drugs can also play tricks with your skin, such as increasing your sensitivity to the sun or discoloring your face so that your cheeks develop tan or brown patches (a condition known as melasma). Taking synthetic estrogen or progestin drugs can mess with your thyroid hormones, lowering them and making you very tired. And numerous studies have shown that a woman's risk for uterine, cervical, or breast cancer is higher if she takes synthetic hormones.

Now let's talk about low sex drive! Have you noticed that after chronic use of the pill, your sex drive crashes? The pill's synthetic version of our hormones squashes the production of testosterone, the big T. No T production, no mojo, and the only thing you want in your bed is a good book. Nobody's getting any. Low testosterone doesn't stop at libido, either. Symptoms of testosterone deficiency that occur outside the bedroom include exhaustion, impaired memory, vaginal dryness, occasional urine leakage or incontinence, bone loss, tearfulness, and depression. If I could tell women only one thing, it would be to tell you that virtually all birth control pills and HRT drugs will deplete this vital hormone, as will chronic stress and grief. I'm betting that some of you ladies have just experienced a major "A-ha!" and figured out what may be causing all those mysterious symptoms lately.

If you deal with these symptoms, it's easy to resolve. First, get your testosterone and estrogen levels measured with a saliva test, so you can correct the imbalances while still enjoying the benefits of your prescribed medications. To get tested, you can have your physician fax his license to Genova Labs and order your test for you, or you can take things into your own hands and order the test kit directly from either ZRT Labs or John Lee's lab (see Resources). Both of those companies sell saliva test kits directly to the consumer. Doctors can prescribe bioidentical creams/capsules for you that contain testosterone or DHEA, the precursor to testosterone. I strongly recommend that you allow your dream doctor to figure out the dosage of these hormones based on your individual test results. Never fool around with hormones. It's important to have balance; just because hormones are OTC or bioidentical doesn't make them safe for everyone.

Other side effects of the pill include abdominal pain and vomiting, which can occur immediately. The more serious side effects may take months or even years to manifest—for example, depression and blood clots. These occur quietly, under your radar, and you may not even connect the devastating conditions to your medication because, "I've been taking it for years just fine!" I've heard this so frequently.

Now here's another secret from behind the counter: Many of the pill's side effects are due to the fact that it's a drug mugger! It "mugs" your body of some life-sustaining nutrients, including such valuable players as magnesium, tyrosine, vitamin C, zinc, and the B vitamins, especially B_6.

Trust me, when your supplies of these essential nutrients run low, you feel sick in all kinds of ways. For one, you can no longer produce adequate amounts of neurotransmitters—the "happy-brain" chemicals that you need to maintain your mood, energy, and feelings of vitality. In addition, friendly gut compounds essential to good digestion (and overall health) go out the window. So do the nutrients you need to preserve your arteries. As a result, women who take birth control pills are at higher risk for depression, heart disease, stroke, and infections. Does this sound like you?

If you do choose to take birth control pills (as I confess I did for twenty years!), or if you decide to take HRT, I have good news. A few easily available OTC vitamins can help turn this whole situation around. I wish every gynecologist who prescribed hormones of any kind told women what they need to do to steer clear of what I like to call "drug-mugging." Luckily, you've got me, so check out my Hormone Helpers below.

Hormone Helpers

Everyone's body chemistry is different, so please bear that in mind as you consider all the suggestions I list in this book. After all, I'm a pharmacist trying to help you by giving you good advice—I'm not trying to diagnose you or treat you. But with all the research I've done, it's clear to me that certain nutrients are helpful to a woman, especially one who has taken hormones in any form, bioidentical or synthetic. So I've put together a list of supplements that I think can help relieve a woman's symptoms of PMS and menopause. I call these my Hormone Helpers because I feel that they can help you metabolize your hormones into safer by-products. This could ease many symptoms you are suffering from and maybe even reduce your risk for estrogen-driven cancers such as cancer of the breast, uterus, cervix, and endometrium. All of the following supplements have a relatively safe track record and a lot of research to back them up.

❋ **DIM Complex by Metabolic Maintenance**—*Take 1 capsule once or twice daily.* Whenever a woman takes an estrogen-containing drug such as birth control or hormone replacement therapy (HRT), cancer becomes a possibility. It's not often, but it does happen and that's partly because of the way man-made estrogens (and progestins) are broken down in the body and eliminated. We need to support our bodies with the right nutrients so that we can safely process estrogen-containing drugs (and the estrogen our own bodies make) into safer by-products that can easily be eliminated. DIM Complex by Metabolic Maintenance is first on my list because it's a multitasking formula and contains various ingredients designed to support estrogen metabolism.

It can help ease all those premenstrual and menopausal difficulties. It's an antioxidant formula that contains B vitamins, C, and citrus bioflavonoids, so it is particularly helpful in lowering homocysteine, sweeping up free radicals, and most importantly, reducing the risk of cancer.

This specialty formula contains DIM (diindolylmethane), a relative of I3C, which is an extract from cruciferous veggies like broccoli and Brussels sprouts. In the body, I3C breaks down into DIM, which becomes a powerful anti-cancer substance. I3C and therefore DIM can help a woman process estrogen into safer by-products and lower her risk of all types of female cancers. And it's not just for gals. Men with prostate problems can safely take this product and expect better prostate health. There is some controversy over whether DIM or I3C is best. I like them equally, but I concur with other researchers who feel that DIM is preferred for people who take acid-blocking drugs (Prilosec, Nexium, Pepcid, Zantac, etc.). DIM is also preferred for older people who don't make much acid, or women with a history of breast cancer.

DIM Complex also happens to contain NAC (N-acetylcysteine), a substance that gets converted in your body and goes on to form a powerful antioxidant and detoxifier called glutathione. Glutathione is known to be a powerful anti-cancer substance, and NAC is the best way to supplement because it penetrates the cells better.

The makers of DIM Complex have also included a naturally occurring mineral called calcium D-glucarate, which actually grabs harmful forms of estrogen right out of your gut and prevents the harmful estrogen from lodging in your reproductive tissues, where it can cause cancer. Studies suggest that calcium D-glucarate may help all kinds of cancers, at any stage. DIM Complex contains 100 mg of it per capsule. For added protection, you could safely take extra calcium D-glucarate, which is sold at health-food stores (*500–1,000 mg two or three times daily*).

So how does one go about getting DIM Complex? It's easy to get confused; there are other formulas on the market that go by that name as well. DIM Complex made by Metabolic Maintenance is a physician-exclusive formula, so I have to tell you that you won't find this one on the shelves at health-food stores very often. The best way to get it is to call Metabolic Maintenance at 800-772-7873 and tell them you've read *The 24-Hour Pharmacist*. Since I'm one of their licensed practitioners, the company has agreed to sell DIM Complex directly to you (mention my name), and they will also give you a 20 percent discount on the retail price, which is about $25–$30. I do not receive any royalties from them, rather, you will get the 20 percent savings instead. www.metabolicmaintenance.com.

You can also ask Metabolic Maintenance if there's a physician in your city who sells it locally. And of course, approved and licensed practitioners can arrange to buy it wholesale.

✳ **CoQ10**—*Take 100 mg every morning.* CoQ10 will support your heart, your arteries, and your circulation; it may also have benefits for your mood.

✳ **Ground flaxseed**—*Sprinkle 1 to 2 tablespoons daily* on salads, cereals, yogurt, or other food. You can pretty much go with any brand sold in your local health-food store. Flaxseed can reduce inflammation, boost mood, and help you process estrogen safely.

✳ **SAMe**—*Take about 200–400 mg once or twice daily.* Try LifeExtension's brand, Nature Made's brand, or any brand that is enteric-coated. SAMe (pronounced "Sammy") is an important amino acid that we need to detoxify our body, freeing it from cancer-causing substances. It can also ease joint pain and can relieve depression. Avoid it if you take antidepressants or have bipolar disorder.

✳ **Vitamin D**—*2,000–5,000 IU per day* can cut your risk of hormonal-related side effects by up to 50 percent. Or just make sure to get fifteen minutes of sunlight each day.

✳ **Probiotic**—Scientists have confirmed that female hormones such as estrogen are not broken down or recirculated properly when the gut integrity is abnormal. Also, lack of probiotics can contribute to pancreatitis, psoriasis and other skin conditions, and lupus. So having a healthy balance is important to your health. *Just follow the dosage on the package for any standard probiotic: Lactobacillus acidophilus, B. bifidum, or Lactobacillus sporogenes.* All of these will replenish the bacteria in your intestines, maintaining your digestion and indirectly reducing your risk of all sorts of diseases, including cancer.

* **Myomin**—*Take three capsules twice daily after a meal for six months to a year.* This formula, created by the Eastern-taught practitioner Dr. Chi, contains four Chinese herbs that promote hormone balance. More specifically, Myomin contains ingredients that improve symptoms of estrogen dominance. Moreover, it lowers the amount of bad estrogens and produces safer forms of estrogen. The product doesn't have large scientific clinical trials behind it, but I can tell you it had some powerful effects on me when I took it to relieve PMS cramping, backache, and an increasingly heavy flow. I noticed dramatic results by my second cycle and have remained compliant. Myomin has been reported to reduce fibroid cysts in the breast, uterus, and ovaries because it helps regulate excess estrogen.

* **Exercise** at least twice a week, because the lower your weight, the less estrogen your body produces.

Shocker #3: You need to watch what you ingest while on the pill!

* **Most antibiotics** reduce the effectiveness of the pill. So use some backup birth control while you're on antibiotics and for seven days thereafter, and replenish your intestinal bacteria (which antibiotics kill) by eating an 8-ounce daily serving of yogurt. If you don't eat dairy, take a probiotic supplement (see my Hormone Helpers). Probiotics are particularly helpful if you're chronically suffering from diarrhea, cramps, or nausea—a likely sign that you're low on friendly bacteria.

* **Certain HIV drugs** become less effective while you're taking the pill (e.g., Agenerase and Lexiva), while other drugs (such as Norvir) negate the effects of the pill. So you'll need a backup birth control method, but of course, if you're taking HIV drugs, you need to use condoms anyway.

✳ **Certain antiseizure medications** significantly reduce the pill's effectiveness, so if you're taking phenytoin, carbamazepine, Trileptal, or Felbatol, use a condom or other backup form of birth control.

✳ **Diabetes meds** can be made less effective by estrogen, so your doctor may need to adjust your dosage.

✳ **St.-John's-wort** makes the pill less effective—so again, use a backup.

✳ **Caffeine-related** jitters and anxiety are intensified by estrogens, so you may need to cut back on the coffee, tea, chocolate, and caffeinated sodas.

✳ **Grapefruit juice** increases some women's drug absorption by as much as 30 percent, which might boost the pill's estrogen-related side effects. So separate your pill and juice intake by one to two hours.

✳ **Vitamin C** also increases your body's absorption of the pill, which may also increase estrogen-related side effects of the pill. Again, separate their intake by one to two hours.

✳ **Mineral oil** reduces the pill's effectiveness. So if you suffer from constipation and are taking the oral supplement "mineral oil" to lubricate your bowels, be aware that it can interfere with the absorption of your birth control pill and separate their intake by one to two hours.

Cervical Dysplasia: The Precursor to Cancer

Sometimes women get a slightly abnormal pap smear, which might indicate a condition known as cervical dysplasia, a possible precursor to cancer. If you're taking birth control pills and you can't activate your B vitamins, you have the perfect recipe for cervical dysplasia.

Lots of research shows that high doses of folic acid can reverse or suppress cancer—try Thorne's 5-MTHF, or Metagenics's FolaPro, *two 800-mcg tablets daily for two months, then go to 1 daily tablet indefinitely.* In addition, try selenium (*100–200 mcg twice daily*) and liquid zinc (*10–15 mg daily until it tastes bitter, then stop taking it: The bitterness means you have sufficient levels*).

Here's another cutting-edge idea I want you to try: iodine! Reproductive tissues, such as the uterus, breast, endometrium, and cervix, need healthy natural forms of iodine (and its sister, iodide) to process estrogens, especially birt control and HRT. The iodine in table salt won't do it, but high-quality supplements can; some are even sold at health-food stores. You may take flack from your doctor about this because iodine is terribly misunderstood, and one poor study sent everyone running scared. But it's a safe, naturally occurring trace element, and we need it for optimal health. Japanese women get 14 milligrams on average each day, while the United Sates Recommended Daily Allowance for women suggests only 150 micrograms! Any doctor can test your iodine levels, if you want to be sure you really need the supplement. If you are low in thyroid, this may be particularly helpful to you; refer to Chapter 1, where there is more discussion regarding iodine in thyroid health. The trace mineral is sold at health-food stores under various brand names; the most popular is a liquid called Atomidine. Be warned, it has a strong flavor, so mix it in juice or something very sweet. Sea kelp is another option, but it has the potential to contain sea impurities. I prefer the complex "iodine-iodide" sold as Iodoral, available at some pharmacies, health-food stores, and at www.illnessisoptional.com. The tablets come as 12.5 mg, but your dosage should be totally dependent on your needs, and your individual need can be assessed easily with a urine test; just ask your doctor. Most people do well on 1 tablet per day, but some need more, some need less. Obviously, follow up with your doctor routinely and make sure that iodine supplementation meets with approval. By the way, the nutrients I've recommended in this section may also work toward correcting deficiencies often associated with epithelial cancer.

Gardasil: The Cervical Cancer Cure?

Gardasil, which was released in 2006, is a series of three vaccinations aimed at women, ages 9 to 26, to reduce the risk of developing cervical cancer later in life from HPV (human papillomavirus) transmitted during sex.

Most parents have noticed a massive (and pushy) campaign to mandate injections for little girls in middle school, ages 11 to 12. These drugs were not tested on little girls, hence, our daughters will become the long-term study group in this human experiment! Even though millions of women have done fine with Gardasil, there are some reports of hospitalizations from adverse drug reactions and a few deaths that are being investigated.

According to the makers (www.gardasil.com): "Gardasil may not fully protect everyone and does not prevent all types of cervical cancer..." and further,

"Gardasil will not treat and will not protect against diseases caused by other HPV types." Let me tell you exactly what this means. Gardasil reduces incidence of infection from HPV types 6, 11, 16, and 18. Types 6 and 11 only cause genital warts (annoying, but not fatal); whereas the 16 and 18 strains of HPV are the strains linked to precancerous cervical cells.

In my opinion, if Gardasil addresses only four strains of HPV, and there are dozens of other strains, why shoot the medical dart? The manufacturer will say that these four strains are the most commonly associated strains of virus linked to cervical dysplasia and genital warts. This is true.

But not everyone with HPV develops cancer; it's an unusual event from a common infection. Those who develop cancer are usually infected with HPV. While Gardasil may be 100 percent effective at eradicating the majority of cervical cancers from type 16 and 18 strains, the risks are too serious to inject your daughter with a drug that doesn't even guarantee immunity. And the potential for deadly side effects should not be ignored. These have already been reported to the FDA since Gardasil's release in 2006: seizures, paralysis, miscarriage, blood clots, Bell's palsy, Guillian-Barre syndrome, and death.

Gardasil contains aluminum—a metal that may be involved in disorders such as ALS (Lou Gehrig's), Parkinson's, and Alzheimer's. If that's true, what will the fallout be in years to come if we inject our daughters now?

HPV could go undetected for years, and vaccinating a woman who's already infected could fuel the development of cervical dysplasia and cancer. The vaccination doesn't guarantee that you won't get cancer either, because other factors come into play. Like smoking. Did you know that smoking, or having sex with a smoker, increases your risk? So does a deficiency in folic acid or vitamin C. Eating poorly will increase your risk of developing any cancer. A healthy immune system will help you deal more efficiently with any virus or bacteria that you encounter. According to cervicaldysplasia.com, "women with normal immune system function can be cured of cervical dysplasia."

So take all this into consideration before you make this big decision for your little girl.

Birth Control DURING the Main Event

✻ **Condom/Rubber**—Of one hundred women whose partners use condoms, about fifteen will become pregnant during the first year of typical use—although that number goes down to only three if condoms are used consistently and correctly. The best-known condoms cover the penis, but you can also buy female condoms that slide inside the vagina. The front end of this latex sheath is open for the guy to enter; the back end is closed to keep his semen from reaching the cervix and uterus. Typically, though, the female condom has at least a 20 percent failure rate.

As you can see, a regular condom plus spermicide is almost as effective as the pill; plus these regular condoms come in all shapes, sizes, and flavors—even chocolate! Can you imagine? If a guy walks into my bedroom with chocolate of any sort, I'm thinking of Godiva, thank you very much! And I'm not exactly expecting it in my vagina. . . . Anyway, use latex condoms to protect against STDs, including HIV/AIDS.

✳ **Spermicide**—You can insert into your vagina a cream, foam, or jelly that kills sperm. According to Planned Parenthood (www. plannedparenthood.org), of one hundred women who use contraceptive foam, cream, jelly, film, or suppositories without any other birth control (such as the diaphragm or condom), twenty-nine will become pregnant during the first year of typical use.

The most frequently used spermicide is nonoxynol-9. Don't count on spermicides to protect you against sexually transmitted diseases (STDs)—they won't (though in most cases, condoms will). The *Journal of the American Medical Association (JAMA)* published a study in 1985 proving that women who use spermicide in conjunction with diaphragms or condoms had a lower risk of contracting gonorrhea. The study included 735 women.

✳ **Withdrawal, or as the kids call it, "pulling out"**—This is birth control the old-fashioned way: The guy withdraws his penis from your vagina right before ejaculation. While this is better than nothing, it's the worst method to prevent pregnancy—according to some experts, it's only 70 percent effective. In other words, for every one hundred women who use this method, thirty will get pregnant during the first year. That's partly because it's often hard to judge just when the guy should pull out, and partly because semen released before climax also contains sperm—and it only takes one marathon swimmer to get you pregnant.

Scientists Have the Best Jobs!

"Rubbers" have been around for thousands of years—and how we know this is because some scientists actually took a magnifying glass to study cave paintings from the Stone Age depicting a man using a condomlike barrier during sex. In Egypt, descriptions of vaginal barriers were found buried with the dead—apparently to prevent an unwanted pregnancy in the afterlife. And in ancient Greece, women used pomegranate halves as diaphragms. Ouch!

Nonoxynol-9 May Be a No-No

Although for years, the CDC promoted spermicides—including nonoxynol-9 (N9)—as a way to stop HIV infection, it pulled a medical one-eighty in 2000, when it released revised guidelines announcing that the frequent use of N9 may actually *increase* the risk of contracting HIV. A study sponsored by the United Nations Program on AIDS (UNAIDS) followed one thousand healthy, uninfected African prostitutes from 1996 to 2000, one group of whom used condoms plus N9 while the other group used condoms alone. The N9 users became infected with HIV at a rate close to 50 percent higher than women using plain condoms.

What do we conclude from this? Perhaps N9 irritates the vaginal wall, increasing risk. As a result, using a spermicide such as N9 has become a heated topic for debate. Some people feel strongly that it reduces risk for STDs, whereas others are leery. The choice is yours, although personally, I suggest using a condom that's spermicide-free because N9 is a synthetic xenobiotic chemical (see Chapter 12) which mimics the effects of estrogen in the body, thus boosting your estrogen load and putting you at risk for hormonal imbalance (for more on the dangers of excess estrogen, see Chapters 12–14). Some good spermicide-free condoms are Durex (produced by SSL International) and Kimono (made by Mayer Labs). And if you're looking for a lubricant to go with that condom, K-Y makes some that have no N9.

Birth Control for "The Morning After"

If your condom breaks or slips off, or if you forgot to insert your diaphragm, an emergency contraception pill called Plan B offers one more chance to prevent pregnancy. Take this "morning-after" pill in an emergency, but don't—repeat *do not*—take it as an alternative to "before" or "during" methods of contraception. The morning-after pill has hormonal doses that are way too high for regular usage.

Plan B will cost you about $25 to $40. Not all pharmacies carry this, so call ahead before you make a trip for nothing.

Plan B—approved by the FDA in 2006 for over-the-counter use among women over 18—contains the progestin known as levonorgestrel, which is also found in many birth control pills. (You can find out more at www.go2planB.com.) The morning-after pill prevents pregnancy in three ways:

1. It tries to stop a woman's ovary from releasing an egg.

2. If that fails, it tries to prevent your egg from hooking up with any sperm looking for action.

3. In rare cases, it prevents an egg—even if it's already fertilized—from attaching to your womb and growing into a fetus. This has been a controversial feature among pro-life groups, so it's important to note that if a fertilized egg *does* implant into your uterine wall, Plan B does nothing to slough it off.

Birth Control of the Future?

We already have a birth control implant drug for women, Implanon, which was approved in July 2006, so it's not a stretch to consider one for men. The *really* good news is that researchers are currently conducting international trials of a male contraception—hormonal injections or implants that would stop the production of sperm! Frankly, I find it amazing that they could even gather enough men who'd agree to let the well run dry, but they did, and we are now very close to drug approval. It's taken longer than anticipated to develop the drug because it's harder to suppress millions of hotheaded sperm than one tiny egg!

When men were surveyed about the possibility, they were remarkably open to the drug. They didn't seem at all concerned about their manliness—or about losing possession of the remote control. But they were worried about STDs and said they might wear condoms anyway.

Side effects of the sperm-squashing pill include weight gain and high cholesterol. Compare that with *our* pill, which carries hundreds of potential side effects. Girls, let's keep our fingers crossed for this!

Oops! What Should I Do *Now?*

Try Plan B if . . .

* you've had unprotected sex of any kind

* the condom broke or slipped off (and maybe get tested for STDs also)

* you forgot to use your diaphragm or it became dislodged

* you've miscalculated your safe day

* he didn't pull out in time

Use a backup condom and/or spermicide for seven days if you forgot to . . .

* take a pill

* apply your patch

* insert your NuvaRing

* or if you're taking an antibiotic along with your birth control pill, patch, or shot

If you've gone more than two days without your pills, my professional advice is to stop taking them and allow your period to begin. Then start a new pack at the end of your period. However, check this with your doctor, who may have different instructions for you.

Sex Myths to Warn Your Daughter About

In my day, boys handed us lines like these, and my teenage sources tell me they're still trying it:

* "If we have sex in a pool or hot tub, the chlorine will kill all the sperm."

✳ "If I wear two condoms—in case one breaks—you *can't* get pregnant. No way!"

✳ "If you douche with vinegar after risky or unprotected sex, you'll kill all the sperm."

✳ "If I drink Mountain Dew right before sex, it will kill all my sperm."

✳ "If I get close to coming and then stop, my testicles will turn blue and I might get sick." (Oh, *puhleeese!*)

✳ "If I pull out right before I come, you can't get pregnant."

Needless to say, every single one of these is FALSE! Knowledge is power, so educate your daughter—*and* your son!

Hormones Can Hurt

Synthetic estrogens can contribute to painful yeast infections because they alter the lining of your gut. At first, the infection shows up as soreness, especially when you urinate, but then you get a painful vaginal itch, a tender rash, and a thick white discharge. (When men get a yeast infection, it's called jock itch.)

Some women suffer from yeast infections all the time because of low immunity, lack of healthy flora in their gut, humidity, tight jeans, and the use of synthetic hormones. Sugar feeds the yeast beast, causing more frequent yeast infections, so eliminate it, and the yeast will start to die off on its own. Sweet!

Now, if you don't have healthy flora in your gut, you could be at greater risk for breast cancer. The reason is that a healthy gut will break down your estrogen easily so that it can be eliminated from your body. A compromised gut—one that is lacking in healthy flora—means that more of that bad and ugly estrogen gets absorbed back into your bloodstream, possibly increasing your risk of cancer. So please, trust me on this, take some healthy probiotics to help clear as much of the bad stuff as possible. You can learn how to pick a good probiotic in Chapter 18. Also, consider those Hormone Helpers listed earlier in this chapter.

If you're comfortable self-medicating, pick up any one of those over-the-counter vaginal creams or suppositories sold in pharmacies or supermarkets:

Monistat, Gyne-Lotrimin, and Vagistat–1. Wise Woman Herbals (www. wisewomanherbals.com) has a nice suppository that contains natural tea tree oil if you want something closer to nature.

By the way, vaginal yeast infections are contagious, so protect your partner by using a condom during sex until you're completely cleared up. And check out Chapter 19 for more tips on how to cure recurrent vaginal yeast infections. You may be surprised at how easy it is.

Suzy's Secrets from Behind the Counter
Emergency Treatment for Yeast Infections

If you're in a pinch—like it's 2 a.m., or you're traveling—and you don't have access to yeast infection meds, dig in your husband's drawers or suit-case and find some antifungal cream, maybe for jock itch or athlete's foot. These products contain the same active ingredients as feminine products, so you could apply them to your sore vaginal area. You need to read the product label. Here are the names of the active ingredients that you are looking for in your medicine cabinet, along with their re-spective brand names: tolnaftate (Tinactin), miconazole (Micatin or Monistat), tioconazole (Vagistat), clotrimazole (Lotrimin), or butocona-zole (Femstat). If you see "hydrocortisone" as part of the ingredient list, along with one of these other antifungal ingredients, that's even better—it helps reduce pain!

12

Monthly Madness

Cramps, Crankiness, and Other
Hormonal Highs & Lows

Does this sound like you?

* Your jeans are suddenly tighter than yesterday and you have to hold your breath to get them zipped, because the bloating is out of control.

* Your husband asks you what's for dinner and you burst into tears.

* You walk into your bedroom to get that, um . . . eh . . . you forgot what you went there for—twice now!

* You have to be very gentle putting on your bra because your breasts are *so* tender!

* You will knock your coworker out if she touches your stash of Snickers or Doritos again. Maybe you'll knock her out anyway—she's really getting on your nerves.

If it sounds like I've been stalking you, I assure you I haven't. Premenstrual symptoms such as bloating, mood swings, brain fog, breast tenderness, and hostility affect more than 40 million women each year. So let's take a closer look at those raging hormones.

The *American Idol* Guide to Your Hormones

Well, first there's **estrogen**, which I think of as the Simon Cowell of the group, even though Simon's a guy and estrogen is, of course, the female hormone. I'm not just calling Simon "estrogen" because of those man-boobs that Ryan's always teasing him about (which, as we learned in Chapter 11, may indeed be caused by estrogen). It's also the fact that estrogen tends to excite your brain, and we all know how excitable dear Simon is. Estrogen helps you think clearly and remember things. It also works your bladder, stores fat from food, controls your thermostat, and generates energy.

Like Simon, estrogen can only be taken in small doses, because it tends to be overbearing. And too much estrogen often produces a type of imbalance known as estrogen dominance, which can lead to PMS, menopausal discomfort, blood vessel damage, and a higher risk of cancer.

Now let's meet **progesterone**, a.k.a. Paula Abdul. Progesterone is a calming, soothing hormone, just as Paula is calmer than Simon—both she and progesterone are very rational, feminine, and pleasant to have around. In fact, Paula complements Simon in the same way that progesterone balances estrogen in our bodies—as she always says, "Opposites attract!" Just as Simon needs Paula, estrogen must be kept in balance with progesterone in order for a woman to burn fat, have luxurious hair, create thyroid hormone for energy, maintain strong bones, and generate sex hormones. Progesterone is so soothing it can even help you sleep.

Sometime after you turn 40, your progesterone levels start to drop sharply. So do your estrogen levels—but progesterone tends to drop faster. Without enough progesterone to calm your estrogen, the way Paula calms Simon, you get all those menopausal symptoms and extra-severe PMS. But progesterone supplements can help. You can buy some forms of supplemental progesterone in an oral form that requires a prescription; you can also buy progesterone creams over-the-counter, or have a bioidentical version of progesterone (one that matches your own body's hormone) custom-compounded for your specific needs. A doctor will need to help you with the custom-fitting process, so call your local compounding pharmacy and ask for some doctors in your area who work with bioidenticals. Either way, though, a small dose of progesterone is all you need, just as a few minutes of Paula can balance half an hour of Simon!

Now, **testosterone**—the male hormone—is the Ryan Seacrest of the group.

Ryan is my favorite metrosexual, and he reminds me of testosterone because he's quick-witted, always in a feisty, playful mood, and sort of sexy with all that stubble! In fact, testosterone helps create facial hair and regulates mood, passion, memory, and sexual appetite.

Like Ryan, testosterone is an essential part of the program. Along with estrogen, it helps maintain cholesterol, blood pressure, heart rhythm, and insulin levels as well as making muscle and boosting your sex drive. Of course, too much testosterone in a woman can deepen your voice, spark acne, incite aggressive behavior, and make hair sprout in places it shouldn't (like your chest) and fall off of places you want it (like your head). You can end up with excess testosterone as the result of some prescribed medications that contain the tricky hormone; it's also possible to make too much on your own, perhaps because you've got cystic ovaries (often related to insulin resistance). So if you're seeing any symptoms of excess testosterone, talk to your doctor right away.

As for **Randy Jackson**, he's "in the dawg house"—the perfect blend of everything, always reasonable, friendly, and fair. He shows us what it's like when all hormones are in their proper balance, a state known in biology as "homeostasis."

Hormonal Highs and Lows: Estrogen Dominance

Actually, there's no such hormone as "estrogen," just as there's no one plant that's a "flower." Three key types of estrogen that we make in our own bodies include estrone, estriol, and estradiol. All three are superpowerful: It takes less estradiol than the weight of a snowflake to transform a prepubescent 9-year-old girl into a full-figured, menstruating woman! But that's not the end of the estrogen story. Here are three other types you should know about:

✳ **Synthetic estrogens**—for example, ethinyl estradiol and lab-created estradiol. These are made in laboratories to mimic the effects of our natural estrogen and then used in meds like birth control pills. Synthetic estrogen is stronger than our own, and it floods all our cells, including our livers. Normally, the liver's job is to filter meds from our system, but synthetic estrogens can be tough to clear. As a result, they hang around in our bodies way too long, causing a wide variety of problems, such as estrogen dominance. Synthetic estrogens feed estrogen-sensitive tissues in your breasts, endometrium, uterus, and cervix, and studies show that the out-of-control tissue growth could increase your risk for cancer.

✴ **Phytoestrogens**—These come from plants and they resemble our own natural hormones pretty closely. Phytoestrogens are high in soy isoflavones and these are easily found in soybean products (like tofu and edamame beans). If we need other sources of isoflavones, then beans, chickpeas, and other legumes are good choices. If you're struggling with PMS or menopause, the isoflavones and fiber will do you good, so try adding some chickpeas to your daily salad, eating hummus, or having a nightly serving of tofu with your veggies—you may be surprised at what a difference it makes.

✴ **Xenoestrogens, a.k.a. xenobiotics**—These are the real bad guys: lab-created chemicals from the petrochemical industry that were never intended for medical purposes (for example, you can find them in plastics, pesticides, additives, preservatives, and other icky places)—that, nevertheless, get into our cells, where they mimic the effects of estrogen in a dangerous way. That's another reason why so many of us struggle with estrogen dominance: We're constantly being exposed to these environmental estrogens that add to our total body burden of estrogen, rather than allowing our estrogen to remain in a healthy balance with our other hormones. (See Part V for a list of some common xenobiotics and what to do about them.)

As you can see, it's extremely easy for your body to overload on estrogen. That's why I want you to be very well informed about any estrogen meds you're taking—contraceptives, HRT, or anything else—because for some women, even a little extra estrogen can have devastating effects. Estrogen dominance can cause painful, fibrocystic breasts, water retention, migraines, varicose veins, osteoporosis, hot flashes, joint pain, dry wrinkly skin, depression, and difficulty losing weight. As if that weren't enough, blood sugar imbalances, low sex drive, brain fog, heavy periods with blood clots (endometriosis), uterine fibroids, thyroid dysfunction, infertility, stroke, and breast cancer (or any "female" cancer) are other potential signs of estrogen dominance.

The Good, the Bad, and the Ugly

All over your body, cells are breaking down estrogen—in your breasts and liver, and, if you're a man, in your prostate, resulting in three key by-products.

There's the *good*: 2-Hydroxyestrone, or "2" for short, which helps prevent cancer.

Then there's the *bad*, 16 alpha-Hydroxyestrone, or "16." This by-product is not all bad, because it helps protect you from osteoporosis, but it also raises your risk for cancer and may spark autoimmune disorders.

And finally, the *ugly*: 4 Hydroxyestrone, or "4," for short. While the good and bad estrogens are easy to measure with simple urine tests, the ugly estrogen is harder to track, although it is also the best marker for cancer risk. Some studies suggest that women with high 2:16 ratios are less likely to get breast cancer than women with low 2:16 ratios; luckily, this ratio is relatively easy for your physician to track. Balance is important, because a high 2:16 ratio is also associated with a higher risk of osteoporosis. So if you *make* too much estrogen, *take* too much estrogen, or are *exposed* to too many environmental estrogens, I think you should take the Hormone Helpers that I suggested in Chapter 11.

Plead Insanity—It's Hormonal!

The reason you want to knock someone out or scream your brains out when you've got PMS may be because higher estrogen increases your levels of copper and thus lowers zinc. You're even more prone to this copper-zinc imbalance if you're taking any type of hormonal contraceptive (including the pill) or hormone replacement therapy (HRT), both of which further erode your mood by lowering your magnesium and B_6 levels. No wonder so many women on hormones deal with unnatural hostility, anxiety, short temper, and a feeling that they are dissociated from reality.

Another factor in PMS insanity is insufficient progesterone. Your brain hoards about twenty times more progesterone than other parts of your body— so if progesterone levels are low, the voice of your estrogen will be "too loud," which will make you kind of cranky. Just as Paula calms Simon, progesterone tames your estrogen—clearing brain fog, calming your inner worrywart, reducing agitation, alleviating depression, and preventing migraines. A 2006 study published in the *Annals of Emergency Medicine* proved that natural progesterone can even help people with disabling traumatic brain injuries, such as those sustained in car crashes, gunshots, and falls. The three-year study, funded by the National Institute of Neurological Disorders and Stroke (NINDS), was the world's first study to show how powerful progesterone could be in humans with brain injuries. The scientists concluded that if progesterone was given to a person soon after a traumatic brain injury, it appeared to cut the risk of death by 50 percent and reduced subsequent disability. So if it can help the brains of those in severe distress, it should certainly be a consideration for women with PMS or menopausal-related cognitive decline.

Conventional medicine usually responds to PMS symptoms by boosting brain chemicals like serotonin or norepinephrine through antidepressants such as Prozac (renamed "Sarafem" to lose the stigma), Zoloft, Effexor, Cymbalta, Wellbutrin, and so forth. These drugs are often prescribed for the two weeks before your period to boost levels of brain hormones that increase feelings of well-being and joy. Even though these medications can help, I think it's even more crucial to bring harmony to imbalanced minerals, which I'll tell you how to do in just a minute.

Natural Relief for Hormones, Hostility, and Headache

In my experience both as a pharmacist and as a woman, I've learned that there are many nutrients that can have a beneficial impact on your hormones and premenstrual changes. The following nutrients—sold at most health-food stores and pharmacies—might have a favorable effect for you, too. Consider any one of them, or a combination that suits your needs:

* **NAC (N-acetylcysteine)**—*300–500 mg, two times a day*

* **Selenium**—*200 mcg once or twice daily*

* **Vitamin B$_6$**—*50 mg twice daily (or 20–30 mg P5P, the active form of B$_6$)*—but back off if you get bad dreams

* **Buffered vitamin C**—*500 mg twice daily*

* **Magnesium chelate or glycinate**—*200–300 mg once or twice daily*—but reduce your dose if you get diarrhea

✳ **SAMe (S-adenosylmethionine)**—*400 mg once daily on an empty stomach upon arising*

✳ **Zinc**—*5–10 mg once with dinner.* Use liquid zinc and when it starts to taste bitter, stop taking it.

✳ **Natural vitamin E**—*500–1,000 IU mixed tocopherol*

✳ **Green tea**—*2 to 3 cups per day*—any flavor is okay

✳ **Rhodiola rosea**—*50–100 mg twice a day*

✳ **Pure USP progesterone cream**—you can buy a transdermal cream at the health-food store, although I strongly urge you to determine your progesterone levels with lab testing because using progesterone can backfire if your hormones are really out of balance. If you choose to self-treat, see Part V for instructions on how to use this cream.

Suzy's Secrets from Behind the Counter
Premenstrual Headache Relief

For premenstrual migraines, try using OTC progesterone cream–*1/8 teaspoon twice daily*–for the ten days leading up to your period. (See Part V for details on how to apply the cream.) If you notice a headache coming on, you can also *dab on a bit of the cream every fifteen to twenty minutes,* rotating areas of application. This commonly requires only two or three applications to abort or at least minimize the headache.

Your Breasts Need a Rest!

Would it surprise you if I told you that breast tenderness—along with many of the other PMS symptoms—are exacerbated by stress and overworking? So many of us lead busy, hectic lives filled with continuous, unrelenting pressure without the rest we need. I call you gals "Juggling Janets," and as a recovering Juggling Janet myself, I can tell you that we "train" our adrenal glands to pump out stress hormones all day long, until we run out of them. Without enough stress hormones to help us cope, we become tired, nervous, depressed, moody, frazzled—and uninterested in sex.

Sounds like PMS and menopause, doesn't it? And when we run out of DHEA, our body automatically forms more dangerous estrogen by-products, lowering 2:16 ratios and increasing our risk of breast cancer. The more adrenally exhausted we become, the worse our PMS and menopause symptoms are likely to be.

So how can we make those tender breasts feel better and ease the rest of our symptoms, too? In many cases, the cure is simple: Slow down the pace! Meditation and relaxation translate to lower cortisol levels, and therefore more pleasant monthly cycles, less frequent hot flashes, and lowered risk of cancer. Book a massage or facial right now, and then read Chapters 1 and 6 on fatigue and anxiety, where I share secrets on reducing tension in your life, sparing your adrenals, and improving your life. Whew!

Premenstrual Relief

For many years now, women have been asking me about which over-the-counter remedies can help relieve PMS-related symptoms. Here are my suggestions based upon both research articles and the dozens of real-life women who came back to thank me:

Bloating and Cramps

* **Calcium citrate**—*500–600 mg twice a day*

* **Magnesium chelate or glycinate**—*200–300 mg once or twice a day.*
    You can also find a good calcium-magnesium combination.

* **Omega-3 EPA/DHA fish oils and ground flaxseed**—*1,000 mg twice daily.* Remember that fish oils may thin the blood, so if you take anticoagulant medications, be warned: Stay at very low doses (500 mg daily) or avoid altogether, whichever your doctor allows.
    Also, sprinkle *1–2 tablespoons of ground flaxseeds* on food during the day; flaxseeds help regulate your estrogen levels.

✳ **Naproxen (Aleve)**—*200 mg two or three times a day;* or else take ibuprofen (Advil or Motrin), *200 mg four times per day.* Either way, take the pills with food to lessen tummy upset. Do not use these medications with uncontrolled high blood pressure or a history of ulcers unless you have your doctor's blessings.

Cravings

✳ **Omega-3 EPA/DHA fish oils *and* ground flaxseed**—Take the fish oils in *1,000 mg doses twice daily,* and sprinkle ground flaxseeds on salads and oatmeal, and in smoothies and baked goods.

✳ **5 hydroxytryptophan** (5-HTP)—*50 mg once or twice daily* will increase serotonin, a "feel-good" brain chemical. 5-HTP also helps release of leptin, our "feel-full" appetite hormone. Stay away from this one if you take prescribed antidepressants.

✳ **Chromium picolinate**—This trace mineral balances levels of blood sugar, helping you to avoid the highs and lows that trigger cravings for sweets. It's also fascinating that a study published in the *Journal of Psychiatric Practice* in 2005 found that 65 percent of those taking chromium (versus 33 percent of the placebo group) had "significantly greater improvements on the depression rating scores," too. So this trace mineral can not only help us quit sugar, but it improves mood. *Try 200–500 mg once or twice daily.*

Tearfulness

✳ **5-HTP**—*50 mg at bedtime* (again, avoid this one if you take antidepressants)

✳ **Magnesium chelate or glycinate**—*200–300 mg per day,* but back off if you get diarrhea

✳ **St.-John's-wort**—*300 mg two or three times daily* (standardized to 0.3 percent hypericin)

Brain Fog

❋ **Lecithin**—Sprinkle a *few tablespoons* of the granules onto your food or into juice each day. It increases sex drive, too!

❋ **Bacopa**—*Take 100 mg three times a day* (standardized extract of 55 percent bacosides). This is nature's "smart pill," and it also induces relaxation and boosts memory.

Breast Tenderness

❋ **Natural vitamin E**—*600–800 IU each day*

❋ **Pyridoxine/vitamin B$_6$**—*50–100 mg per day* (or P5P—*20 mg per day*)

❋ **Pure progesterone cream**—*1/8 teaspoon twice daily* applied to breasts, chest, or inner arms. Choose a different site to apply the cream each time you put it on—and stop if your symptoms worsen.

❋ **Iodine-iodide**—This supplement is sold over-the-counter as Iodoral at www.illnessisoptional.com. *Dosage is 12.5 mg every morning,* but back off if you experience an unpleasant brassy taste, runny nose, or acnelike skin lesions. It's a good idea to take fish oils while on iodine to keep things in balance, about *500–1,000 mg daily.*

Suzy's Secrets from Behind the Counter

Avoid the Booby Trap!

Where your breasts hurt matters. If they hurt around the sides and armpits, it may be a sign that ovulation just occurred. If they're sore everywhere, or just in the front around the nipples, it may mean high estrogen and low progesterone. Apply progesterone cream (see Part V for complete instructions), and you might also *take three capsules daily of Myomin.*

Xenobiotics: Bad for Your Breasts

As we saw earlier, xenobiotics are chemical sneaks that fake out your body, going into all the cells where your normal estrogen would go. As a result, you're at risk for breast, uterine, and endometrial cancer, while your man is at risk for prostate cancer.

Xenobiotics are everywhere now, so don't drive yourself totally crazy trying to avoid them. Do be aware, though, that they're in foods; everyday household items such as cleansers; spermicides (yes, nonoxynol-9); and many medications. They're also in marijuana, so if your son's breasts seem to be getting bigger, "grass" may be part of his diet! (Hey, this conversation about breasts reminds me of Simon for some reason!)

Unlike real estrogen, xenobiotics don't break down; they just linger in your body until you excrete them with other waste products. They also linger in the hormone-treated meat we eat—farmers like them because they fatten up their cattle, but are those xenobiotics the reason that we're facing increased risk of estrogen-related cancers while sperm production has dropped by 50 percent over the past forty years? Xenobiotics from industrial waste and other types of pollution are definitely the reason some of our sea critters now have male and female sex organs. Seriously! And if a mom-to-be is exposed to xenobiotics, the embryo she carries is hit hardest of all, because its sex glands are still developing. My suggestions?

✳ Put a filter on your water taps or set up a special water filtration system called "reverse osmosis." Pollutants can seep into your water supply even if you're using a well—they travel through the rain and the groundwater—so I advise filtering, just to be on the safe side.

✳ Use natural pesticides on your lawn—your local pest-control agency or chamber of commerce can tell you which companies in your community sell such products.

✳ Buy "certified organic" foods, which are free of harmful chemicals and pesticides.

✳ Minimize dry cleaning—the chemicals can be xenoestrogenic.

Balance Your Hormones with the Anticancer Diet

✳ Cook with fresh rosemary, garlic, and turmeric spice, all of which have anticancer properties.

✳ Sauté or steam some greens every single day—turnip greens, mustard greens, kale, chard, or spinach.

✳ Say NO to all fatty or fried foods.

✳ Choose hormone-free meat, poultry, dairy products, and eggs. Well-designed trials prove that breast cancer is associated with animal fat intake, so try to eat more fish, tofu, and vegetable proteins while cutting back on animal foods.

✳ Prunes can increase your 2:16 ratio.

✳ Berries of any color contain anticancer nutrients.

✳ I also want you to eat fresh onions and garlic. No cheating—I said fresh produce, *not* the powdered spices!

✳ Eat cruciferous veggies, which are best for your breasts and for your guy's prostate. Cabbage, Brussels sprouts, broccoli, radishes, and cauliflower are naturally rich in Indole-3-carbinol (I3C), and your body converts I3C to a chemical known as diindolylmethane, or DIM, helping you to make more of the good estrogen and less of the bad and the ugly. As with any compound, data conflicts and isn't always positive, but the vast majority of studies have found that I3C can protect against cancer. Numerous studies have been done in animals and humans, and some are quite fascinating. Studies on lung cancer indicate that I3C is powerful and can reverse DNA damage caused by cigarette smoke. By turning metabolism toward less powerful metabolites, I3C helps reduce levels of "strong," cancer-promoting hormones in the body. This helps reduce the potential for the development of hormone-related cancers. Studies of DIM suggest that it may be even better than I3C because it may work in the presence of low acid, a condition common among women and people who take acid blockers.

Suzy's Secrets from Behind the Counter
Do You Need an Adjustment?

I learned about this trick from my husband, who's a chiropractor. He manipulates my spine (called an adjustment) on the first or second day of my period, which shortens my cycle by a couple of days and helps reduce pain and cramping. Call me a coward but I like his "Activator" method, which employs a gentle handheld tool that applies pressure without any "cracking." It's not just me—studies confirm that chiropractic adjustment can reduce prostaglandins, chemicals that cause pain and inflammation.

Bounce Your Breasts

If your breasts are lumpy and painful, it could be that your lymph is not draining properly. Lymph is a clear fluid that circulates throughout your body, cleansing all your tissues of toxins and impurities. The clean lymph travels through your arteries; the "dirty" lymph is supposed to drain away through your lymphatic system, assisted by your lymph nodes, which act as filters.

Now here's something most people don't know: Any fluid that travels through your arteries is pumped along by the beating of your heart—but the only thing that helps your lymph to drain properly is movement. So if you're a sedentary person, you may have sluggish lymph—lymph that collects in your lymphatic system without draining as quickly as it should. And since lymph contains such toxins as dead or cancerous cells, waste products, fat, viruses, and heavy metals, you want it to drain as quickly as nature intended.

So how do you get your lymph moving again? First, burn all bras that are tight, restrictive, or underwired. Don't worry about droopy breasts; bras don't prevent that. The sag happens because the musculature weakens; it's a myth that bras prevent sagging. Tight bras—or constant use of bras—are not that good for you. That's because tight cleavage-producing bras can actually hamper the lymphatic system, which causes stagnation. A Harvard study, published in the *European Journal of Cancer* in 1991, discovered that women who go bra-free have lower rates of breast cancer, about 60 percent lower!

In 1995, Sydney Singer and Soma Grismaijer of the Institute for the Study of Culturogenic Disease published their book, *Dressed to Kill: The Link Between Breast Cancer and Bras* (Avery Press). Their study included almost 4,600 women. The group was split half and half between women who had breast cancer and women who did not. The researchers noticed that the more hours per day spent in a bra, the higher the rate of breast cancer. According to their study, women who did not wear bras had a dramatically reduced rate of breast cancer. It could be that the lymph doesn't flow properly because bras create constant pressure and are restrictive, raising breast temperature, too. The results are shocking and very controversial, and many other scientists think they are hogwash. But it's not so easy for me to dismiss statistics like this, found in *Dressed to Kill*:

✳ If you wear a bra more than 12 hours a day, your risk goes up dramatically for breast cancer, fibrocystic breast, tenderness, and pain.

✳ If you wear a bra 18 to 24 hours a day, your risk for developing breast cancer goes up 100 times than if you were bra-less.

So ditch the bras made of thick polyester padding in favor of 100 percent cotton bras or camisoles—and go bra-less when you can. Because if you let all your lymph fluid drain properly, that may not only ease your breast pain, it can generally boost your health. (Now, don't throw out that black lacy push–up number—just save it for a special occasion!)

Here's another thing you might do: Bounce your breasts! Bouncing helps you drain the lymph, so it's especially good for those of you who are too big to go bra-less—say, for example, you're a D cup, so your breasts weigh in somewhere between 15 and 23 pounds. During exercise or bouncing, breasts move a vertical distance of about 6 to 8 inches. Join a gym or buy one of those small personal trampolines (about 3 feet wide) and jump for 10 minutes a day to pump out that stagnant lymph. Bouncing improves immune function, repairs injured cells, and helps you circulate more oxygen throughout your body. It may also lower blood pressure and help certain types of headaches. Some people find that bouncing induces a sense of euphoria—always a good thing!

I think you should massage your breasts too—just 30 seconds a day will get the lymph flowing. You'll notice a difference within a week. The trick is to massage the sides near your armpit as well as underneath, where sluggish lymph hangs around. (Remember, the lymph drains only by the movement of your muscles, so if you're sedentary, lymph tends to move slowly or not at all.) I prefer doing a quick breast massage in the privacy of my shower—but hey, if your man catches you, invite him in to lend a hand!

Hormonal Horrors

Endometriosis is a painful condition that causes severe pain around each period as the endometrial lining is irritated and bleeds excessively. It may be related to a number of factors, including iodine deficiency or insulin sensitivity. You can ease and perhaps even prevent this condition by balancing your estrogen with progesterone, slowing down the production of those "bad and ugly" by-products.

If you are headed for surgery, why not consider my Hormone Helpers (see Chapter 11) first? You can try them for one month and see if they help. I want you to make one adjustment, though: *Take two or three capsules of Myomin three times daily, after each meal,* and sprinkle ground flaxseeds on everything. You should notice some improvement after your next cycle. Then, by the third month, drop your Myomin dose to *one or two capsules twice daily* and continue for a few more months. Please make sure you get lab testing done to make sure that you do not reduce your estrogen too much! This supplement, like many others I've recommended in this book, really works well, and you may find yourself at the other extreme of too-low estrogen.

Now, for most women, there is also an insulin connection, so you might also cut out any kind of white-flour product, including bread, cakes, and pasta as well as all other sweets and starches. Please read Chapter 16 on Diabetes to learn how to normalize your blood sugar.

A little iodine-iodide may help too (brand name Iodoral)—it creates safer estrogen by-products. For this reason, scientists have studied its role in the breast, and yes, it appears to reduce cancer risk—the worst hormonal horror of all! You can buy some at your local natural health-food store, but I have to warn you, iodine is terribly misunderstood and some doctors don't advise it. I myself have read a lot of research about it, so I personally am comfortable suggesting it for your consideration, since iodine and iodide play crucial roles in our health, particularly breast health. If you do decide to supplement, it's best to use a complex that includes both iodine and iodide rather than plain iodine. Iodoral is a brand that is sold on various websites, including www.illnessis optional.com. You can also see if your physician will prescribe some Lugol's solution for you. Otherwise, OTC forms of iodine derived from organic Asian seaweed are available. You might see these sold as "kelp." Some of you may recall that years ago, iodine was highly recommended by Edgar Cayce, the world-renowned psychic channeler.

So if your physician approves, try *Iodoral 12.5 mg each morning.* If you don't notice significant relief by your third cycle, you could apply pure progesterone cream as another option. Stay on the Myomin; consider the first day of your period as Day 1, and wait until Day 6 to apply ½ teaspoon pure progesterone cream every night until Day 26, rotating sites of application. (See Part V.) Repeat the procedure each cycle, and you'll probably notice some relief within two or three months. You can also take Nu-Iron—an easy-on-the-gut form of iron, sold OTC, which will offset any iron-deficiency anemia that happens when you bleed so much. Take the iron for no more than 60 days—that should be plenty. (Iron may cause a harmless discoloration of the urine or feces.)

Fibroid tumors are another hormonal horror—firm, round, benign lumps that form in the uterus. They can lead to painful sex, heavy periods, and irregular bleeding. Conventional medicine's answer is sometimes surgical—a hysterectomy followed by synthetic HRT for years. Not in my book! Don't let them cut anything out of you until you at least try my Hormone Helpers (see Chapter 11), but again with an adjustment: *Take three capsules of Myomin three times daily, after each meal.* You should notice some improvement after your next cycle, but if you're still very uncomfortable, bring in the progesterone cream. Most women don't need it, but if you do, begin it on Day 12 (counting the first day of your cycle as Day 1). And absolutely take the iodine-iodide that I recommended above.

13

Surge Protection
for Your Hot Flashes

*Y*ou're dripping with sweat one minute and freezing the next. You haven't had a good night's sleep in months, you occasionally lose bladder control, you want to bite everyone's head off, and you feel as though your insides are drying out. Welcome to menopause!

It was eighteen years ago, but I'll never forget the time Kathy fretfully leaned over my pharmacy counter and begged me to help her deal with her hot flashes. She could hardly get the words out, stating that she had been up all night—again!—and she was fighting with her husband about it (apparently he didn't empathize with her enough), and she was getting no help from her current medication, either.

As a brand-new pharmacist, I was schooled in all the latest drugs and their benefits. I'm sort of an encyclopedia, so I began parroting everything I knew from pharmacy school, eagerly informing Kathy about the newest estrogens that could cool her off and the strongest sleep aids available. She left with a laundry list of products that she was going to ask her doctor to prescribe, and I was pleased that by most clinical assessments, I'd given her the perfect pharmacy consultation.

Even though it's been years since this incident happened, I've thought of it often, mostly because now, our conversation would be so different. I'd tell Kathy not to take lab-created versions of hormones when bioidentical, natural hormones exist, some that she could buy without a prescription. I'd walk her down the supplements aisle and show her several natural, safe ways to cool off, calm down, and fall asleep—no doctor required. Oh, if I could only turn back time!

Well, maybe I can't go back and help Kathy—but, ladies, your 24-hour pharmacist is right here for *you*!

What "Everybody Knows" About Menopause

1. Hot flashes and other uncomfortable menopausal symptoms are a normal part of aging, as our estrogen drops to nil by the age of 50.

2. The best remedy for menopausal symptoms is prescription hormone replacement therapy (HRT).

3. All those natural supplements touted for hot flashes have never been proven to work.

Well, guess what? What "everyone knows" is wrong! If you'd like to be one of the lucky few who know the truth, read on!

Is It Hot in Here or Is It Just Me?

For most women, it starts with a kind of "aura," or feeling—perhaps a rapid heartbeat—to signal that a power surge is imminent. Then you feel a surge of heat, your face may turn beet red, and you could break into a sweat as your heartbeat races. Perhaps your chest tightens as you feel anxious and then cold.

Or perhaps you're one of the lucky women who breezes through menopause, never getting a single hot flash? If so, count your blessings, because other women may get hot flashes or night sweats as often as ten to twenty times a day!

Here's what's going on beneath your skin. When your body heats up—from hot salsa, a hot drink, or a session on the Stairmaster—your brain's thermostat kicks into gear, saying, "Uh-oh, this woman is heating up. I'd better discharge some chemicals to widen her blood vessels so she doesn't explode right there in the gym!"

Normally, this type of temperature regulation goes off without a hitch many times a day for many years, since your body can tolerate about a degree and a half change. Estrogen levels go from being steady for decades, to crazy ups and downs during menopause. Things settle down after two to five years, which is why hot flashes eventually stop. But during menopause, your brain thermostat doesn't like this estrogen roller coaster and gets soooo touchy! Suddenly a tiny rise in body temperature—even less than a single degree—sets off your "hot" button and voila, a hot flash! It's not just women who get them, by the way. Guys do, too, especially if they're taking prostate medications, like Lupron, for example.

So let's clear up Myth #1 right now: When estrogen levels eventually even out after menopause, they don't always drop to nil. In fact, many menopausal women are able to maintain some level of estrogen. That's good news and bad news: It means that even after menopause, you can suffer from estrogen dominance (too much estrogen relative to your progesterone), especially if you're overweight.

Erratic estrogen during menopause is one stressor on your mental thermostat—adrenal burnout is another. If you live a life of chronic stress—and what woman doesn't?—you keep asking your adrenal glands to release stress hormones. Overuse will burn out your adrenal motor, which in turn damages your brain's thermostat—and you end up with lots of hot flashes.

So the little-known key to reducing hot flashes is to nourish and repair your adrenal glands. That's because stress exhausts your adrenal glands and also reduces your progesterone output, which tilts your estrogen-progesterone ratio to create estrogen dominance. And what are the symptoms of estrogen dominance? Insomnia and anxiety—which stress you out more, which tax your adrenal glands, which lower your progesterone levels—yes, that's what we call a vicious cycle! And medications can't fix it.

A hot flash is your body's way of crying out and saying, "You're burning the candle on both ends—cool it!" The more exhausted your adrenals, the more severe and maddening your hot flashes are likely to be. By the way, the more adrenal fatigue you have, the more likely you are to suffer from testosterone deficiency—creating even more problems.

So let me repeat myself, because this is huge news to women with hot flashes: If you want to alleviate or prevent hot flashes, start taking care of yourself. Make time for your body to rest and don't sweat the small stuff—and please find ways to decompress after your hard day's work. (Check out Chapter 1 to find out more about nourishing your adrenals.)

Suzy's Secrets from Behind the Counter

Medicine Can Make You Sweat, Too!

Did you know that more than 70 medications can trigger a power surge in either men or women? Common offenders include antidepressants like Effexor, Cymbalta, Prozac, and Sarafem; triptan migraine meds like Maxalt; aromatase inhibitors like Aromasin, Arimidex, and Femara; the SERMs Evista and tamoxifen; and Boniva, used to treat osteoporosis. If you think you're getting hot flashes from these or any other medications, ask your doctor about lowering your dosage or switching to an alternate drug.

 Do NOT stop taking prescribed medication without consulting your doctor. Some meds have to be weaned slowly!

Let's Talk About Surge Protection

Most conventional textbooks teach that hot flashes are related to low estrogen levels, but that may not be the case. Consider this: If hot flashes were *only* caused by low estrogen levels, women would be having them for the rest of their lives. But after a few years, hot flashes do finally go away, with or without the meds. That's because estrogen isn't the only issue: Other factors include lifestyle, diet, coping skills, rest, and how much support you get in your life—and the big one, progesterone levels.

So now let's clear up Myths #2 and #3: that only HRT works and that natural alternatives don't. People believe those myths because they hear only about the studies funded by major medical companies and pharmaceuticals, but there is proof behind some natural remedies, too. Here are a few ways to help end the misery—no doctor required!

⁂ **Black cohosh (*Cimicifuga racemosa*)**—belongs to the buttercup family. In 2001, the *American College of Obstetricians and Gynecologists* agreed that black cohosh may be helpful for hot flashes if taken for six months or less. It is also thought to help with bloating and vaginal dry-ness. The consensus is that black cohosh behaves like estrogen but with-out the dangerous side effects. Some research has also shown that it may even have an antidepressant effect.

Some studies have compared black cohosh to estrogen. In a 24-week study, 60 women who were post-hysterectomy were treated with either black cohosh or various estrogenic compounds. Black cohosh was found to decrease symptoms similarly to the estrogen.

Because black cohosh hasn't really been studied for very long, and published studies are generally 6 months long or less, we don't really understand the long-term effects of the herb. I'd like to see more data trickle in because it's possible that, since black cohosh is estrogenic, it may have some negative effects on the uterus, endometrium, or breast tissue, but again, this has not been clearly defined.

It also might cause upset stomach and headaches in sensitive women, so use it with care. If you want to try black cohosh to see how you re-spond, and how well you cool off, try the most popular OTC brand, Remifemin, taken as a *20 mg tablet twice daily* or Triple Whammy's brand called Menopause Transition with Black Cohosh, *1 tablet twice daily*. This brand has been used in clinical studies with good results. There are many other quality brands with varying doses sold at health-food stores, though I wouldn't take a product with less than 2.5 percent triterpene glycosides.

Warning: Black cohosh may cause stomach discomfort and head-aches and, rarely, liver damage.

> *Pregnant women should not self-medicate with black cohosh, but some women do take it under the supervision of their fam-ily physicians.*

* **Flaxseed**—These super little seeds should be a staple in everyone's diet, and they're also proven to help reduce symptoms of menopause. Flaxseeds have about one hundred times more lignans than any other food, and if we have lots of friendly flora in our gut, we can convert certain lignans into powerful anticancer compounds. Ground flaxseed is rich in protein, minerals, and fiber, and it's a fabulous natural way to combat hot flashes, breast tenderness, erratic cycles, and other PMS and menopausal discomforts. Lignans can help you get that great head of luxurious hair, lessen acne, and, in men, nurture prostate health. Flax is rich in essential fatty acids, similar to those found in fish oils, so they're great for your heart and cholesterol ratios.

You can buy seeds and grind them up yourself; I like this way best because they are freshest. You can also buy them in a bag already ground up. On the other hand, I'm not so crazy about flaxseed oil, which is not the best form if you are trying to squash menopausal symptoms—it goes rancid quickly, and it has barely any lignans, anyway. In fact, even the seeds might go rancid if you don't store them in the fridge, preferably in a dark container that protects them from light. I sprinkle these wonder seeds on pretty much everything, *1 or 2 tablespoons a day.* Since flax is a fiber, drink lots of water!

✳ **Vitamin E and citrus bioflavonoids**—This is a very powerful combination that some people consider a super flash-buster. Again, proven! Bioflavonoids come from fruits and vegetables, and in combination with supplemental vitamin C and vitamin E, they may be able to relieve anxiety, irritability, vaginal dryness, and mood swings as well as hot flashes. Try *500–1,000 IU mixed vitamin E along with 1,000 mg bioflavonoids twice a day.* You can boost bioflavonoids by eating lots of intensely colored fruits and veggies—carrots, squash, tomatoes, berries, broccoli, and greens—or you can buy a supplement in your pharmacy or health-food store. The most important bioflavonoid is called hesperidin, so make sure your supplement contains that. Thorne makes an interesting variety of hesperidin, HMC Hesperidin, that is easier for the body to utilize.

✳ **Progesterone**—This powerful hormone helps us minimize hot flashes. It, too, has been proven to work, according to many studies, basically because it makes your brain less sensitive to the erratic behavior of estrogen, stretching out the rails and making that roller-coaster ride less crazy. A perimenopausal woman in her late thirties or early forties who is dealing with progesterone deficiency or estrogen dominance can also use progesterone.

Natural progesterone products look exactly like your own

progesterone—and that's true even of the products sold over-the-counter. But doctors have been perpetuating Myth #2: that the best remedy for menopausal symptoms is prescription hormone replacement therapy (HRT), like Provera (medroxyprogesterone). Provera and other HRT meds are not natural: They're drugs cooked up in a lab, and though they may ease your hot flashes, they are hardly the *best* remedy! Provera, for example, comes with over a hundred different side effects, not to mention huge risks—including death. So why not take natural progesterone instead, which should protect against cancer instead of causing it? When discussing HRT, it's important to understand that there's an exception in the pharmacy. Not all prescribed hormonal medications are synthetic. For example, there's Prometrium. This drug is a form of natural **progesterone** and it is derived from peanuts (you can't take it if you have nut allergies). Prometrium capsules are an "oral micronized progesterone" derived from a natural source and Provera (medroxyprogesterone) is a synthetic progesterone wannabe made in a laboratory.

Your doctor may try to frighten you into taking HRT drugs by telling you there are no head-to-head studies comparing synthetic hormones to bioidenticals. Well, duh, synthetic drugs have multibillion-dollar companies behind them—plants don't! Just because no one has done head-to-head studies doesn't mean that the plants *haven't* been studied—as we just saw, some of them are proven to work very well indeed.

If you're taking natural progesterone in any form—prescription or OTC—dosage is important, and so I urge you to work with a savvy doctor and pharmacist who understand bioidenticals and can test you to be absolutely sure you're taking the right amount for your needs. Please don't overdo those OTC creams, which should be used sparingly and at the lowest effective dose.

If you insist on self-medicating, keep a diary of your symptoms, noting how they alter with each week and each cycle, so that you can adjust your dosage. For now, you can follow the guidelines I've prepared for you in Part V, but please make an appointment with your dream doctor today. (To find your dream doctor, see Part V.)

✳ **Chaste tree extract (*Vitex agnus-castus*)**—Here's another proven plant extract—this one inspires your brain to produce a hormone that causes ovulation (which is why it's also used for infertility). When you ovulate, you produce more estrogen and progesterone, giving your body better balance, making that roller-coaster ride much smoother—and leaving you with less sweat on your face! Obviously this won't work if you've had your ovaries surgically removed. One more note of caution: If you have endometriosis, uterine fibroids, or cancer of the breast, ovaries, or uterus, chaste tree berries could worsen your symptoms because of its hormonal properties.

Chaste tree is usually found in multitasking formulas, such as Enzymatic Therapy's AM/PM Menopause Formula or Life Extension's Meno-Relief 1650, so read the labels. It's better if your chaste tree is in a combination formula, but if you buy chaste tree on its own, use your own instincts to determine the dosage. A good range would be *100 mg two to four times daily.*

Other Ways to Banish the Furnace Blast

✳ Sleep in light clothes—you don't want to sweat at night.

✳ Apply a cooling gel patch to your forehead, neck, or chest. Be Koool's Hot Flash gel sheets can be carried in your purse till you need one. You peel off the adhesive backing and apply the gel sheet wherever you want for immediate surge relief that lasts for several hours. The Head Spa Massager, available at Drugstore.com, Rite Aid, and Walgreens, is another innovative choice that can help alleviate some of your pain. It feels like a thousand fingers massaging your scalp. The company offers a 30-day return policy just in case you are not thoroughly pleased. Cost: $50 (www. gadgetuniverse.com or 800-429-1139).

✳ Steer clear of people and situations that trigger strong emotions—or find ways to manage those emotions differently.

✳ Limit or eliminate hot foods, caffeine, and nicotine.

✳ Take up yoga or meditation, or get regular massage: All these stress relievers reduce cortisol and other stress hormones to help your body's thermostat heal itself.

> We make estrogen in our ovaries until menopause; then it's produced in our fat cells and adrenal glands. So a heavy postmenopausal woman may be at greater risk of estrogen dominance than her skinny menstruating sister–and at greater risk of estrogen-driven cancers.

✳And for an instant relaxer—close your eyes and take three breaths. That instantly changes your brain waves to a slower, more relaxed state. It's amazing how calming that can be!

Soybeans: Sinner or Savior?

Although more than half of all U.S. women suffer from hot flashes, hot flashes are very rare in Japan. There are lots of theories about why, including the fact that Asian women don't eat a lot of red meat, helping them avoid all those hormones to which we Western carnivores are exposed. But another factor is almost certainly the fact that Asian women also eat significantly more soy foods than we do.

Soy is a source of natural estrogen, a.k.a. plant estrogen or phytoestrogen. Although phytoestrogens are indeed natural, they're not bioidentical—that is, they are not an exact replica of our own hormones. Still, their soy consumption probably means that Asian women don't have to go on our Western-style crazy estrogen roller-coaster ride—all that soy keeps their estrogen levels more stable and makes their "hot button" far less sensitive.

When this comparison became widely known, the soy industry tried to convince us that their little bean could reverse all our menopausal symptoms, but in my experience, it just ain't so. One study I read recently showed that women taking soy supplements reported a 50 percent decrease in the severity of their hot flashes—but the placebo group enjoyed a 35 percent decrease, and the frequency of hot flashes remained the same.

For sure, soy can be good for you (unless you're suffering from an estrogen-driven cancer, in which case, opinions are mixed). But you can't necessarily depend on it to give you the relief you're looking for. Still, if you do want to beef up your soy intake, supplement with *50–100 mg isoflavones per day*; the label will likely say "genistein" or "daidzein," referring to soy's active ingredients. Don't take too much: It could cause confusion or forgetfulness. Or—my preference—eat real soy foods as Japanese women do. Miso soup is one of my favorites, and it protects against cancer. Natto is another Japanese favorite—it's a fermented soy food that feels like sticky mashed potatoes, though it tastes quite strong. You really have to acquire a taste for that one! Edamame beans, tempeh, soy sauce (try the low-sodium variety), and tofu are also great soy sources, and other healthy isoflavones can be found as well in chickpeas, dried beans, peas, and other legumes.

Even with healthy forms of soy, don't overdo it. Soy can act like one of those drug muggers, stealing zinc and magnesium from your system. The effect is clinically insignificant unless your diet is based entirely on soy, but if it is, you could lower your thyroid production, causing fatigue and other symptoms of hypothyroidism.

Oops! Where's the Restroom?

An article in the *Journal of the American Medical Association (JAMA)* offers more coverage of the Women's Health Initiative—a fifteen-year study still in progress of some 161,800 women. Apparently, women who used the hormonal products Premarin and Prempro experienced more embarrassing leaks—the kind that happen when you cough, sneeze, laugh, or lift heavy things. In fact, the study showed that women who didn't even have leakage before taking the hormones were more likely to become incontinent, while women who suffered already saw their condition worsen over the course of a year.

Using Bioidentical Hormones: Tests Are the First Step

Bioidentical hormones are plant-derived and then morphed in a lab to look precisely like human hormones. As a result, I feel that they're safer to use and cause fewer harmful side effects than synthetic estrogens/progestins—though that doesn't mean they are risk-free. For sure, we need more clinical data to prove their safety and effectiveness, but I'm using common sense: Since they resemble your own body's hormones so closely, I can't help believing they're our best choice.

Bioidentical hormones come in all strengths and combinations: Some are taken orally; some applied vaginally; some—including the over-the-counter forms—rubbed into the skin. The beauty of these creams is that they allow more progesterone to work for you, but less progesterone by-products to hang around and cause side effects such as drowsiness (which could be a good thing for sleep-deprived women!) or bloating.

If you want to switch from prescribed HRT to bioidenticals, you can theoretically do it on your own (since you've got the OTC option)—but I strongly advise that you don't. Hormones are powerful—your hot flashes should tell you that!—and you need proper dosages and adequate monitoring, no two ways about it. So the best thing to do is to find your dream doctor—someone who understands bioidenticals—and have him or her do some tests on you, first to determine a starting dose, then to keep making sure that your hormone levels are in a healthy range.

There is a lot of debate about which test is best: saliva, blood, blood spot, or urine. (Please refer to my Resource section for a list of premier labs.) Now, here's what I think in a nutshell:

✳ **Saliva tests**—Good for people who apply hormones right onto the skin. Make sure that you draw saliva levels midway between your application times. For example, if you apply your progesterone cream around 10 P.M. each night (to help relax you before bed), do your spit test around 9 or 10 A.M.—right between two 10 P.M. doses. If your levels come back very high, you are probably using too much—or else testing at the wrong time. (See why I want you to work with a doctor?)

✳ **Capillary blood spot**—This is also a good test if you're using the skin creams. It's just a painless finger prick, but it shows a very accurate picture of what is happening in your cells. It's much better than a typical blood test, which could show an artificially low level of hormones, leading your doctor to prescribe too high a dose.

✳ **Blood test**—Some doctors use this, but it isn't so good for people using topical hormone creams because, again, the levels come back relatively low. That's because the hormone in a cream goes through your skin into your blood, then leaves your blood rapidly to go right to its target cell. As a result, traditional blood tests aren't quite as accurate as the other kinds.

* **Urine testing**—I like urine tests because a 24-hour measure of urine mirrors pretty closely what's happening with the hormones inside your cells. However, these particular tests work better when you're taking oral forms of hormones; they aren't as accurate if you're using hormone creams.

Custom-Fitting Your Hormone Meds

Physicians who test your hormone levels can take bioidenticals a step further by customizing a medication to fit your particular needs. For example, some estrogen creams include a smidgen of DHEA to jump-start your adrenals—the perfect recipe for the adrenally spent, tired menopausal woman with too many power surges during the day! Another specially compounded formula (a formula custom-created by your pharmacist according to your physician's specifications) might include estrogen along with testosterone cream, which would not only relieve vaginal dryness, but also add some fireworks to your bedroom fun.

As you can see, even if you've been suffering severe symptoms for a while, there is hope for you—so call your local compounding pharmacy (a place where they prepare their own meds) and ask them for the names of the closest physicians who prescribe bioidentical hormones. (To find a local compounding pharmacy, check the yellow pages under "pharmacy" or call the International Academy of Compounding Pharmacists—contact information is in the Resources section.)

Love Your Liver

A damaged liver can't break down estrogen properly, so your estrogen may be approaching dangerously high levels, increasing your risk for cancer. Check yourself out: If your tongue has branching veins underneath it; or if you have bad breath, experience fatigue, or see tiny red spots on your abdomen, your liver may be overworked. Check with your doctor and take my Hormone Helpers from Chapter 11. And here are some liver-loving supplements you can try:

* **Milk thistle,** a.k.a. silymarin, improves your liver's filtering capability. *Take 150 mg three times per day,* standardized to 80 percent silyma-

rin. It's sold everywhere, but there's an extra-potent form called Siliphos, which is available from Thorne, Phytosome, and Natural Factors.

✳ **Liver Chi** gives your liver a break by reducing the toxic by-products that your liver is supposed to filter out of your system. *Take three capsules two or three times daily before meals.* Visit www.chi-health.com.

✳ **SAMe** (S-adenosylmethionine) helps your liver detoxify estrogen. I recommend *200–400 mg once or twice daily on an empty stomach.*

> *If you're taking hormone replacement drugs, DO NOT suddenly stop taking them. When you take these drugs, your body's own hormone production slows down, so you need to come off the meds slowly, over the course of a few months, under a doctor's supervision, so that your body can resume production of its own natural hormones.*

part IV

And Everything in Between

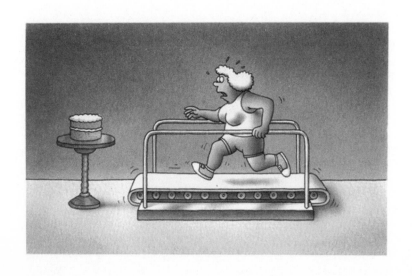

14

Lose Fat While You Sleep . . . When Pink Elephants Fly!

Sometimes I think we are cash cows for the medical industry. Think of it: Obesity causes us to have a higher risk for coronary heart disease, hypertension, type 2 diabetes, gallbladder disease, osteoarthritis, stroke, cancer, and infertility. And in the last few decades we've seen a whopper of an increase—over 127 million people are overweight! What's worse is that our younger generation has plumped up too—the number of obese children has tripled since 1980. We're pouring billions and billions of dollars into the medical industry—and it all starts with what we eat.

You can't imagine how many thousands of people I've seen over the years come to the pharmacy and peruse the aisle for all those big-ticket weight-loss products that provide little benefit. Well, this chapter is to help you navigate through all those confusing products so you can stay away from the useless and dangerous ones. Later on, I'll take you by the hand and help you find products that actually work.

Don't Diet Anymore—Just Edit What You Eat

If you're holding on to unwanted weight, your body is being tricked, because the foods you eat are sending toxic messages to your cells:

✳ "Gee, there are no nutrients here, and I'm still hungry—even hungrier than I was before. Guess I'll eat something again soon!" (That's the voice of potato chips, French fries, or pretty much any type of greasy fast food.)

✳ "Holy cow, that's a lot of sugar! I'll store it as fat, 'cause I don't need that much energy right now." (Now you're hearing white-flour baked goods and sugary items such as bagels, bread, pasta, soft drinks, cake, and candy bars.)

✳ "Whoa, this stuff is sweet, I'll treat it the same as I do sugar and store some fat!" (Despite being calorie-free, artificial sweeteners can trigger fat-storing messages in the brain, according to some studies. These include NutraSweet, Equal, Sweet'N Low, and Splenda, among others.)

Now, where do diets fit into all this? When most people diet, they basically just eat less of what they normally eat. But that's an artificial way to live, and besides, cutting back what we normally eat may not help if those "fattening" messages continue, albeit at a slower pace. I don't like diets because they are not maintainable. Eventually, you get off the diet and a vicious cycle begins.

On the other hand, when we eat healthy foods, we send our brains a positive, healthy message. So be choosy about what goes into your mouth, because it could go straight to your hips. If you take the word "diet" and rearrange those letters, you'll see the word "edit," and that's exactly what I think you should do. *Don't diet—edit what you eat.*

Here's how:

✳ Instead of artificial sweeteners, use natural sugars, honey, stevia, maple syrup, agave syrup, or evaporated organic cane juice. (For more on stevia and agave syrup, see Chapter 6.)

✳ Instead of soda, drink water, preferably alkaline water.

✳ Instead of clear vegetable oils, use coconut, grapeseed, avocado, or olive oil.

✳ Instead of white-flour products, choose dark ones like whole wheat, rye, or pumpernickel.

✳ Instead of French fries, how about a baked potato?

✳ Instead of greasy beef burgers, eat fish, bison-buffalo (preferably free-range), lean turkey, or chicken.

✳ If you like juice, cut it with some water or even club soda so it's not so sweet.

✳ Instead of milkshakes, why not juice some fruits and veggies or make a nonfat yogurt smoothie?

✳ Instead of salads all the time, steam some greens—the fiber will fill you up and you'll get more nutrients.

Now if you really get into this and make the commitment to editing what you eat, take a look at the book *Eat This, Not That!* by David Zinczenko and Matt Goulding (Rodale, 2007). It will teach you cool things like why it's better to eat a Whopper Jr. (hold the mayo) versus a BK Big Fish. These two Burger King entrées are quite different in nutritional makeup. I thought the fish sandwich was better for me until I learned that the Whopper Jr. has only 12 grams of fat, compared to the BK Big Fish's 52 grams of fat! Avoiding fast food is ideal; however, if you are going to indulge in it, choose wisely.

Suzy's Secrets from Behind the Counter
Amazing Almond Flour

Did you know that diabetics and people on low-carb diets can eat almond flour? It's gluten-free, and since it's a nut flour, there are virtually no carbs!

I get excited to tell people with Crohn's, colitis, and other inflammatory bowel conditions that this flour can really help you! Almond flour is (obviously) made from almonds, which are rich in protein, vitamin E, and phosphorus (good for your bones). Almonds don't have cholesterol—but they do contain cancer-fighting antioxidants. That's no small feat for a tiny nut! The good news is that ground-up

Some drugs give you the munchies: sedatives and tranquilizers, antidepressants, allergy pills, female hormones, and diuretics. Alas, there is no antidote (though you might try a large cheese pizza!), but at least if you find yourself ravenously hungry, you'll know why—and you might ask your doctor to switch you to another type of medication if you're concerned about weight gain.

almond flour confers all these benefits as well. You can buy small bags of it at the health-food store, but I really like the flavor and texture of the brand sold by Lucy's Kitchen Shop at www.lucyskitchen.com (888-484-2126), $65 for 10 pounds, and it lasts for months in the fridge. There are delicious recipes and guidelines for this "Specific Carbohydrate" diet at www. breakingtheviciouscycle.com.

Stay Away from Diet Scams!

The bitter truth is that almost none of those magic pills, potions, meal plans, energy bars, or drinks will melt fat away permanently if you don't continue taking them. Diet scammers know that if you're desperate, you'll buy anything without verifying its authenticity, purity, or manufacturer—which could be located in a dirty garage. You won't lose weight but you will lose money—and possibly your health. And am I being dramatic if I say your life is at stake? Some products—even reputable ones—contain ingredients that can jack up your heart rate, cause your blood pressure to skyrocket, and damage your kidneys—a lethal combination for people with weak hearts or multiple medical conditions.

Now, let me introduce you to some popular products on the market:

✴ **Zantrex-3**—a "jolt" pill to boost fat burning. This little dynamo has the same amount of caffeine as 3 to 4 cups of coffee. You'll see ingredient names like yerba mate and guarana seed as well as caffeine itself. Yes, this one will help suppress appetite and you might lose some weight, but taking high-energy stimulants can be very dangerous if you suffer from heart disease, high blood pressure, diabetes, or anxiety. Why take a chance, even if you're healthy? Weight-loss effects are temporary, and the risks are cold sweats, a racing heart, jitters, stomachache, and diarrhea.

✴ **NeoForm-3000**—You might have seen this as a mailbox stuffer with no ingredients listed, no phone number, and no real address. The model is drinking wine and eating French fries. I feel healthier just thinking about it! I say, pass quickly on this and any other "stuffer" that is just intended to soak you.

✳ **TrimSpa**—Ah, yes, the late Anna Nicole Smith's pet product. The story behind this one is almost funny: A stage hypnotist trying to sell more TrimSpa was charged by the New Jersey Attorney General in 2005 with deceptive advertising practices. He and his associates would lure people to seminars to learn about nondrug approaches to weight loss and then do a sales pitch for TrimSpa. The maker was forced to pay $750,000 for this indiscretion. As for product contents, it contains a synergistic formula that will help you drop the pounds, no doubt, but it contains stimulants, so it may be harmful if you suffer from high blood pressure, anxiety, heart disease, kidney problems, or diabetes. And once you go off the product, the weight creeps right back on.

✳ **SBM-GIGA-MAGTAB**—Just soak me by the pound, please! I read one of their advertisements for the "fruit acid" supplement (which, by the way, is completely different from the mineral sold by the same name for magnesium supplementation) and it said, "Eat what you like, whenever you like" and "You won't regain weight." Yeah, right, when pink elephants fly. Their website was more conservative, saying that you might lose "up to a pound a day." When I called Canada to pretend to order this, a woman said the price was based on how many pounds I wanted to lose. So I told her "ten to twenty pounds," and she said I'd have to give them $98 plus shipping—every twenty days! The audacity of that! When I called again three days later, the price had changed to $75 for a two-month supply. Hey, maybe if I wait another few days, they'll pay me to take it! I say, "Pass."

✳ **ThermoSlim**—Makers had to pay $1 million in consumer redress to settle allegations that they had made false or ridiculous claims during their infomercial, such as saying that you could lose "95 pounds in 60 days"; that you could eat all the hamburgers, French fries, milkshakes, and cheesecakes you want and still lose substantial weight; and that "this is the safest . . . product available for weight loss." Safe? What makes anyone think rapid weight loss is safe—it's downright dangerous! You need to lose weight gradually—2 or 3 pounds a week *at most*—or you'll risk flooding your body with all the toxins stored in your fat, not to mention stressing your liver, kidneys, and heart.

✳ **Body creams and gels**—Don't be naïve, there's no such thing as a cream that dissolves fat or gets rid of cellulite. Cellulite happens because little fat deposits settle into the tissue, so it's partly a problem of circulation. Creams simply don't penetrate deep enough to dissolve fat globules, so don't believe those pretty labels with the sexy airbrushed thighs. When you see ridiculous claims, put the product right back on the shelf. I think these creams are basically moisturizers, sold to unsuspecting people who believe deceptive ads. Not you, I hope!

✳ **Patches**—I'm guessing there isn't a single active ingredient in those things that authentically burns fat or removes cellulite; plus, they can be irritating. Hydrogel slim patch has already been shut down, and numerous fraudulent companies have been cracked down on by the Federal Trade Commission (FTC). Remember the infomercial, "Peel Away the Pounds"? The makers of the seaweed patch featured in that one had to settle $1 million dollars in suits for claiming that it can melt away three to five pounds of weight per week. Hey, if I'm going to be near seaweed, it's going into my mouth, in the form of a sushi tuna roll with spicy mayo and ginger!

✳ **Abdominal gadgets**—My husband, who is a chiropractor, calls these "muscle twitchers"! You strap them to your waist and they supposedly melt 4 inches in thirty days and give you a set of six-pack abs just like the paid model (who doesn't even own the product). As if! Sorry, ladies, the only way to build up your muscles is to sweat—but you probably still won't look like the model unless you're genetically blessed, eat like a bird, and make exercise your full-time job. Yeah, and you'll probably still need liposuction. C'mon people, just say NO!

Fat Starts in Your Brain

And no, I'm not calling you a fathead! I'm saying that your brain simply isn't sending out the proper signals to tell you to stop eating because you are full. That chemical signal is called "leptin," and it's a stop sign. If you wolf down your meals, you don't get the stop sign in time because you need about ten to fifteen minutes for it to become activated. That's why people who eat quickly tend to be plumper than those who take their time and savor every bite. If you're short on vitamin D because you don't get enough sun, you also don't get the leptin stop sign. So, supplementing with D (about *1,000 IU per day*) can indirectly cause weight loss.

Even if fat starts in your brain, it eventually lands on your seat cushions. The best way to reset your fat-burning thermostat is to exercise. According to one study, just 45 minutes of daily exercise will eventually make you eleven to eighteen pounds lighter than you'd be if you were sedentary. Exercising allows your body to burn fat even when you're in rest mode because it changes the way your cells process the molecules you eat.

Has Your Doctor Uncovered Everything?

Some of us have trouble losing weight or maintaining a healthy weight because our metabolism is out of whack. We eat less and less—but still, the weight stays on or even increases. To turn things around, we need to restore a healthy metabolism.

The most obvious place to look for metabolic problems is in the thyroid. Most doctors can measure your thyroid hormone levels with a simple blood test. (For more on thyroid function, see Chapter 1.)

Another likely place to find metabolic misfiring is with a woman's hormones. Many women make too much estrogen or they take estrogen-containing medications that might cause them to retain water, hang on to fat, or develop low thyroid, which further contributes to weight gain. Balancing hormones and maintaining healthy levels of estrogen are important, so read Chapters 11–13.

Another obscure reason for stubborn weight gain is inflammation. Dangerous inflammatory chemicals such as Reactive Oxygen Species, C Reactive Protein, and homocysteine are signs that your body is dealing with inflammation, a condition that has lots of health risks and can also translate to you tipping the scales. Luckily, your next move is simple: Ask your doctor for a blood test to see how you weigh in with these inflammatory markers. If your levels are high, you can work with your doctor on bringing those numbers down and therefore improving your health in every way.

One easy way to do this is with OTC supplements like B vitamins and the acid betaine hydrochloride, which can reduce inflammation. I found a combination product that contains body-ready absorbable forms of B vitamins and the betaine—all in one: Thorne's MethylGuard. Just follow the directions on the label. If you can't find this, or you can't tolerate acid (betaine), then get a high-quality B-Complex 100 and take it daily. Also, SAMe (S-adenosylmethionine) is essential, especially since this amino acid can also help you with joint pain and depression. Dosage: *200–400 mg twice daily on an empty stomach*. I like Life Extension and Nature Made brands, but there are many others sold at pharmacies nationwide.

A Walk Down the Aisle

Now let's take that walk I promised you—down the aisles of my pharmacy to help you find the products that might actually help you lose weight—no doctor required!

* *Hoodia gordonii*—This natural appetite suppressant comes from a South African cactus and will reduce your appetite without the jitters. Residents of the bush have eaten it for centuries, and they look fit and trim to me! I love this one because it tricks the brain into feeling full, so we lose interest in food and eat less. Even though there aren't large studies to back Hoodia, pharmaceutical companies think a lot of it anyway: They are trying to patent the active ingredient P57 so they can sell it to us at a premium. For now, hoodia gordonii is over-the-counter, and it's a safe option for people to try, along with diet and exercise of course. Some people claim it gives them a sense of well-being. Buy only good products that are authenticated by independent labs (there are lots of fakes out there), and make sure that what you buy has a Convention on International Trade in Endangered Species (C.I.T.E.S.) certificate dated within six months and that the company offers a phone number as well. Some of the better products so far include HoodiThin and HoodiSpray liquid extracts and two oral supplements, Desert Burn and Hoodia Gordonii Plus. The dosage is different with each product, so just follow product guidelines.

* **L-carnitine**—This amino acid is able to pick up fat from your bloodstream and shuttle it over to muscle cells, where you can burn it off. That's good if you're overweight because you probably have addi-

tional fat cells, high cholesterol, and extra triglycerides that clog your blood vessels. Having carnitine around helps clear the body of these fats, which ultimately gives you more energy even as you lose weight. It's not a stimulant at all, though you may feel less fatigued. Yeah! Even better, carnitine is attracted to muscles, including the heart muscle, making this a heart-healthy supplement. *Dosage: 500–1,000 mg three times daily.*

✳ **Glucomannan**—Extracted from the yam family, this is a water-soluble dietary fiber just like the ones you find in the laxative aisle. You've got to buy this product at a health-food store, though. As a fiber, glucomannan makes you feel full, so you'll eat less. Besides weight loss, take glucomannan for constipation and heart disease. Take it with plenty of water, and don't overdo it—this product swells inside your body to a size much bigger than typical fibers. The dosage varies greatly, so please follow the directions on the labels. Two good brands are made by Nature's Way and Natrol.

✳ **Omega-3 fatty acids**—Fish oils are rich in omega-3s—and they speed up the rate at which you burn fat. People sometimes write to my syndicated column asking if fatty acids will make you fat. Absolutely not! In fact, you need good fats like these in order to eliminate bad fats. *Dosage: 1,000 mg once or twice daily.*

✳ **Dandelion (*Taraxacum officinale*)**—This plant extract supports the liver to eliminate toxins, including those that gather and form cellulite. It's a diuretic, so it should also reduce your water weight. Don't pick the yellow flowers out of your yard; get the real deal from a fresh market. Eat a few raw leaves in your salad, or else drink the tea. I don't like the supplements because this herb has the potential to interact with too many medications for diabetes, gallbladder disease, heart disease, and high blood pressure. So eat a few leaves, but that's it.

✳ **5-HTP (*5-hydroxytryptophan*)**—This helps shut down your carb craver; it also helps with mood and insomnia. 5-HTP is the precursor to serotonin, a calming, feel-good brain chemical. When I take this wonder supplement, I can walk right past an oven full of baking brownies and not even care. The supplement chromium picolinate claims to do this and it might be helpful, but it gets mixed reviews from my patients (whereas most people thank me for the 5-HTP tip), so I'm going with my patients! Just be aware that 5-HTP may cause drowsiness—so start with small doses and work up, and be aware that it can enhance the effect of tranquilizing meds. Also, please avoid it if you take SSRI antidepressants like Prozac, Zoloft, or Paxil. *Dosage: 50 mg two or three times daily.*

✳ **Guggul (*Commiphora mukul*)**—Used in Ayurvedic medicine, guggul could help control cholesterol while improving your ratio of good to bad cholesterol. Weight loss is possible, too, but not if you continue to eat cheeseburgers. In a clinical trial testing 103 adults with guggul, the scientists concluded that guggul offers little or no benefit (even at very high doses) if used while eating a typical Western diet. So it may not be a miracle supplement, but it may be of some assistance if you make healthful dietary and lifestyle changes. Also, here's a warning if you have thyroid disease: Guggul seems to increase TSH (thyroid stimulating hormone), so take guggul only with your doctor's blessings and routine monitoring for thyroid hormone. And finally, this supplement is capable of thinning your blood, which is considered a good thing; however, this can be dangerous for certain people who take anticoagulant medications (warfarin, Plavix, aspirin) or herbs (ginkgo, ginger). *Try 1 or 2 grams twice daily* or as directed on the product label.

✳ **Coenzyme Q10**—This powerful antioxidant makes your cells burn food more efficiently, making it a simple, safe way to reset your metabolism and assist your body in its quest to lose weight. It also happens to resuscitate suffocating cells in people who are fatigued all the time, or who suffer from cardiovascular disease, high blood pressure, or liver disease. *Try 50–100 mg every morning.* I like Jarrow, Country Life, Healthy Origins, and Vitamin World.

✳ **Adaptogens**—If you are under tremendous stress, then your hormones are out of balance. You might have high or low cortisol, low progesterone, low DHEA, or many other imbalances, any of which might cause you to hang on to weight. Adaptogens help nourish your adrenal glands (please read Chapter 1), and when your adrenals are healthy, your cortisol levels normalize so that you can burn up fat. I recommend finding ways to relieve stress with yoga, with other breathing techniques, or with meditation, but you can also take such adaptogenic herbs as Panax ginseng, Ashwagandha, Eleuthero, licorice root, rhodiola, and Cordyceps. I like combination formulas, including Thorne's Phytisone and Metagenics's Adreset, but you either have to buy these brands from a participating physician or call the companies directly (see Resources). Some brands that may be easier to find include Gaia Herbs's Stress Response, Herb Pharm's Adrenal Support Tonic, and Nature's Sunshine's Mineral-Chi Tonic. Those last two are liquids, so they are particularly easy to get down, especially if you have trouble swallowing.

Excellent Enzymes

You don't see enzymes promoted heavily because they are not an immediate fix to obesity. But since enzymes help you process your food efficiently, they will ultimately help you lose weight. You'll feel full and satisfied; your brain will have everything it needs to make "feel-good" chemicals; and your metabolism will rebalance and function more efficiently. If you were going to take just one supplement (in addition to your daily multivitamin), it should be enzymes. I believe that America's overall health would improve dramatically if people made high-quality enzymes a part of their daily routines.

They're so important that if you are deficient in enzymes, you could end up with stomach gas, indigestion, bloating, heartburn, flatulence, and many other diseases throughout your body. Some studies have shown that enzymes ease psoriasis, chronic inflammation, high blood pressure, diabetes, fatigue, acne, allergies, arthritis, infections, depression, anxiety, vertigo, and asthma. You'll see some benefits within a week, though it takes about three months for the full benefits to kick in.

It's best to get your enzymes by eating lots of raw or slightly steamed veggies. Don't overcook: Heat is the enzyme's enemy. If you do decide to buy enzymes in a supplement form, look for products that contain such key enzymes as lipase (to digest fat), amylase (to digest carbs), lactase (to digest milk sugar), and protease (to digest protein).

All enzyme products should be avoided in people who have gastritis or ulcers (gastric or duodenal). Specifically, protease enzymes can irritate and further inflame the stomach and duodenum.

You'll see all kinds of other terrific enzymes in high-quality blends including pancreatin, papain, bromelain, trypsin, and chymotrypsin. Here are some good choices. Choose one of these supplements; don't take all of them together!

✳ **Wobenzym N**—*three capsules twice daily taken at least forty-five minutes before meals*

✳ **Enzymedica's Digest**—*one to three capsules before each meal*

✳ **Thorne Research's B.P.P.**, which stands for betaine, pepsin, and pancreatin: *one or two capsules with each meal.* (This brand contains a little acid along with the enzymes.)

My Own Diet Picks

People always ask me what diets I recommend. Of the ones I've studied, I really like the following. Besides liking them all for weight loss, I know they can bring health and wellness in so many ways: Any one of these could help you reduce your risk for heart disease, cancer, and stroke, while also helping you fight inflammation, pain, autoimmune diseases, and fatigue.

✳ The pH Miracle Diet—www.phmiracleliving.com

✳ Mediterranean Asian Diet—www.mediterrasian.com

✳ Dean Ornish Diet—www.ornish.com

✳ Barry Sears Zone—www.drsears.com

✳ Specific Carbohydrate Diet—www.breakingtheviciouscycle.com

✳ Vegetarian Diet—no specific diet, but see www.goveg.com for some good ideas

The Skinny on Cellulite

The dimpling of skin—the most common sign of cellulite—happens more frequently in women than men. It's because some tissue is pulling down on your skin while fat cells and those holding water are pushing up: The combination causes that orange-peel look. It's not just in overweight people, either; skinny women have cellulite too.

There are many theories as to why cellulite forms, but I think it has to do with reduced circulation. Connective tissue beneath the skin becomes weak and deformed, and so the buildup begins. That's why diets and exercise have only a minor effect on cellulite, because it's not a result of fat, but rather of poor circulation. This also explains why younger, healthy women don't have much cellulite—whatever their weight—while older women seem to get it more. Check out Chapter 2 to learn how to patch up your blood vessels and improve your circulation, because most creams, lotions, wraps, and potions won't help.

Before you resort to buying a pair of body-shaping Spanx (which do work well), try brushing your cellulite away. You want to get rid of the stuff right, not just conceal it until your unsuspecting partner finds out the truth. Dry skin brushing improves circulation of the lymph, and this could level the lumps, but of course, you also need to eat a healthy diet. Buy a body brush for about $10—a soft-bristled brush sold in health and beauty stores. Brush your extremities in short strokes (or circular ones), starting at your feet. Work your way up, always moving in the direction of your heart: up your legs, inward on your arms. Your goal is to brush all your blood towards the heart, so that your heart can process it and recirculate your lymph. One warning: Don't body brush if you have any type of cancer.

Body brushes and loofahs are such nice exfoliators, so try doing this in the shower with your favorite shower gel. If your guy wants to get into the act one evening, have him use one feather-light brush stroke, then one hand stroke in the same place. Have him do this all over—it feels great on your back!

Fat-Blocking Pill May Cause Unsightly Side Effects

Alli, the only FDA-approved diet pill, is an over-the-counter fat blocker that works exactly like the prescription drug Xenical (orlistat). Alli is basically

Xenical, but half the dosage. The drug prevents about one-quarter of the fat in your meal from getting absorbed, so if you eat four slices of pizza, you'll incorporate the fat of only three slices. This would be a good time to remind you that if you're trying to lose weight, then you should be on a low-calorie (low-pizza) diet!

It's shocking, but currently, approximately 65 percent of U.S. adults are overweight or obese, according to the National Institutes of Health.

In a 2006 study of adolescents ages 14 to 18 years old, orlistat did not significantly reduce body mass index in comparison to a placebo group after six months usage. In comparison with the placebo group, the orlistat group had increased adverse events, usually occurring in the gastrointestinal tract.

Orlistat is not a miracle pill; it's an assistant to a bigger plan that includes diet, exercise, and willpower. It only modestly outperforms dud pills, but the upside is that it won't rev you up, speed up your heart, or interfere with sleep. Side effects that could ruin a night out, or an airline trip, include loose and unexpected (!) stools or gas. Vitamin deficiency, especially of the fat-soluble vitamins such as vitamins A, D, E, and K, could occur with long-term use. People who take blood thinners or have diabetes or thyroid disease should consult their doctors before taking Alli.

Visit www.myalli.com or most pharmacies/retailers.

15

Botox and Other Ways to Cheat Father Time

I f you're like most women, you probably have drawers and drawers full of half-empty bottles, tubes, creams, and lotions that promise to give you radiant, younger-looking skin and "dramatic," "never-before-seen" results. Most of these products are nothing more than moisturizers that contain a multitude of unpronounceable ingredients and synthetic chemicals that might even age you faster!

Certainly there are many wonderful products out there, but I believe that truly gorgeous skin, hair, and nails begin on the inside. Good stuff in, good stuff out! So in this chapter, I'll clue you in about some of the best-kept nutritional secrets and products to help you turn back time. And you won't have to spend huge amounts of money to feel pretty. It starts from the inside, one healthy cell at a time.

Tick-Tock, Tick-Tock . . . the Free Radical Clock Is Ticking

Why does the clock seem to tick faster for some women? Why do some women look terrific, while others the same age have deep wrinkles and saggy skin? It could be the result of damage by free radicals—highly charged molecules that are buzzing around like crazy among your cells. The free radicals grab partners—other cells that were just sitting around doing nothing—and it riles them up too, creating a chain reaction in your skin: a squad of wild cells firing randomly and killing off perfectly innocent "bystander" cells and tissues.

Long story short: Free radicals age you! They must be stopped and there's only one thing that can do it: their nemesis, antioxidants. So first, you've got to avoid free radicals, and then, when they do invade your system, you've got to neutralize them as soon as possible.

Foods That Cause Wrinkles—Sugar, breads, pasta, coffee, processed foods, artificial sweeteners, MSG.

Wrinkle Busters—Water, salmon, olive oil, grape seed oil, blueberries, orange juice, green tea, kale.

It's best to eat a diet rich in healthy foods that have plenty of antioxidants, but feel free to supplement, too. It may take months, but the effects you'll get will go beyond beauty because antioxidants improve your health in so many ways, lifting your mood, supporting heart health, boosting your energy, and fighting cancer, to name just a few.

Skin Revitalizers That Can Turn Back Time—No Doctor Required!

Here are my favorite ways for you to look beautiful—for less than $10 a month!

1. **Silica**—Every strand of hair on your head, every fingernail, every tooth, and every square inch of skin contains silica. You see silica in the form of sand on the beach, but other forms of it keep our hair shiny and nails strong. A deficiency in silica (which happens as we age) can lead to dull, dry hair, brittle nails, and osteoporosis. It's okay to try out those fancy-shmancy shampoos and nail-hardening products—but if you stick to the silica, you'll get way better results!

Your first step to "silicizing" your diet is to focus on such vegetables and grains as oats, millet, onions, whole grains, and potatoes. You can also take silica supplements, but be sure to take only 100 percent pure aqueous extract, derived from spring horsetail (*equisetum arvense*)— that's a superb source of silica that will also give you some calcium. It's interesting that silica is used to form collagen, so it can help repair torn ligaments, and help ease hemorrhoids. I like Cellfood's Essential Silica *(15 drops twice daily)* and Natural Factors's brand *(500 mg three times a day)*.

   2. Vitamin E—Vitamin E is a terrific wrinkle buster. I like vitamin E because it's sort of "oily," so it slides into the fatty skin cells where other antioxidants can't. Don't worry, it won't make your skin oily at all. On the contrary, taken daily, it can soften skin, make your hair shiny and thick, and smooth out fine lines. E is a powerful beautifier that also helps protect your heart, your vision, and your immune system while reducing PMS symptoms. This is definitely your supplement if you want to minimize scarring. For little wounds and even minor surgical areas, just puncture a capsule (*800 IU*) and squeeze it right on, or apply the vitamin E oil sold in pharmacies and health-food stores nationwide.

   3. Vitamin C—Vitamin C is your antisag supplement—it keeps your skin from drooping, and it's your best defense against the free radical clock. Unlike E, which is "oily" in personality, C is slippery like an eel. It is water-loving and gets into most cells of our bodies to have profound impact. Taking C (and applying eye creams with it) lightens those dark circles by patching up the broken capillaries that cause them. C makes you happy, energetic, and focused, too, because it is used to make happy brain chemicals. You can find vitamin C in fresh citrus fruits, strawberries, peppers, spinach, broccoli, and tomatoes. The better Cs are either buffered or sustained-release with a ratio of 2:1 ascorbic acid: bioflavonoids. Take about *500 mg twice daily*.

   4. Alpha lipoic acid (ALA) or R-lipoic acid (RLA)—ALA is another powerful wrinklebuster that is capable of reducing lines by up to 50 percent, according to one small study. And everything alpha lipoic does, R-lipoic does better. These nutrients grab deadly free radicals and unwanted metals and help clear them from your system. That's a plus, because such heavy metals as mercury, cadmium, and lead are associated with diabetic neuropathy, high blood pressure, Alzheimer's, and liver disease. And this is supercool: Both ALA and RLA regenerate four other antioxidants that are even more powerful: vitamin C, vitamin E, Coenzyme Q10, and glutathione. So if you take either ALA or RLA along with these, you get much more bang for your beauty buck!

Dosage: Alpha lipoic acid: 100 mg every morning; you can find it at health-food stores and some pharmacies. *Or try R-lipoic acid: 50 mg once daily*, available from Thorne Research (www.thorne.com) and in some health-food stores.

5. **B-complex**—The B stands for "beautiful hair"! All the Bs are good for your lovely locks, but biotin is the star working with its sisters (folic acid, thiamine, B_6, B_{12}, riboflavin, and the rest) to protect against premature graying, greasy hair, dandruff, and poor hair growth. The Bs fight fatigue, too—how beautiful is that? Now if you have dry skin, lesions, muscle twitching, poor coordination, or insomnia, you may be deficient in Bs. Some 40 percent of dermatitis sufferers are also deficient in B. Estrogen-containing drugs—like birth control or HRT—are drug muggers, so if you're on those meds, be sure to supplement! (See Part V for other drug muggers that steal your Bs.) *Take 50 mg B-complex every morning.*

6. **Omega-3 fatty acids**—Essential fatty acids called omega-3s come from fish. I know it's weird to think of omega-3s as skin supplements because fish have such awful scaly skin, but trust me, the "fishy" extracts called omega-3 fatty acids (sometimes called EPA/DHA) will make your complexion glow. They also add shine to the hair and prevent your skin and hair from getting dry and brittle. This is *the* supplement if you have psoriasis or eczema. The fish oils story gets even prettier because omega-3s improve digestion and will help you lose weight. Make sure your brand is of high quality (I like Nordic Naturals). *Take EPA/DHA 1,000 mg once or twice daily.* If allergies mean that you simply can't take fish oils, there is an algae-derived source of essential fatty acids—krill oil—and even though it's

Coconut oil is nourishing to really dry, scaly, cracked skin on your hands, elbows, or heels. Pick up a bottle from the health-food store and massage it in twice a day for a few weeks.

still marine-derived, many people do just fine on this. Take the same dosage, *1,000 mg once or twice daily*. Neptune, Twinlab, Thorne Research, and other quality companies make this.

Plant-Based Antioxidants

Plants, especially berries and vegetables, contain powerful antioxidants too. There's no reason why you can't take a plant-based antioxidant along with the vitamins and nutrients I've listed. In fact, I absolutely would. The nutrients in them have wide-reaching effects throughout the body and protect every cell. Check out Thorne's Plantioxidants (www.thorne.com) or Enzymatic Therapy's Doctor's Choice Antioxidant (sold widely at most pharmacies).

You can also try some of the many delicious juices packed with these sorts of antioxidants, like pomegranate juice, blueberry juice, and specialized tropical juices like Noni, Goji Juice, or Mangosteen (the last three are sold at most health-food stores).

Itchy, Irritated Skin

Here's an easy solution for you if you have eczema or dermatitis, two names that describe really itchy, irritated skin: Try taking evening primrose oil (EPO), a dietary supplement of essential fatty acids that is rich in GLA (gamma linoleic acid). Research from 1993 proved that babies with eczema had low levels of these essential fatty acids, probably because their mothers were deficient. Children and adults with these skin conditions respond dramatically well to GLA-rich supplements such as evening primrose oil, sometimes in as little as four weeks.

Supplements are sold as gelcaps with the words "evening primrose oil" on the label. You'll also see other words on the label such as "linoleic acid" or "other fatty acids." This is fine. Take EPO with meals to minimize any stomach upset, and do not overdo it because excessive amounts of GLA can create inflammation in the body.

Goin' Natural

Let's face it, it's hard to decipher all those ingredients on the labels. But it pays to be careful, because some so-called "beauty" products for our hair, skin, and nails contain toxic chemicals that studies have shown to be harmful when they penetrate our skin.

For example, many shampoos and cosmetic products are laden with synthetic colors and fragrances (which may contribute to cancer); diazolidinyl urea (which can release the dangerous preservative formaldehyde); sodium laurel sulfate (some controversial studies link it to headaches and nerve damage); propylene glycol (which may cause liver and kidney damage, and eczema); and parabens (which are xenobiotics—substances that act like estrogen in your body, adding to estrogen dominance and everything that goes with it). And don't get me started on lipstick and makeup—I don't have enough pages in this chapter!

The point is, if you are trying to be health-savvy—which I always recommend—please look for safe and natural alternatives that are eco-friendly and people-tested. Start by visiting www.safecosmetics.org, where you'll find every single company that has signed a document promising to "not use chemicals that are known or strongly suspected of causing cancer, mutation, or birth defects in their products . . ." As of April 2008, about five hundred companies had signed, and the website continuously adds to its list. You may be surprised: As of this writing, most of our big beauty names were missing, including Estée Lauder, Lancôme, Procter & Gamble, Revlon, L'Oréal, and Avon. I am pleased to tell you that the Sally Hansen brand has agreed to remove from its nail polish three nasty chemicals linked to cancer and birth defects.

Even though I'm attached to a few big-name products in my makeup drawer, I am doing my best to tilt my own beauty regimen in favor of holistic, natural companies that put in extra time and money to make sure that consumers are safe and protected from harmful chemicals. Some companies that did make this pledge include Aubrey Organics (www.aubrey-organics.com); The Body Shop, found in many malls (www.bodyshop.com); Hugo Naturals (www.hugonaturals.com); Juice Beauty (www.juicebeauty.com), Naturopathica (www.naturopathica.com); The Purist Company (www.purist.com); and Sheer Mineral (www.sheermineral.com). You can sometimes find these and other natural companies at health-food stores, some pharmacies, retailers like Sephora, and online.

Check out another cool website called Skin Deep, where you can actually type in a product name and find out how safe it is. Since the FDA has assessed only about 11 percent of the 10,500 ingredients found in our cosmetic products, it should interest you to use this website to evaluate how safe your products are. I was absolutely stunned when I looked up one of my favorite facial cleansers and found that it contained five ingredients linked to breast cancer, and five other ingredients thought to be potential "endocrine disruptors," which could affect all hormone systems as well as fertility. I won't even begin to tell you what I found in my self-tanning gel, which I promptly threw out. Trust me, you'll not only become more savvy after you visit this website, you'll also be more choosy about your personal care products. That's a good thing because every little thing you do now to preserve your health comes back to you later. Don't naively slather on poisons! Check out how safe your products really are and switch brands if necessary. It's so simple; get online today and visit www.ewg.org/reports/skindeep.

Get Rid of Granny Hairs

✳ If hair grows all over your face, have your hormone levels checked. (You may have too much testosterone.) I like ZRT and John Lee's labs for hormonal testing because they sell reliable home test kits directly to the public.

✳ To get rid of unwanted facial hair, consider Vaniqa, a prescription cream clinically proven to reduce the growth of unwanted facial hair in women. You get results in about two months. Any doctor can prescribe it for you, and more information can be found at www.vaniqa.com.

✳ You could consider electrolysis if you have just one or two stubborn granny hairs, but my friends who've tried it tell me that for any more than that, this procedure can get pretty uncomfortable. Still, some people find the results worth the discomfort.

Unpuff Your Eyes

Ooh La Lift by Benefit instantly depuffs and firms the eye area. You put it on and the tightening botanicals and light-reflecting pigments help you look as though you slept all night—even if you didn't. It's applied underneath your eyes as though it were concealer. It fades in and after a minute you feel a pulling or tightening sensation as ingredients like raspberry and algae extract, chamomile extract, and vitamins A, D, and E go to work to depuff your eyes and hide the fact that you were up all night with your baby or studying for those finals. Apply it throughout the day, even over makeup. Available online at www.sephora.com or www.benefitcosmetics.com.

Suzy's Secrets from Behind the Counter
Homemade Moisturizers from Heaven

Many fancy moisturizers are unaffordable—some tiny jars cost more than $200! Fortunately, you can make a fantastic anti-aging moisturizer at home that will hydrate your skin, prevent moisture loss, and soften fine lines. Purchase a fragrance-free moisturizing lotion or cream. Try to find one that contains antioxidants, such as vitamins A, C, or E; it will help reduce environmental damage from free radicals. For a 2 ounce jar of cream, add 10 drops of pure essential oil of rose and 2 drops of German chamomile. If you don't like the scent of rose or the price tag of this highly prized essential oil, try 4 drops of ylang ylang and 8 drops of lavender. For a 4 ounce bottle of lotion, add 20 drops total of one of these pure essential oils or a blend of essential oils. Either way, you can make a homemade moisturizer for your face or body that is wonderful for your skin and smells heavenly!

Magic Masks

For a nice pick-me-up and fix-me-up, try a refreshing mask.

✳ **Biore Cleansing Mask**—What's blue and hot and clean all over? The Biore Cleansing Mask, which cleans and purifies your skin as it heats up on your face. Within seconds you feel like you're getting a spa treatment (or maybe a hot flash?). The warming mask opens your pores and absorbs excess oils and dirt. You can buy it at most pharmacies. Cost: $8. But please stay away if you have very sensitive skin, or don't like chemicals.

✳ **Silica Mud Mask**—Straight out of Iceland's famed hot spring, the Blue Lagoon, this mask contains natural silica to bring out your skin's inner glow. It deep-cleanses and exfoliates, shrinking your pores and making your complexion smooth and radiant. I also like their mineral bath salts, which help with eczema and psoriasis. I don't consider myself high maintenance, but these are both gotta-haves on my list, even though neither one is cheap—they each cost approximately $50. www.bluelagoon.com.

✳ **Dermalogica Anti-Bac Cooling Masque**—If you are acne-prone, this masque can help reduce the frequency of breakouts. It contains cooling menthol; zinc to fight bacteria; and green tea and licorice extracts to calm angry inflamed skin. You almost want to eat it! It also contains natural tea tree oil and essential oils of rosemary, sage, and orange to aid in skin repair. Dermalogica is sold at fine salons nationwide, at Sephora, and online for about $35. You can find product information at www.dermalogica.com.

Beauty with Botox

Beauty in one shot! The potent poison actually is quite effective at reducing frown lines that make you look angry, deep forehead wrinkles, or those cute crow's feet which bother some people. Botox is the number-one cosmetic procedure in the United States, with almost 4 million treatments in 2005. After a few shots administered in a few minutes for a few hundred dollars, you can expect to drop ten years off your age. You'll need to wait three or four days after your injections before you see results, but then they'll last four to six months.

The key to good Botox treatments is finding a doctor who has an artistic flair. You need to be choosy because not all doctors are as skilled (or as handsome) as Sean and Christian on *Nip/Tuck*. Bad Botox jobs are all over Hollywood, giving some of our celebrities and news anchors that expressionless, deer-in-the-headlights look.

If you're not fond of needles, ask your doctor to numb you with an anesthetic cream and an ice pack. After a few minutes, you won't even notice those shots going in. Be careful about meds that can interact with the Botox: certain antibiotics (gentamicin, clindamycin); the heart medication quinidine; and some medications used to treat Alzheimer's and Myasthenia Gravis. Cost: $200–$800 per session, depending on how much is injected, what area(s) of your face is treated, and what city you live in. For more information, go to www.botoxcosmetic.com.

Depending on where it's injected, Botox can help relieve migraines, low back pain, excessive sweating in the armpits or hands, and possibly interstitial cystitis—a maddening urge to pee.

My Lipstick Is Bugging Me!

You may feel like an unwilling participant on *Survivor*, but bugs go into the making of almost all lipsticks on the market, and even some of our food! Some people are sensitive to the color, while most people are simply grossed out. It's shocking, but FDA-approved colorants include ground-up powdered red beetles. No company would dare put that on the label. They disguise it with these names: carminic acid, carmine lake, cochineal extract, C.I. 75470, crimson lake, Natural Red 4, E120, "added color," or "natural color."

These dyes impart the pretty pinkish red color to almost all lipsticks. (Yes, even natural ones. Aren't insects natural?) They're also used in red-colored drinks, ice cream, popsicles, candy, and yogurt. If I want pink yogurt, I'll add strawberries, because in my house, I chase bugs down with a broom, not a spoon!

While there is a yuck factor involved with insect coloring, you have to weigh out the risks of synthetic dyes that could trigger allergic reactions, produce cancer, or affect your brain. It's been estimated that women eat about four to nine pounds of lipstick in their lifetimes just by licking their lips or eating while wearing lipstick.

There are about 20 million vegetarians in the United States, and certain forms of the Jewish or Islamic religions who avoid animal-derived products, so I researched and called dozens of cosmetic companies. I learned that lipsticks can be colored with minerals or with flower petals. Some companies create lipsticks without harming animals, and/or without gluten, parabens, lead, or petroleum-based ingredients. Here are a handful of companies that produce lipsticks that are carmine-free:

* **Zuzu Luxe Lipstick and Lip Gloss**—Lead-free, these come in gorgeous colors and feel very moisturizing. The case looks very high end. The product is vegan and free of carmine, beeswax, and synthetic FD&C colorings. Colored with minerals, they go on silky smooth.

* **Beauty Without Cruelty**—This company's lipsticks are vegan, with no animal-derived ingredients or testing and no synthetic fragrances. The packaging is contemporary with slim cases. There are a wide variety of colors available, tinted with synthetic colors and easily found in health-food stores. These lipsticks go on fairly smoothly, they do not feel sticky, and they won't get on your teeth. For more information, www.beautywithoutcruelty.com

✳ **Real Purity**—Colored with minerals, these lipsticks are moisturizing with sweet almond oil and pynogenol. There are many color choices to pick from, and the cases make them look high end. Colored with minerals, the entire product line is free of preservatives, petroleum products, and solvents of any type. Vegan friendly. www.realpurity.com

✳ **Beauty Wise Lipstick**—These lipsticks are vegan, colored with minerals, and contain essential oils. www.holisticbeauty.net (Click on "Cosmetics" on the left-hand side, and then click on "Lips" in the center of the page.)

Revive with Restylane

Restylane is an injection just like Botox, also done at a skilled and trained dermatologist's office. The procedure, which knocks a decade off your face, can be completed in an hour and it's pretty popular: It's been used in over seventy countries and over 3 million treatments have been done.

How does it work? Restylane is a filler that softens or erases those deep facial wrinkles, especially laugh lines that go from your nose to your mouth. Some women use the filler to plump up their lips or fill in sunken areas beneath the eyes.

Typical side effects include temporary redness or swelling, which could last up to a week—and, of course, some people do have allergic reactions. The procedure costs about $400–$600 and must be repeated two to four times a year. www.restylane.com.

Saving Face

✳ Make sure he or she is a medical doctor with an active license.

✳ Find out if the doctor is "board certified" in plastic surgery or dermatology by calling the American Board of Medical Specialties at 866-275-2267 (866-ASK-ABMS) or look online at www.abms.org.

✳ See if he or she has a website—another level of authenticity, but not necessarily a guarantee.

✳ Talk to his staff to see if the doctor has done similar work on them, so you can see it.

✳ Bedside manner matters—you want to feel comfortable.

✳ Check out the before and after photos—but make sure they're his or her own. Doctors can purchase premade photos!

✳ Ask if the doctor is open to giving you anesthetic cream. Even if you don't need it, you want to know up front whether your doctor is sensitive to your needs.

✳ Find out if the doctor has had any board disciplinary actions taken by a state medical board—those records go back forty years. Now, don't concern yourself if the doctor has been penalized for something petty, like a failure to report a change of address. What you're looking for are serious disciplinary actions for such infractions as chemical dependency, incompetence, negligence, and any type of felony conviction, such as illegal or Internet prescribing—or murder. (Shudder!) You can find this out quickly over the Internet for about $10 at www.docinfo.org. If you don't have online access, call 817-868-4000, and they can send you the records you request by mail.

Suzy's Secrets from Behind the Counter
You Can Buy Retin-A Without a Prescription

Well...almost! Women love Retin-A and Renova (tretinoin), which boost the skin's collagen content, smooth out wrinkles, and help with acne. After a treatment, your skin will appear more vibrant, firmer, and even-colored.

But since that pricey cream is simply vitamin A, try these possible alternatives: SkinMedica's Retinol Complex, which contains three different compounds that work like Retin-A, $45 and RoC Retinol Correxion for under $20.

You can buy growth hormone in a tube! Kinerase lotion contains kinetin, a growth hormone derived from plant and animal DNA. Use it on your skin for a few months and watch the wrinkles recede. Cost: $120. www.kinerase.com.

Don't Pass on the Pearly Whites

Tooth whiteners are a fabulous way to sass up your smile, take years off your age, and remove those coffee, tea, and wine stains. I love these products, which are easy and comfortable to use. Crest Whitestrips and Simply White work in less than two weeks, and the WhiteLight system works in about thirty minutes. For less than $20, you get visible results.

But please, don't get too obsessed with whitening your little pearls, because the bleaching chemical can hurt your gums if you are sensitive or if you overuse these products. Remember, they work because they contain a bleaching chemical, too much of which is not good for you. And remember, this is *not* a substitute for flossing and routine dental visits!

Awaken Your Eyes

Who wants dark circles? They make you look like you've been up all night! They can be the result of dehydration, adrenal exhaustion, insomnia, allergies, trauma—even some medications and herbs that increase circulation, such as blood pressure pills, aspirin, or ginkgo biloba. The skin under the eye is very thin, and when blood passes through the vessels beneath it, you see a bluish tint. Plus, the capillaries that move blood around the eye area are very delicate, and when they break, you see darkness beneath the thin skin under the eye.

But don't despair: Hylexin can lighten up those dark circles by patching up the leaks and flushing out stagnant blood. You can get it at fine retailers (Saks, Macy's, Bloomingdales, or Sephora), at www.hylexin.com, or by calling 800-621-9553. Cost: $100. It should "awaken" your eyes within two to three weeks. When I stayed up too late working on this book, I actually tried it—and it worked!

Dab age spots with apple-cider vinegar and lemon juice (50:50 mix) several times each day. This could take months, but it's effective. Or have your doctor order you a prescription gel called Solaraze.

Better Than Botox?

Well, that's the claim that the producers of StriVectin-SD make in their ads for the product. Lots of women and metrosexual men are finding that this product can diminish fine lines, wrinkles, and crow's feet, all without Botox. StriVectin-SD has been shown to visibly reduce the appearance of stretch marks and was sold for that purpose. Then people began putting it on their faces and noticed that wrinkles would disappear. The product contains a variety of substances that firm the skin, while adding elasticity and moisture.

The product is very expensive—about $135 for a 6-ounce tube—but some women apparently don't mind paying because it's still cheaper than one Botox shot. I bought a tube of this and I couldn't see any difference, but some friends tried it and they were happy. It is not going to work as well as Botox in my opinion, but it's worth a try if you are needle-shy, although I'm partial to my Skin Revitalizers listed on page 230. www.strivectin.com.

Make Your Genes Young Again

Dr. Stanislaw Burzynski has bottled the fountain of youth. His innovative cosmetic lotion and cream works on a genetic level and shuts off your "aging" genes while simultaneously turning on your antiaging genes. The effect? To mimic the genetic sequence of your youthful years. When you shut off "wrinkling" or aging genes, you slow down the process of aging and everything that goes with it. His cosmetic products offer a unique perspective because they work on your DNA, penetrating well beyond the skin surface where most cosmetics stop.

Dr. B's product can be used in conjunction with any other cosmetic or facial product because it works on a different pathway. One of the ingredients in his skin product is tamanu oil, which the Polynesians considered sacred as they used it for centuries for healing and protecting their skin. Tamanu oil is also antibacterial, antifungal, and anti-inflammatory. When taking this product along with Dr. B's oral supplements, you might get even more of an antiaging effect and, of course, systemic protection.

I've tried Aminocare cream around my eyes while also taking Dr. B's Aminocare A10 oral supplements for two months. I noticed more energy, better sleep, improved digestion, and a reduction in fine lines, especially around my eyes, so now I'm a believer! For more information, visit www.aminocare.com or call 800-856-8006.

If You Don't Like to Shave . . . Zap It!

Laser hair removal is big business these days as women flock to have their follicles deadened with low-level laser treatments. Frankly, I don't want to kill anything I was born with, but laser zaps are certainly a cool option for men and women who don't like shaving, waxing, or using those smelly creams.

The laser pulse feels like a rubber band snap every time it pulses on you. Quality companies will cater to their patients' needs, so if you're sensitive to the discomfort, they can numb you beforehand. You might need to spread your treatment sessions over the course of a year or two, and prices vary. For example, upper lip treatments are about $600, while lasering your lower legs runs anywhere from $3,000 to $4,000. The cost of a Venus razor and some gel? $10—and there's no zapping.

Suzy's Secrets from Behind the Counter

An Antidandruff Tea

If you have dandruff or seborrhea, think of the herb rosemary. You can drink one cup of rosemary tea each day, and you can also put a few drops of pure rosemary essential oil into your favorite shampoo. (Don't ever drink essential oils—it is very dangerous.) Either way, the rosemary can improve most scalp problems by bringing excessive oil secretions back to normal. Because rosemary stimulates circulation, it could stimulate hair growth too.

16

Natural Approaches to Diabetes: How Sweet It Is!

Diabetes sneaks up on you. In fact, many people are shocked when their doctors give them the diagnosis at a routine checkup when they've had no symptoms.

The medical community has different opinions about what causes diabetes, and all of its complications such as blindness, infections, painful foot and leg ulcers, nerve damage, kidney failure, cancer, and stroke. Not that long ago, people who were given the diagnosis of diabetes were basically told to cut out sweets and lose weight. With the advent of injectable insulin and, now, oral medications, diabetes has become a much more treatable disease. Actually, you can live a healthy, normal life!

Back in the 1980s, about 30 million people worldwide had diabetes. Today, the International Diabetes Federation says diabetes affects 246 million people worldwide, and millions more are unaware they have the disease. By 2025, the number of people who are affected by diabetes is expected to skyrocket to 380 million!

If you're dealing with a diabetes diagnosis, read on. In a few minutes, you are going to be armed with lots of information that will help you find some sweetness in your life again.

It's easy. I'll show you how.

Sweet Pee

Diabetes mellitus literally means "sweet urine." Before we could prick a finger with cool devices such as Accu-chek, Freestyle, and One Touch that measure blood levels of glucose, docs of olden days used to taste a drop of urine! I think this is why they stopped doing house calls. A diabetic with this sweet-tasting urine can put a few drops of it out on the driveway and watch the ants collect for their lunch buffet. You can try it, but if you get caught for indecent exposure, don't snitch on me.

Too High, Too Low? You Need to Know

The amount of sugar in your blood changes all the time, from minute to minute.

Too low—Too little sugar in your bloodstream is called "hypoglycemia." The scary symptoms include dizziness, shakiness, sweating, racing heartbeat, confusion, headache, and crankiness. If you don't eat or drink something sweet quickly enough, you could pass out or have a seizure. Carry a packet of honey, or my personal favorite, a tube of cake frosting—any flavor you like.

Too high—Too much sugar in your bloodstream is called hyperglycemia. Constant hyperglycemia is usually labeled a disease—diabetes! Symptoms such as fatigue, chronic yeast infections, slow healing of cuts and scrapes, dry skin, dry mouth, erectile difficulties, polycystic ovaries, or blurred vision fly under the radar. But if you experience these symptoms, in addition to extreme hunger and constant thirst (and therefore frequent potty breaks), then you have a blood sugar problem.

Pancreas 101

When you eat, your pancreas squirts out two primary hormones (insulin and incretin), both of which have one primary purpose—to break down sugar. The pancreas is also responsible for releasing digestive enzymes, which you need to break food down into teeny-tiny particles. Think of insulin as a key which "unlocks" doors on the surface of your cells. When the doors open, blood sugar is allowed inside. This is good because your cells turn this sugar into energy for you. If insulin can't unlock the doors, then all that sugar loiters outside—in the bloodstream—and you develop hyperglycemia or diabetes.

It's worth noting that most glucose (sugar) is turned into energy, but some of it gets stored in the liver and muscles so you have energy to draw upon later. And whatever sugar is left over gets stored as fat (!) and, of course, it collects around the parts where we want it least, like our bellies, thighs, and butts.

Know Your Diabetes

✳ **Type 1 diabetes**—Kids usually develop this type, hence its other name, "juvenile diabetes." The global incidence of type 1 diabetes in children and adolescents is increasing annually by about 3 percent. It occurs because the body can't make enough insulin, so the cells stay locked up, and blood sugar builds up in the bloodstream. Currently, insulin injections are the gold standard of treatment.

✳ **Type 2 diabetes**—Most Americans who develop sugar problems get type 2 diabetes, and being sedentary or overweight is a risk factor. It results from "insulin resistance," which simply means that your pancreas makes enough insulin but your cells snub their noses to it, having lost sensitivity to its effect. This means that the carbs and sugar in your meal break down to glucose (because you have plenty of insulin), but the sugar loiters in the bloodstream and eventually gets stored as fat.

✳ **Gestational diabetes**—About 4 percent of all pregnant women get high blood sugar. The placenta may be responsible because the hormones it makes help the baby grow, but may block insulin's action in mom.

✳ **Pre-diabetes**—In this condition, a person's blood sugar is higher than normal (80–120 mg/dl), but not high enough to qualify for diabetes. There are 54 million Americans who have pre-diabetes, also termed "dysglycemia," and, folks, a diagnosis like this should be your wake-up call.

✳ **Syndrome X**—A cluster of conditions that includes diabetes, high blood pressure, and high cholesterol. You can bet that people with big love handles either have it, or are on their way to it. The condition results in part from unusually high levels of inflammatory chemicals, and it's harder to resolve than diabetes. Experts sometimes refer to this as "metabolic syndrome" or "metabolic syndrome X." People with this triple threat are obviously more likely to die of a heart attack and stroke than if they had diabetes alone. Because excessive weight is always involved, and many people refuse to give up the foods they love, can I convince you to get your blood flowing? You don't have to exercise yourself to death, just get moving!

A 2007 study called STRIDDE, which was funded by the National Institutes of Health and published in the American Journal of Cardiology in December 2007, proved that walking is better at reversing syndrome X than is running. So don't stress yourself out and think you have to wear spandex and run on the treadmill at 10 miles per hour! Just take a brisk walk each day in nature. It will do your body and soul a lot of good.

Natural Cures: What Can You Take?

✳ **Fenugreek (*Trigonella foenum-graecum*)**—Fenugreek, the food with the funny name, grows well in the Middle East. The seeds contain fiber as well as other highly active compounds that lower blood sugar, boost the release of insulin, and increase your body's sensitivity to insulin. Fenugreek can lower cholesterol and triglycerides, too, so it's the perfect natural remedy for someone with blood sugar issues and high cholesterol or heart disease (yes, syndrome X). (Another interesting tidbit about fenugreek: It can stimulate milk flow in breastfeeding mothers!) You can buy it at any grocery store and cook with it or juice it. Some people prefer supplements because fenugreek is somewhat bitter-tasting at first but it has a sweet finish so it's often used to flavor imitation maple syrup. The dosage varies tremendously, depending on the product you choose and the way it is cultivated so follow package directions.

Safety warning: Taking excessive amounts of fenugreek (about 100 grams or more) may cause gas, bloating, or diarrhea. Individuals with peanut allergies should use fenugreek with caution or avoid it completely because fenugreek is in the same family as peanuts and chickpeas. Women who are pregnant or anyone taking blood thinning medications should stay away.

✳ **Gymnema sylvestre**—The Hindu name of this herb, which has been used in Ayurvedic medicine for centuries, translates to "sugar destroyer," which explains its use for treating syndrome X as well as type 1 and type 2 diabetes. It's a remarkable herb because it tries to normalize blood sugar and cholesterol, and—the best part—it's a craving-killer for sweets. Among other things, gymnema jump-starts the pancreas, creating the cells that secrete insulin. Also, gymnema makes your cells hungry for glucose, so all that sugar doesn't build up in your bloodstream. Therapeutic effects for people with gout and rheumatoid arthritis have also been seen. I have been a pharmacist for two decades and can't name one drug in my pharmacy that is this revolutionary. *Dosage: 300–800 mg with each meal or shortly thereafter (not before).*

Safety warning: Make sure that your supplement uses leaf extract because the leaves contain the active ingredients.

✳ **Bitter melon extract or karela (*Momordica charantia*)**—In the United States, we call it *bitter melon,* but in India, it's called *Karela,* and in Japan, it's called *Nigai Uri.* I'm betting that bitter melon has never made it to your grocery list, even though it has some rather delicious benefits. Almost 100 studies prove that bitter melon can lower blood sugar. Some of its compounds behave just like insulin, while others increase the effect of your own circulating insulin. Special focus should be given to polypeptide-P, a plant insulin found only in bitter melon that behaves like animal insulin. Just like fenugreek and gymnema, bitter melon can improve cholesterol ratios, so it's great for either type of diabetes and syndrome X. You can buy the fruit if you want; just wash the skin, remove the seeds in the center, slice it thinly, and stir-fry it to reduce bitterness. There are plenty of recipes online. It's also sold as tea and capsules; one popular brand name is "Charantea" (www.charanteausa.com). You can *drink one cup of tea after each meal, or take two 500 mg capsules after each meal.*

Safety note: Bitter melon lowers blood sugar, so you want to take this on a full stomach, preferably after meals, or you could develop hypoglycemia. Follow the recommended doses on the label because too much even of a good thing can cause stomach upset. Bitter melon is not for pregnant women or children under age 7. It may also increase menstrual flow in some women.

✳ **Chromium, vanadium, selenium, and zinc**—Trace minerals make insulin work more efficiently so it can unlock more cells, and therefore better help your body process carbs, proteins, and fats. Vanadium actu-

Coffee Lovers May Have a Latte to Celebrate

Java junkies may have something to cheer about. Older studies said that caffeine was contraindicated in diabetes; however, a Lancet study in 2002 discovered healthy, beneficial chemicals in coffee that offset the damage done by caffeine. According to the study, people who drank seven cups a day were 50 percent less likely to develop type 2 diabetes. Seven cups?! That's a bit much for my liking, and I can't recommend that to you, as much as I like coffee. But the good news is that people with diabetes can look at a cup o' Joe with fresh eyes. Go for one or two cups a day, and maybe choose decaf. Definitely skip the frappaccino loaded with sugar and cream, and please monitor your blood sugar until more data percolates in.

ally mimics insulin and zinc, which helps the pancreas make insulin, squash free radicals, and improve sensitivity to insulin. These trace minerals can help with any form of diabetes as well as syndrome X. Many people with diabetes are deficient in zinc. Because modern manufacturing and agricultural techniques have stripped our soils of trace minerals, our food supply is deficient in these vital nutrients. Using a good trace mineral supplement can help you control blood sugar levels, and maybe even lose some weight. You can find capsules and liquid supplements made by various manufacturers; they're just called "Trace Minerals."

Natural Cures: What Can You Eat?

✳ **Fish**—The more cold-water seafood you eat, the lower your risk for heart disease. People with diabetes usually have an unhealthy ratio of bad dietary fats (such as trans fats) to good, healthy fats, so offsetting that with good fats is important. Because it's hard to eat enough fish high in these healthy essential fatty acids (EFAs)—such as fresh, wild-caught cod, salmon, mackerel, and herring—most people supplement with fish oils or krill oil. *Try about 1,000 mg two or three times daily with food.*

✳ **Foliage**—Yes, foliage! Plants contain chlorophyll, a dye that makes them green. I'm not asking you to go munch on your houseplants, but do start eating more greens each day. Good choices include chard, kale, turnip greens, mustard greens, celery, spinach, and broccoli. You can sauté them with fresh garlic or try juicing them, adding a few mint leaves for flavor. Chlorophyll in greens (or in supplements) can eliminate bad breath, plus it alkalizes the body, enhancing the health and efficiency of all your organs, including your pancreas. When this happens, your medication dosages will need to be reduced. There is more discussion on greens, including how to supplement with them, in Chapter 18.

❋ **Fiber**—Fiber is the part of plants that your body cannot digest. It's actually a carb, but the calories don't count because fiber just passes through you. Fiber is not found in animal foods, only plant-derived foods such as fruits, vegetables, whole grain breads and cereals, legumes (kidney beans, chickpeas, lentils, and so on), and seeds and nuts. Fiber is a great natural cure for people who need to normalize blood sugar and lower their risk for heart disease. Don't "diet," but rearrange the letters in that word to spell "edit." It becomes much easier to get fiber in your meals if you edit what you eat.

❋ **Whole grain breads**—Choose these over white breads, and make sure that "whole grain" is the first ingredient in your bread, not "whole wheat flour" or "bleached" flour.

❋ **Brown rice**—This is superior to white rice because white rice is stripped of the fibrous bran layer.

❋ **Fresh fruits and vegetables**—Leave the skin on—it contains fiber. Wash it very thoroughly to scrape off pesticide residue, or buy organic produce.

❋ **Dried beans and peas**—Don't just open a can; buy dried beans and peas and soak them overnight in a bowl of water. This breaks down the complex sugars within, so when you cook them (in fresh water, of course), you maximize nutrition and minimize gas.

Suzy's Secrets from Behind the Counter

Sugar and Spice Make Everything Nice

This is not an excuse to eat gooey cinnamon rolls, but did you know that the active ingredient in cinnamon, called MHCP (methylhydroxy chalcone polymer), mimics insulin and increases insulin sensitivity, therefore lowering your blood sugar? In one study, it also lowered levels of bad cholesterol and squashed free radicals! Just half a teaspoon of cinnamon a day significantly reduces blood sugar levels, so sprinkle away. It's also okay to soak a cinnamon stick in your coffee or tea, or to supplement.

Some Drugs Do Diabetics a Disservice

That's right, look in your medicine cabinet to see if you could be dealing with a drug that has raised your blood sugar, versus the disease of diabetes. It's true that many popular medications raise blood sugar; here are just a few:

* water pills (diuretics) that lower blood pressure (bumetanide, furosemide, HCTZ)

* blood pressure pills (captopril, bisoprolol, atenolol, lisinopril, metoprolol)

* steroids for asthma, arthritis, and allergies (cortisone, dexamathasone, prednisone)

* Prozac (fluoxetine)

* estrogen-containing drugs (such as birth control and hormone replacement therapy)

* HIV drugs (indinavire, lopinavir + ritonavir, ritonavir, squinavir)

There's an Arsenal of Diabetic Drugs Available

Please listen to your doctor's advice to work out and lose weight, because medications are not fun. Many of you probably already take meds right now, so before you combine those with dietary supplements, get your physician's approval (and monitor your blood sugar routinely) because it's possible that the combination could reduce your blood sugar too much. Because so many of you take oral meds, I've included the following section of medication categories to help you learn about your meds. I've made up catchy names for these, but I've included the technical term for these meds in parentheses so that health-care practitioners who use my book as a reference can follow along.

Insulin Drivers (Sulfonylureas)

Type 2 diabetes: These oral medications help drive the production of insulin from your pancreas, but they work 24/7, so you run the risk of hypoglycemia. There are older "first-generation" drugs such as chlorpropamide and tolbutamide, but the newer "second-generation" drugs work just as well with fewer side effects, such as weight gain. These include Glucotrol (glipizide), Diabeta or Micronase (glyburide), and glimepiride (Amaryl). You should not drink alcohol with these medications or take them with blood thinners. Tell your doctor if you are allergic to sulfa drugs.

Muscle Magnets (Biguanides)

Type 2 diabetes: These meds make your muscles take up more glucose so it's not hanging around your bloodstream. They also put a clamp on your liver so it doesn't dump out too much sugar. The most famous muscle magnet is metformin, sold under the brand names of Glucophage, Fortamet, and Riomet (a liquid form). This drug has several advantages: It doesn't cause weight gain or dangerous blood sugar lows, plus it's a good choice for someone with heart failure. It even helps relieve polycystic ovarian disease. Please note, however, that metformin is a drug mugger for B_{12}, so supplement with about 1,000 mcg three times a week while on this medication. A deficiency of B_{12} can lead to neuropathy, confusion, memory loss, depression, mouth sores, and fatigue.

Sugar Busters (Meglitinides)

Type 2 diabetes: These are quick-fix drugs taken about 30 minutes to an hour before meals. They rapidly raise insulin while you're eating, which is when you need it most to bring down sugar levels when they're highest. Common ones include Prandin (repaglinide) and Starlix (nateglinide). Weight gain is possible.

Glucose Gobblers (Glitazones or Thiazolidinediones)

These drugs help make better use of the insulin you have, so that the doors on your cells unlock, allowing the cells to gobble up glucose that is hanging around. Many people used Rezulin until its recall in the 1990s due to liver fatalities. Two popular medications today include Avandia (rosiglitazone) and Actos (pioglitazone). Avandia came under fire in 2007 when an article in the

New England Journal of Medicine reported that data pooled from dozens of studies suggested that Avandia caused a 43 percent higher risk of heart attack.

Starch Stallers (Alpha-Glucosidase Inhibitors)

Type 2 diabetes: These drugs slow down the breakdown of starch and carbs in the small intestine. By stalling that process, glucose from your meal enters your bloodstream more steadily, rather than spiking all at once. This is good because insulin is able to keep up with the pace. These meds include Glyset (miglitol) and acarbose, which is sold under the brand name Precose in the United States and Glucobay in Europe.

Incretin Increasers (Incretin Analogs)

These medications act like the hormone incretin, which, you may recall from the beginning of this chapter, acts like insulin and seeks to lower blood sugar. Incretin is actually released along with insulin from your pancreas. People with diabetes are usually deficient in incretin, so having this med on board helps you reduce the glucose spike while you eat. This means it will help reduce your appetite, thereby helping you lose weight, which are great benefits for those with syndrome X, too. Available as Byetta injections and Januvia tablets. Side effects may include dizziness, flu-like syndrome, and headaches. Note that the FDA approved Janumet in April 2007, which combines Januvia and Metformin.

Pancreas Pushers (Amylin Analogues)

Type 2 diabetes: Amylin is a natural hormone that is made in the same part of the pancreas that makes insulin. Pancreas pushers are drugs that trigger the release of amylin and therefore lower blood sugar. Symlin (pramlintide) is an injectable drug that is used along with insulin in very hard to treat cases of type 1 or type 2 diabetes.

Bread Is No Longer Out of Bounds

If you use almond flour, you can eat bread to your heart's content. Since it's a nut flour, it has virtually no carbs and it's sugar free. Almond flour is just ground-up nuts. You can do it yourself by grinding some nuts using the pulse mode of your food processor. Voila, the flour is yours to bake with, and the consistency is similar to cornmeal. Be aware that almond flour doesn't rise very much, even with the addition of baking powder; you'll have to get used to the heavier texture of the bread. You can read more about almond flour in Chapter 13.

Specific Symptoms and Treatments: Are We Doing Enough?

Diabetes is often accompanied by a host of other often troublesome symptoms. If you are plagued by one of these complications and haven't been able to find relief, read on for some tips and suggestions.

✳ **Painful neuropathies**—For many years, you may barely notice the pain, which usually starts out as a "pins and needles" sensation in a finger or toe. Later on, as the nerve damage progresses, you might feel a burning sensation or experience tinnitus (ringing in the ears), changes in digestion, or blisters on your feet. If you experience this "diabetic neuropathy," try this:

✳ *Alpha lipoic acid*—Dosages vary, *try 100–200 mg two or three times a day.*

✳ *Vitamin B₁₂—500–1,000 mcg per day.*

✳ *Vitamin B₆—50 mg daily, or 20 mg daily* of its activated form, P5P.

✳ *Folic acid*—This dose may seem high, but *take 2–4 mg daily in the morning for 90 days, then reduce to 800 mcg daily.*

✳ *Fish oil—1,000 mg three times daily with meals.*

✳ *Huckleberry leaf tea—Drink one glass of tea per day.*

✳ **Vision loss**—If the little capillaries in the eyes lose circulation, your vision can suffer. You might develop cataracts, or a condition known as "diabetic retinopathy," which can lead to blindness. If you are slowly losing your sight, try this:

✳ *Taurine*—It protects the retina, lens, and the nerves of the eye. *Try 500 mg twice daily.*

✳ *Bilberry*—Similar to blueberries, bilberry fruit contains antioxidants that protect the tiny capillaries in your eyes and provide support for the retina and cornea, preserving your vision. *Twice daily, try taking 80–160 mg of bilberry extract (berry) standardized to 25 percent anthocyanosides.*

✳ Lycopene—Eat salsa! Tomatoes contain a lot of lycopene, which protects your eyes.

✳ **Kidney damage**—If your doctor has told you that your kidneys are suffering as a result of your diabetes, try the following:

✳ *Taurine—500 mg twice daily.*

✳ *Melatonin—About 1–3 mg at bedtime.*

✳ *Proanthocyanidins—Drink 2 tablespoonfuls of cranberry juice daily.* It contains proanthocyanidins—chemicals that protect the kidneys and reduce risk of infection.

✳ **Heart damage**—If you've been told that you have heart disease in addition to diabetes, start by reading Chapter 2. Then try the following recommendations:

✳ *L-arginine*—This amino acid improves insulin sensitivity and opens up blood vessels, improving blood circulation and increasing energy and a feeling of warmth. Try the extended release form, Life Fitness Arginine TR, which is sold at CVS and online.

✳ *L-carnitine*—An amino acid, l-carnityl protects the muscles, improves oxygen and blood flow, and reduces risk of heart failure. It also squashes free radicals and eases neuropathies. *Try 500–1,000 mg twice daily.* Vegetarians are often deficient.

✳ *Hawthorn*—Drink hawthorn tea, *one cup a day.*

Refresh with Red Bush Tea (Rooibos Tea)

Some of the most frequent and painful complications of diabetes are those that occur in the tiniest vessels of the body, the "microvascular" pipeline. When free radicals damage this delicate pipeline, complications occur such as

Sweet Alternatives

Avoid artificial sweeteners—after all, they're artificial! It's best to use natural sweeteners such as stevia, agave syrup, brown rice syrup, and honey. Your body recognizes these from Mother Earth and knows how to break them down and eliminate them, unlike lab-created chemicals which can harm you.

cataracts, blindness, painful sensations in the hands and feet (peripheral neuropathy), facial nerve pain, and stroke.

People with diabetes should stay focused on reducing free radical damage, and one way to do this is with an herbal tea called Rooibos or African red bush tea. It's naturally sweet, so depending on your tastes, you may not even need to add honey or stevia. Even better, it doesn't contain any oxalic acid, so it won't aggravate kidney stones like most teas can. Rooibos contains quercetin, which increases the strength of capillaries, improving circulation and preventing those microvascular complications.

Cool Products for Diabetics

1. **GlucoBoy**: This is a highly precise glucose-monitoring system for children or adults who are young at heart. It's fashioned after a Game-Boy, so you'll be more apt to comply with insulin injections. For more on this device, visit www.glucoboy.com.

2. **Rx Crocs:** These funky-looking plastic shoes are cushiony and roomy so toes can wiggle. The Rx Crocs are lined with antibacterial material to prevent infections.

3. **Medi-Fridge**: A portable tiny refrigerator that plugs in anywhere. It can hold insulin or injectable pens and is ideal during travel or cruising. The Medi-Fridge measures 8.5 x 2.5 x 4.25 inches and costs about $60. For more information, log on to www.medi-fridge.com.

4. **Frio Cooling Wallet:** A wallet that allows you to travel with insulin or insulin pens. To activate the gadget, you have to wet the inner

Know Your Numbers

Normal fasting blood sugar (FBS) is 70–120; this is the amount of glucose in your bloodstream at resting level. The number goes up significantly after a meal. The FBS gives you a snapshot of time and is a good screening and monitoring test.

Another blood test known as Hemoglobin A1C is more reliable because it tells you how your blood sugar has behaved over the last three months, accounting for all the hills and valleys. If your A1C is high, it's a good bet you have insulin problems. The American Diabetes Association recommends that your A1C be 7 percent or less.

compartment with tap water. The crystals form a cooling gel that stays cold for about three days straight. Can be used over and over. $25—$40 To learn more, go to www.frious.com.

Fanfare for Your Feet

Foot wounds are among the most common and severe complications of diabetes and are now the most frequent cause for diabetes-associated hospitalization. It starts out very innocently with a cut or scrape, probably because your shoes are too tight. But people with diabetes have reduced circulation, so your toes don't get enough oxygen, and when that happens, the tissue suffocates, dies, and turns black. Black tissue on your toes or anywhere on your skin indicates gangrene. If you spot any redness (a sign of infection) or blackness on your legs, feet, or toes, see a podiatrist. (Don't go to your pharmacy looking for Neosporin or some other antibiotic salve—it will not help!) Since there is usually little, if any, pain associated with this condition, many people ignore it, but it could cause life-threatening osteomyelitis—an infection that starts in your foot and winds up in your bone. Even worse, some infections could cost you your limb. Yes, I mean amputation. Find a good podiatrist near you by logging on to www.podiatrynetwork.com and plugging in your zip code.

17

More Jiggle, Less Joint Pain

What You Can Do About Arthritis

Dear Suzy:

I am in such terrible pain, I can hardly walk anymore and I take four different pain medications for my arthritis. My doctor says that I will be in a wheelchair within a year, and I am desperate. Please, Suzy, do you have any other advice? I don't know what else to do!

That question and others like it come to me every day from readers who are suffering with debilitating joint pain that no longer responds to prescription medicine. It breaks my heart to read these cries for help, so this chapter is for those of you who feel like your "quality of life" has ended and you are stuck in a body riddled with pain. *You're not*—so don't give up hope!

True, arthritis is the nation's leading cause of disability, resulting in about 750,000 hospitalizations and 36 million outpatient visits every year. But pain relief can come in strange forms that your doctor would never think of, including chili peppers, bee venom, pineapple, shellfish, green-lipped mussels, and worms! Sounds like a buffet menu off *Survivor*, but I am serious. Let's start with the basics: why you're in pain in the first place.

Why Does It Hurt?

The word "arthritis" means "joint inflammation"—and it's the inflammation that causes pain and stiffness in your joints. We tend to associate arthritis with aging, but two-thirds of the people who suffer from it are actually younger than 65.

There are two major types of arthritis, "osteo" and "rheumatoid." Osteoarthritis, the most common form, can occur in any joint—knees, hips, fingers, and spine. It's basically just caused by wear and tear on the joints. That's why you tend to hurt more when it's cold outside: The cold weather increases stiffness in your already stiff joints. So it makes sense that hot humid summers increase flexibility and bring relief to your achy bones. If you don't happen to live in a swamp like I do, then buy yourself a moist heating pad for instant relief.

Whereas osteoarthritis confines itself to painful joints, rheumatoid arthritis is a sign that your immune system is out of whack. Even though these two types of arthritis have different causes, the treatments are sometimes the same—though I'll let you know about a few important exceptions.

With either type of arthritis, you have to correct the underlying cause in order to prevent irreversible damage to your body. That's where things get sticky, because drugs focus on relieving symptoms and come with some risk. That's awesome when you hurt—but please think of these meds as only one slice of the pie. Some other slices might be herbs (to reduce inflammation); dietary supplements (to add more jiggle to your joints); rub-on creams (to numb the pain); and massage, acupuncture, and chiropractic (to enhance your flexibility and untie those knots in your muscles). I think you should try a bit of everything—because after all, who wants just one slice of pie?

Suzy's Secrets from Behind the Counter

Baby Your Hands, Flatter Your Feet

To soothe your aching hands and feet, take a wax paraffin bath! Not your whole body, silly—just your hands or feet. Just dip your hands or feet into the warm wax a few times; then let the wax solidify on your skin as you wear mitts or booties for deep heat penetration. The more wax dippings you do, the more heat penetration—and the more relief! After five or ten minutes, you peel the wax off to reveal smooth, silky hands or feet and, best of all, less pain for a few hours!

You can preview what this feels like by going to a nail salon and getting a hand wax for $5 or $10; or sometimes it's included in spa manicures or pedicures. Chiropractors' offices may offer it, too. Or you can just buy a paraffin bath—it's about the size of a toaster and it costs anywhere from $40 to $200, depending on the brand. Go to any pharmacy, beauty store, or retailer (Target and Wal-Mart have some fine, inexpensive choices). I bought the Spa Petite by Therabath (www.therabath. com) because it has a variable temperature control and it uses a high-quality paraffin wax, plus the manufacturers are committed to quality and have been manufacturing a professional version of this product since 1962. Cost: $70.

Pain Relief from Unexpected Sources

Standard prescription pain relievers are taking a lot of heat. Blockbusters like Vioxx and Bextra have been taken off the market because they were found to cause fatalities. And serious doubts continue to shroud Celebrex and other NSAID (nonsteroidal anti-inflammatory drugs) such as naproxen and ibuprofen. In the wake of these controversies, I've felt compelled to look for pain relievers that didn't come from behind my counter.

Commitment is key for these nontraditional pain relievers: Stick with the program and you'll see some powerful results. You may have to wait several weeks—even months—to reverse the years of damage to your joints. It's time for you to think outside the pill now—*way* outside—because these treatments are astonishing, and no doctor is required!

1. **Hot chili peppers, a.k.a. capsaicin—*recommended for both osteoarthritis and rheumatoid arthritis.*** Don't worry, you don't have to eat anything that will make your eyes water! I'm talking about the over-the-counter creams and patches that contain capsaicin (pronounced "cap-SAY-sin"), the ingredient that puts the "hot" in hot chili peppers. Products such as Zostrix, Salonpas, and Capzasin all relieve muscle aches and strains with two or three applications. With arthritis, you need repeated applications. The pepper extract relieves arthritis pain by faking your body out and training it to become less sensitive to the

pain. The pain doesn't really go away, but you think it does because your nerve endings get numb. As my teenage son says, "That bangs!"

Be sure to massage the capsaicin in well, two or three times daily. These are pepper creams, don't forget, so any burning or stinging sensations are considered "normal" and should disappear after a few days of continuous treatment. Some people don't even notice, but when others take a shower or walk outside into a steamy summer's day—then, yikes, it gets hot!

Immediately after application, wash your hands with soap and water at least twice so that you don't accidentally touch sensitive areas (like your eyes) and hurt yourself. Of course, if you're trying to relieve arthritic pain in your hands, then leave the cream on for thirty minutes, being very careful not to touch your eyes, mouth, or any other sensitive part of your body. Do your private business in the bathroom *before* applying pepper creams! After half an hour has passed, wash the cream off really well.

If you find you just can't tolerate pepper creams, consider Tiger Balm. This cool (and smelly) rub-on salve was originally made for Chinese emperors. Apparently their backs hurt (from too many romps in the sack, or so the story goes), and the formula was born. Tiger Balm doesn't contain capsaicin but still needs to be washed off compulsively, as it will tingle way more than you want it to if it gets in your eyes or on other sensitive areas.

2. **SAMe (S-adenosylmethionine)—*recommended for both.*** This substance is formed in our body out of methionine, an amino acid found in eggs, fish, meat, and milk. It's one of the best supplements you can take—it addresses so many different conditions, including fibromyalgia, migraine, depression, and, of course, joint pain. In 2002, scientists got together and reviewed eleven randomized trials on SAMe. They looked at outcomes such as pain level, improvement in joint function, and adverse reactions associated with the dietary supplement, which, by the way, was promoted in European countries for decades before it was sold in the United States. The scientists examining all these studies (called a meta-analysis) came to their own conclusions and decided that those who took SAMe fared as well as those who took NSAIDs (such as

ibuprofen), but had fewer side effects than those taking drugs. Start with *200 mg twice daily—taken on an empty stomach upon arising and in the evening.* After two weeks, you can begin gradually increasing your dosage until you've worked your way up to *1,200 mg daily*—if you can afford the pricey pill. Cost: $200–$300 per month.

 Don't take this one if you have a bipolar disorder.

3. **Pineapple—*recommended for both.*** A powerful extract of this tropical fruit—bromelain—works pretty much like a drug but better, because serious side effects are slim to none. The effect isn't immediate as with drugs, but you should see results in a few weeks. Bromelain relieves joint pain by squashing the production of chemicals that cause pain and inflammation. It's a proteolytic enzyme—an enzyme that "eats" protein for fuel; or rather, it eats "protein gunk." Think of it as a Pac-Man rushing through your body, chomping down on clots, cysts, and dangerous plaques. Game over, and you win!

Bromelain is one of the best researched anti-inflammatory enzymes. There are lots of terrific brands sold nationwide at health-food stores, pharmacies, and online. *Dosage: 500–750 mg three times a day between meals, on an empty stomach.*

4. **Shellfish—*recommended for osteoarthritis only.*** From the shells of crabs, lobster, crawfish, and shrimp comes glucosamine, a powerful substance that we also make in our own bodies to use for tendons, ligaments, and cartilage. Unfortunately, our production declines as we age, so taking high-quality supplements could add more jiggle to our joints. It actually builds up the shock-absorbing quality between our joints, so there's less friction there. It's the friction that causes the pain.

5. **Glucosamine—*recommended for osteoarthritis only.*** It is not a painkiller, but it does address the underlying cause of pain—a huge slice of your healing pie! Not all the studies for glucosamine show benefit, but some do—enough for me to take notice. The best part of glucosamine is that it won't poke holes in your gut the way NSAIDs can, nor damage your liver as acetaminophen may. And of course, unlike

COX-2 meds (e.g., Celebrex or Mobic), sudden death is not one of the risks.

Glucosamine is sought after because many studies show that it outshines acetaminophen, ibuprofen, naproxen, other NSAIDs, and even some prescription drugs. I'm impressed by the famous GAIT study—the Glucosamine/Chondroitin Arthritis Intervention Trial—a six-month research project that was published in the *New England Journal of Medicine* in 2006. It involved 1,200 people and proved that the combination of high-quality glucosamine and chondroitin (a supplement derived from cow cartilage—usually from the cow's windpipe) relieved moderate-to-severe knee pain better than Celebrex did. If you think perhaps a supplement company funded that study, think again—the $14 million project was funded by the National Institutes of Health—the largest, placebo-controlled, double-blind clinical trial ever conducted on glucosamine and chondroitin. You don't have to hit *me* over the head—I'm convinced!

Some scientists think that "glucosamine sulfate" is better than "glucosamine hydrochloride" because their research shows better performance with the sulfate form. If you're allergic to "sulfa," don't stress: Sulfa is a drug; sulfate is a natural compound—they're completely different. However, most glucosamine is marine-derived, so if you're severely allergic to shellfish, glucosamine could spark an unwanted reaction—but don't worry, you have other choices.

Besides allergies, some people don't want shellfish-derived glucosamine because of religious convictions, personal preferences, or fear of all that pollution in our oceans. If you prefer not to ingest shellfish products, you can get chicken- or cow-derived products—just check the label. There are also vegetarian supplements containing glucosamine that are derived from corn. One popular brand is Source Naturals's Vegetarian Glucosamine sold at most health-food stores. *The dosage is 500 mg three times a day or 750 mg twice a day.*

> *Some data points to glucosamine as raising blood sugar, but I don't think it's clinically significant. If you are diabetic and monitor your blood sugar, pay attention to the "bumps." Worst-case scenario, your doctor ups your diabetes meds slightly, but you experience significantly less arthritic pain. Sounds like a no-brainer to me!*

6. **MSM (methyl-sulfonyl-methane)**—*recommended for both.* This super nutrient gets such mixed reviews, but I still believe in its virtues. I tried it when I was bothered by knee pain (a result of too much aerobic dancing), and it worked very well for me. I even noticed less "crackling" of my joints, more energy, and faster-growing hair.

MSM breaks down in the body to provide us with sulfur, an element that's essential to life because it eliminates impurities and allows for healthy joint function. When MSM is taken alone, *try 800 mg three times a day with meals to prevent tummy upset.* If MSM is taken in combination with glucosamine, shoot for *300–400 mg three times a day, again with meals.*

7. **Gum Resin from the Boswellia Serrata Tree—Boswellia** (pronounced boz-wheel-ia) **Serrata**—*recommended for both.* This has been long used in Ayurveda, India's traditional system of medicine. It's well studied, extremely effective, and reduces inflammation and pain better than most commonly prescribed NSAIDs, including ibuprofen and naproxen—without the NSAIDs' nausea, acid reflux, stomach pain, and ulcers. However, in some rare cases, Boswellia can produce diarrhea, skin rash, and nausea.

Research shows that Boswellia helps people with asthma, Crohn's disease, and ulcerative colitis as well as those who suffer from either type of arthritis. This botanical works like a 5-LOX inhibitor, a technical term that means it reduces inflammation by reducing leukotrienes. This is a different way than NSAIDs or COX-2 inhibitors work, so you can safely take it along with most other arthritic drugs.

There are lots of good brands; just get one that's been standardized to about 60 percent Boswellic acids. Dosage varies widely, so you'll have to experiment to see how much you need to relieve your pain: *Try anywhere from 400–1,000 mg two to four times daily.*

8. **Omega fish oils**—*recommended for both.* Fish oils are another alternative that's compatible with almost any other supplement or prescribed medication. They have a natural anti-inflammatory effect on the joints because they reduce prostaglandins—nasty chemicals that cause swelling and pain. Fish oils are fundamental to good health. Taking

1,000 mg four times a day with meals should provide some relief over the course of a few months.

> Since fish oils can thin the blood (usually considered a plus) please take only 500 mg once or twice a day *if you're also taking heparin, Coumadin (warfarin), or any other blood thinner. Keep an eye out for easy bruising or nosebleeds, a sign of superthin blood, and, of course, get routine blood work at your doctor's office so you can be monitored properly.*

9. **Niacinamide—*recommended for both.*** This form of vitamin B₃ may be particularly helpful for painful knees. It's found in most multivitamins, but joint pain sufferers sometimes want an extra boost. Careful, though, things could get hot and sweaty: This powerful nutrient causes your capillary vessels to expand quickly, leaving you temporarily hot, itchy, and blotchy in the famous "niacin flush."

The best way to take this supplement is in the clever form of inositol hexaniacinate, which will also help you avoid that flushing effect. Besides arthritis, you might see benefits for Raynaud's disease, diabetes, tinnitus, and cholesterol reduction. *Dosage: 500 mg inositol hexaniacinate three times a day.* Work your way up to this dosage gradually, though, starting with, say, *250 mg three times a day and gradually increasing by 50 mg per dose every few days.*

10. **Serrapeptase—*recommended for both.*** Silkworms produce this enzyme when they eat their own silk and become butterflies. Like bromelain, it's another protein-eating "proteolytic" enzyme. Because Serrapeptase can reduce inflammation with repeated use, it's a terrific pain-buster. People have been using it for more than twenty-five years throughout Europe and Asia, and it may work for you, too, instead of aspirin, ibuprofen, or NSAIDs.

I like to recommend this product to people with fibromyalgia pain and to athletes with sports injuries. According to some research, serrapeptase can also "digest" blood clots and arterial plaque, making it a powerful nutrient for those with both heart disease and arthritis. Get an enteric-coated brand to make sure that it gets past your acidic stomach and down to your intestines, where it gets absorbed. There are many good brands; I like Physician Formula's Serrapeptase and also SerraEzyme. *Take 200–400 mg (also stated on the label as 20,000–40,000 units) once or twice a day.*

11. Green-lipped mussels (*Perna canaliculus*)—*recommended for both*. Sure, you can eat these little guys if you want to—I like them drenched in hot garlic butter sauce. But the pain-relieving quality comes from their extract, which has been studied in humans and dogs with great results. Perna canaliculus contains a natural antihistamine and omega-3 fatty acids (both of which calm inflammation) as well as a little glucosamine (which helps to build shock-absorbing cartilage between your joints). I like Natural Life's Green Lipped Muscle Extract, because they take it from unpolluted waters, and their product is listed with the Australian Register of Therapeutic Goods. I also like Lyprinol by Dr. Ray Sahelian.

> Avoid foods from the nightshade family, which can make either type of arthritis worse: Say no to tomatoes, potatoes, eggplants, peppers, and—surprise!—tobacco. Also avoid pesticides, which, like nightshades, overstimulate your nerve endings.

 Since this product is marine-derived, it may cause allergies for people who are allergic to shellfish.

Chondroitin: Not All It's Cracked Up to Be

You may be wondering about chondroitin, a supplement that's gotten a lot of press as a joint reliever. I'm not so excited about it: In my opinion, research results for glucosamine are far more impressive and consistent. Although some people swear by chondroitin, others don't notice much of an effect. That's probably because chondroitin is such a big molecule and has so much trouble squeezing through the doorway of your cells when taken orally. It's okay to take chondroitin if it's in combination with other supplements, but if you're just going to pick up one item, I personally think you're better off with the other choices on my "top eleven."

The Simplest Solution

Are you feeling overwhelmed? Confused? Or simply worried about spending all that money? We can make it simple! Here's what I would do if I were suffering from either type of arthritis:

* ✳ I would begin with hot pepper cream and try it for four weeks.

* ✳ At the same time, I would begin taking the omega-3 fish oils because most Americans are deficient in essential fatty acids, which are natural anti-inflammatories.

* ✳ If those two steps didn't provide enough relief, I'd buy AR-Encap, a product made by Thorne Research that contains numerous arthritis-busters, including glucosamine, MSM, Boswellia, turmeric, and also Devil's Claw, a painkilling herb. It may take a few weeks to see results.

* ✳ If I was still in pain, I'd bring in the Serrapeptase. Again, it may take a few weeks to see results.

* ✳ If I still needed something more, I'd add bromelain and SAMe.

Try that sequence—but be ready to play around because the other supplements from "Unexpected Sources" are very valuable, too. Go with your intuition, because what works for one person may not work for another. That's as true for prescription drugs as for alternatives—so be patient, be optimistic, and don't give up.

Rheumatoid Arthritis Sufferers: Don't Take Glucosamine or Chondroitin

This is a hot topic, but my own opinion is that people with RA should avoid glucosamine and chondroitin. That's because those two supplements are used to build cartilage within the joints—helpful for osteoarthritis sufferers, who struggle with a deficit of cushioning material, but not for people with RA, who have an immune system that views this squishy cushion in between the joints as an enemy! (Check out Chapter 4 to find out how gluten sensitivity may be involved.) With RA, the more cartilage you have, the more of an "enemy" your immune system sees—and attacks. So stay away from the glucosamine and chondroitin—why create more trouble for yourself? Once you put the fire out in your immune system, it may be okay to bring in joint builders like this, but do so only under the advice of your rheumatologist.

He Said, She Said, NSAIDs—What Is the Bottom Line?

As your 24-hour pharmacist, I'm going to give you a checklist detailing the order in which to try conventional pain relievers if you're suffering from osteoarthritis:

* **Tylenol**—It's cheap and sold everywhere without a prescription. It's known as acetaminophen in the U.S., and paracetamol in most other countries. Don't use too much, though, or it can damage your liver, especially if you also drink, have liver disease, or take other liver-stressing meds. Standards say that the maximum dose is 4,000 mg per day, but in light of its liver-damaging potential, I think it should be lower—say, *2,500 mg total per day*—just to be on the safe side. Bottom line: It's a good first choice to relieve pain unless you have liver damage from other medications or alcoholism.

* **NSAIDs (nonsteroidal anti-inflammatory drugs)**—I like these drugs in low doses for short-term treatment of pain, including body aches, toothaches, PMS cramps, and, of course, joint pain. Popular ones include Aleve (naproxen) and Motrin and Advil (both ibuprofen), all of which are available by prescription in higher doses. These drugs temporarily reduce pain, but their side effects are potentially serious—ulcers, kidney problems, and gastrointestinal (GI) bleeding. People with ulcers or intestinal perforations should run from these drugs. A trick to buffering the nausea, stomach upset, and heartburn that these drugs produce is to take them with food or a tablespoon of Maalox. Bottom line: These drugs are okay in low doses for short-term pain relief in most adults—and very handy for PMS cramping!

* **COX-2 drugs like Celebrex (celecoxib) and Mobic (meloxicam)**—These you get by prescription only. Vioxx belonged to this group, but was yanked in 2004 due to the fatalities it seemed to cause. They work well

and don't rip up your GI tract like some NSAIDs; however, they do affect your cardiovascular system by slowing down your kidneys and causing greater risk of swelling, spikes in high blood pressure, heart attack, and stroke. They're best if taken at low doses and with some of the supplements I suggest in "Pain Relief from Unexpected Sources." Bottom line: They're effective, and even okay if you have gastrointestinal (GI) problems, but dangerous for people with high blood pressure or heart disease.

✳ **Ultram (tramadol is the generic)**—The drug is a prescribed pain reliever that has the added benefit of boosting your levels of serotonin, a "happy-brain" chemical that lifts mood and reduces sensations of pain. Side effects include GI problems, headache, drowsiness, and dizziness. This drug can also potentially lower your seizure threshold. Bottom line: I think this med is safer than NSAIDs and COX-2s, but it's not for everyone, especially if you take other medications that lower your seizure threshold, including such SSRI antidepressants as Prozac, Paxil, or Zoloft.

✳ **Painkillers**—These are for serious pain: Darvocet (propoxyphene/acetaminophen); Vicodin or Lortab (hydrocodone/acetaminophen); or oxycodone (the strongest of them all). These effective pain relievers are also addictive—but if you're genuinely suffering every day, your doctor should show some compassion and prescribe them for you. Find a pain specialist who will if your general practitioner is hesitant to take you out of pain. They won't reverse the damage, but honestly, no one should be in pain all day simply for fear of addiction! Side effects include nausea, constipation, dizziness, and drowsiness, so please, hand over the car keys while you're taking this stuff. Bottom line: The key thing is to get yourself out of pain and enjoy some quality of life—but of course, you'll also need to take some "Pain Relief from Unexpected Sources" to eventually wean off the drugs.

✳ **Steroids**—Last on my list because, even though they are not addictive, they've got too many side effects and little or no curative power. In my book, they're terrific for a quick boost only, such as with an episode of gout, carpel tunnel syndrome, asthma, an allergic reaction, or a bout of rheumatoid arthritis. Problems such as nausea, weight gain, canker sores, or crankiness may not sound so bad, but if you stay on prednisone or a similar drug for too long, you may have to reckon with such horrors as insomnia, psychosis, seizures, chronic infection, pancreatitis, and Cushing's syndrome.

Never suddenly stop taking your steroid medication—while you've been on the meds, your body has stopped producing its own natural steroids. Stopping your steroids suddenly is the equivalent of hitting a wall when driving 70 miles an hour! If you decide to get off them, taper off very slowly, under your doctor's care—PLEASE.

Suzy's Secrets from Behind the Counter

Get into Those Medicine Bottles

If those child-resistant caps on your medicine bottle are giving you grief, ask your pharmacist for easy-open caps that just pop or twist off. Because of laws designed to protect children and minimize household poisonings, you'll have to sign a little waiver at your pharmacy—but that's it. Then all of your prescriptions will come with easy-open caps—unless your pharmacist forgets. (Hey, we're only human.) So check your bag each time you pick up a prescription, and remind your pharmacist to make the switch if he or she forgets.

What's the Buzz About Bees?

You can't be bug-phobic for this arthritis treatment: real live bee venom, injected by the bee's own stinger! Don't try this in your garden, please . . . you have to find a medical doctor who is familiar with "apitherapy." The doctor will warm up a few bees that have been temporarily frozen—maybe even blowing on them to agitate the critters. Then they let the bees sting you on the area of pain—such as your knee—and the super-duper anti-inflammatory chemicals in the bees' venom do all the work. Wasps and hornets are starting to cash in on the action too.

Honestly, this works better than cortisone, relieving pain and inflammation within minutes. In fact, some athletes use this type of therapy right on the field instead of cortisone! You *must* work with a specially trained physician, though, because if you're one of those people who's allergic to bee stings, you could die from anaphylaxis—a life-threatening allergic reaction that puts you into shock and stops your breathing. So your physician needs to have a shot of epinephrine ready, just in case. (To be fair, anaphylaxis is possible with any drug, additive, or food product.)

Good Ideas to Beat Gout

Uric acid is a natural and normal compound in our bloodstream, and it's usually fully dissolved. But when our blood changes chemistry, the uric acid doesn't dissolve fully, but rather forms a precipitate. That's a big word for an undissolved glob of something, and in this case, uric acid forms sharp crystals. It seems to concentrate in the big toe for some reason, waking and tormenting sufferers in the wee hours of the morning. They can't get up that easily, and walking creates a horrific sense of pain, like walking on needles or sharp pieces of shattered glass.

During an attack of gout, you might also have a fever. Gout occurs in men most of the time, and the condition can spread to other joints as the amount of uric acid increases in the body. The condition is associated with kidney stones, too. If you wake up in the wee hours with a gouty attack, doctors usually recommend ibuprofen (Motrin or Advil) or naproxen (Aleve)—not aspirin, because aspirin can make it worse.

Even though the pain is usually in your big toe, what you put in your mouth really matters. Especially if it's cherries, but I'll get to that shortly. Because gout is the result of excessive uric acid crystals in the body, avoiding foods high in uric acid is important. Meats, especially organs (liver, heart, kidney, brains), are high in uric acid, increasing your risk for gouty attacks and kidney stones. You can further help yourself by reducing your intake of or eliminating sugar and caffeine products. Also, go easy on these: anchovies, shellfish, mackerel, mushrooms, and yeast (baker's and brewer's).

At some point, you should also look in your medicine cabinet. Some drugs and supplements increase your risk for symptoms of gout. The following medications can contribute to causing your gouty attacks:

* insulin

* Levodopa (for Parkinson's)

* aspirin

✳ niacin (found in supplement and in the drugs Advicor and Niaspan)

✳ vitamin A

✳ Cyclosporine (calms the immune system)

✳ diuretics (water pills used for high blood pressure)

Drinking alcohol matters, too—did you know that your first attack may occur after a drink? And as long as I'm giving you pointers to avoid these terribly painful attacks, please don't overeat, and limit your stress. Bumping your toe has been reported as a factor in gouty attacks as well.

Colchicine is the prescription standard in treating gout, and there are anti-inflammatory drugs your doctor can prescribe. Quercetin, which is found in green tea and apples, as well as bromelain, which is found in pineapples, are potent anti-inflammatories that can prevent gouty attacks. Another simple supplement is a *plant-based* antioxidant, sold by your local health-food store. Antioxidants and those popular juice drinks that contain the extracts from fruits and veggies are very helpful at reducing inflammation and painful attacks.

Obviously, if you have gout, life may not feel like a bowl of cherries, but eating them can help tremendously. According to a popular folk remedy, you should eat a large cupful of fresh or frozen cherries every day. This whole idea began in 1950, when a small study involving twelve people showed that their symptoms improved after eating cherries. Fresh cherries contain potent antioxidants, so if you want to follow this folk remedy, try eating a bowl of cherries every day, or drinking a cup of cherry juice each day. The stream of anecdotal reports from people all over the country piqued the interest of the Agricultural Research Service, who in May 2004 published their own findings about cherries. They found ten healthy women, ages 22 to 40, and had them eat a big bowlful of Bing cherries in the morning, making sure that they did not consume other fruits or beverages that could confuse the results. On the morning of the cherry breakfast, the scientists measured levels of inflammatory chemicals in the women's bodies, such as C reactive protein and nitric oxide, two chemicals that would go up in a person if they had a gout attack. The study found that these chemicals were lower than before the women ate the cherries, a sign that cherries could, in fact, reduce inflammation in the body.

18

Go Blow Your Nose—
Just Not Near Me!

Bedtime Stories That Will Boost Your Immunity

I t's terrible, lying there sick as can be . . . your nose is stuffed, there's a box-ful of crumpled Kleenex on the floor by the bed, you can't swallow, you're shivering with chills, and your chest feels like it's going to pop if you cough one more time! Awww, I feel so bad for you, I wish I could comfort you the way I did my kids, but I'm a bit of a germ freak, so how about I tell you a bedtime story instead.

Once upon a time there were seven dwarfs . . .

✿ *1. Dopey . . .*

. . . a.k.a. cough suppressants, which usually contain dextromethorphan, a chemical that gets into your brain and may leave you feeling, well, dopey. Still, you can take these if you have a nonstop dry, hacking cough—but not a wet one because in that case you want to cough up the phlegm (it could be danger-ous to suppress it). Wet coughs, accordingly, require an expectorant—some-thing that helps you bring fluids up. Take expectorants with plenty of water to break up chest congestion.

I like plain cough suppressants, and plain expectorants—but I don't like the combination formulas, because the two ingredients work against each other: Cough suppressants shut you down, while expectorants make you spit phlegm up. There are many good products out there, but two that I like are Delsym for a cough suppressant and Mucinex for an expectorant. These are sold at pharmacies nationwide.

✺ 2. Happy . . .

Decongestants, which unstuff your nose, make me instantly happy, especially the nasal sprays like Afrin or Neo-Synephrine, because I can get air into my stuffy nose in less than five minutes. I just love that, but don't use nasal sprays for more than three consecutive days or you'll start to find that you get a "rebound congestion" and can't clear your airway again—a condition known as *rhinitis medicamentosa.*

You can also find nonmedicated saline sprays to thin out the thick mucus—especially helpful for babies who are all stuffed up. Don't worry, these nonmedicated saltwater drops/sprays are safe to use anytime, as often as you like, because they *don't* cause rebound congestion.

Decongestants also come in the form of oral tablets that contain phenylephrine or pseudoephedrine, which give you energy—another reason to be happy. These energy-boosting substances are actually related to amphetamines, and so some pharmacies hide these products behind the counter—because druggies buy them to make speed. I'm not saying not to take them, but you should be aware that oral decongestants can raise blood pressure, make pinpoint pupils, increase heart rate, and cause palpitations and anxiety.

✺ 3. Sneezy . . .

If you're feeling sneezy, try some of the older antihistamines, such as Benadryl (diphenhydramine), Tavist (clemastine), and Chlor-Trimeton (chlorpheniramine). As they dry you up, they also get rid of your itchy, watery eyes and scratchy throat—even your hay fever. These antihistamines sit at your cells' doorways to keep your cells from dumping histamine and misery-causing chemicals into your bloodstream.

Of course, there's a down side: The drying effect of antihistamines can also cause dry mouth, dry eyes, and sometimes even vaginal dryness; not to mention dizziness, blurred vision, and diarrhea. The older ones make most people drowsy and should not be taken while driving. Some multitasking products like Contac, TheraFlu, Vicks, and NyQuil—good for coughs, sneezes, runny nose, and a host of other symptoms—also contain sedating antihistamines, so just take them at night and sleep through the side effects.

For a nonsedating antihistamine, try one of the new second-generation antihistamines such as over-the-counter Claritin (loratadine or Alavert) or prescription drugs Allegra and Clarinex. The FDA approved the over-the-counter use of Zyrtec which began selling like hotcakes in early 2008. It makes some people sleepy. Just be sure to consult your doctor if you've got narrow-angle glaucoma or urinary or prostate problems.

✺ 4. Sleepy . . .

Suppose fever and achiness are making you feel sleepy—but a runny nose or a bad cough are keeping you awake. Then you want to take a sedative to help you sleep—with my blessing—but I do want you to be careful doing it. Most cold sufferers reach for over-the-counter sleep medications like Sominex, Nytol, or Unisom, but these may not be ideal for you: Some actually contain the same sedating antihistamines that are found in many cough/cold remedies, so you could fall prey to a deadly duplication.

You're better off doing one of two things. Either take a combination product like NyQuil, in which all the different meds are already combined properly "so you can rest"; or, if you don't want a multitasking product, just take one of those sedating antihistamines (such as Benadryl) and cover both bases.

✺ 5. Grumpy . . .

Who *wouldn't* be grumpy with all those achy muscles—and the headache! Tylenol (acetaminophen in the U.S., paracetamol elsewhere) is the most popular pain reliever in the world, and it also works well to reduce a fever. But don't take too much—it can damage the liver. In fact, the pharmacist I saw while vacationing in Iceland was only allowed to sell me a handful—and even then, it was hidden behind the pharmacy counter. Contrast that with our pharmacy shelves, which boast pain-reliever bottles by the hundred, sometimes by the thousand!

Other good pain relievers include ibuprofen (Motrin, Advil) and naproxen (Aleve), both of which also reduce inflammation. Aspirin is another choice, but it thins the blood, so seniors who take prescription blood thinners (Plavix, warfarin, heparin, Lovenox) need to be especially careful and stop using it if they notice easy bruising. Finally, take all these pain relievers with a light snack to minimize tummy upset.

☸ *6. Bashful . . .*

You have to get naked for this next type of medicine, so I hope you're *not* bashful! SudaCare Shower Soothers are foil-wrapped tablets that you can buy at any pharmacy. Just unwrap the sealed packet, drop a tablet onto your shower floor, turn on your shower, and step in. In a minute, you're surrounded by a steamy vapor of eucalyptus, menthol, and camphor to comfort you and open up all your passageways. (Just don't touch the tablet or even get too close to it: The tablet gets hot after it's activated, and it's an eye irritant.)

☸ *7. Doc . . .*

Because you have to know when to call the doctor! Enough is enough sometimes, so call your doctor if . . .

✳ your cold doesn't clear up in a week to ten days

✳ you develop a rash

✳ you have a very painful sore throat or see white patches

✳ your fever is very high (over 102° Fahrenheit) or lingers at 101° for three days

> Please get a new toothbrush after a cold—you don't want to reinfect yourself. Or you can dip your toothbrush in grapefruit seed extract for a few minutes, then rinse it off.

✳ you have pain in your ear(s)

✳ you are wheezing or short of breath

✳ you have swollen lymph glands

✳ you are spitting up yellow and green stuff

Antibiotics Don't Help Colds and Can Make Them Worse

Colds are caused by viruses. More than 200 different species of virus have been identified that can cause the common cold, but not one of those strains will be cured by an antibiotic. Antibiotics can help you get rid of infections by killing bacteria, but colds are caused by viruses—a completely different critter. When I wrote about this in my column, the response was overwhelming. That's one of the biggest "secrets" from behind my counter: *Antibiotics don't help colds.* If you catch a cold and get relief from a prescribed antibiotic, it could be a placebo effect or your natural ability to get better on your own sooner or later. In fact, antibiotics can weaken your immune system by destroying friendly flora in your gut—the good bacteria that your immune system needs to stay healthy. When you destroy the good bacteria (the natural flora), you make a nice, comfy environment for the virus to take over and continue to infect you. It can't set up camp in a healthy environment, can it?

That's why reputable doctors won't prescribe antibiotics for a cold—but I'm a pharmacist, so I know all my patients' secrets, including the way some people stash their leftover antibiotics and then take them later. Bad idea! I also know many doctors who write prescriptions because patients insist on it, even though the doctors would readily admit it's not quite the right treatment.

I'm particularly sensitive to the overuse of antibiotics because I grew up in a household where antibiotics were prescribed for me if I so much as sniffled. As a result, my immune system was weakened because it didn't have enough practice fighting off infections on its own. On a global level, the overprescribing of antibiotics leads to resistance: Bad bugs learn how to outwit once-useful antibiotics by morphing into more deadly forms, so that otherwise simple, controllable infections can now potentially kill us.

What can you do? Only take antibiotics if you're sure you have a bacterial infection—and only when your doctor prescribes them. If your doctor hasn't done some kind of a culture or swab of the infected area, he or she is just guessing—maybe it's viral, in which case the meds will do you no good and may be more harmful in the long run. So make sure that the antibiotic ordered will indeed kill the specific bacteria that you are infected with. Doctors have a tendency to make educated guesses, and sometimes they guess wrong.

And please don't pressure your doctor for antibiotics—use some restraint and encourage your doctor to use some as well. Finally, if you ever do have an antibiotic prescription, I want you to promise me that you'll finish the whole course. If you stop taking the antibiotic when you feel better, you might get sicker than you were before, because the leftover bacteria in your body can grow out of control.

When It Hurts to Swallow

* Use a steam vaporizer or cool-mist humidifier in your bedroom.

* Gargle with warm saltwater (½ teaspoon salt, ½ teaspoon baking soda in an 8-ounce glass of water).

✳ Drink warm tea or hot water with grated ginger and honey.

✳ Use zinc lozenges (Cold-EEZE) for healing and pain relief; other numbing lozenges include Cepacol, Cepastat, Ricola, Halls, and Chloraseptic.

Try Vicks ointment. Yes, I know it's a chest rub, but I like to put it around my nostrils when they're sore from too much nose-blowing because it makes them feel cool. Another feel-good option is Carmex lip balm, sold in most pharmacies, which has the same moisturizing yet cooling effect.

✳ Take a little Tylenol (acetaminophen) if you need it.

✳ Alkalol is the brand name of a product that was developed by a pharmacist in 1896, a natural rinse solution containing salt, baking soda, eucalyptus, and other ingredients that cool off sore, scratchy throats and help heal mouth sores! Check out www.alkalolcompany.com or look in your local pharmacy.

✳ Hold the OJ and the carbonated soda—they won't feel good going down.

✳ Gargle with UlcerEase, a unique anesthetic that is wonderful for people with mouth ulcers, canker sores, or an achy tongue.

Oscillococcinum

This homeopathic substance with the strange name is pronounced o-sill-o-cox-see-num. It's non-drowsy, easy to take, and supposedly abates your flu symptoms if you take it at the onset of your illness. (It won't help much if you take it later on.) If I'm the jury, then the jury's out: Some studies say oscillococcinum doesn't do much for you, but other research shows that it can shorten your misery and ease your aches and pain.

I can tell you this: Many of the people who use this homeopathic product—which is sold in forty-three countries—come back for more. In France, this med is covered by the national health-care system, and it's that country's best-selling flu remedy. If you want to try it, it's sold over the counter in the U.S. at virtually all pharmacies. You can take it safely along with other cough and cold remedies or prescribed antibiotics.

Have a Drink!

No, not the alcoholic kind, I mean fresh water. Sorry, no coffee either: Caffeine and alcohol can dehydrate you, when what you should be doing is loading up on water so you can flush all the germs out of your system. And when you're sweating with a fever, hacking up sticky, slimy stuff, or blowing mucus from your nose, then you're losing fluids that way, too. So replenishing your body with fresh water is crucial.

Get this, not all water is created equal! The more alkaline, the better, because these waters have a normal-izing effect on a sick body—and if your body is sick, it's more "acidic." Some of the waters available these days are enhanced with antioxidants and minerals, and they are also ex-

Chicken soup actually is good for you—at least, if you make it with garlic and onions. These powerful antioxidant vegetables really do boost your immune system while killing bacteria, fungi, and viruses. Put them in your soup last so they don't overcook.

tremely pure. Because of my sleuth tendencies, I actually stuck a pH strip into them to verify their alkalinity. These are my top picks (but of course there are others): Fiji (www.fijiwater.com), Essentia (www.essentiawater.com), Zephy-rhills (www.zephyrhillswater.com), and Evamor (liveacidfree.com). It's great if you can drink these all the time, not just when you're sick.

Once Upon a Time, There Were Three Little Pigs . . .

Here's another bedtime story for you, about how you can build up your long-term immunity to prevent colds and flu. Remember how each of the pigs built his house from a different material in his efforts to withstand the huffing and puffing of the big bad wolf? And remember how some materials worked better than others? Well, I'm going to tell you how that relates to your immune system—no doctor required!

Straw

The following nutrients are terrific, no doubt about it, but they're only a small part of building immunity. Like a straw house, they'll give you some basic protection, but by themselves they aren't enough to stand up to the wolf's assaults.

⁕ **Foods**—Eating well is the easiest way to build immunity. I believe our health starts with the stomach, and what we put into it: After all, the gut is where half of your immune system lives. One great first step is to eliminate white sugar from your diet. Some experts believe that just one teaspoonful of sugar can shut down your immune system for about an hour. And if you've got an insatiable sweet tooth, you might have an overgrowth of candida, which in turn exacerbates infection, fatigue, jock itch, vaginitis, and brain fog. So stick with fewer sweets and processed foods, while you consume more fresh foods like vegetables, fruits, nuts, and seeds as well as—of course!—fresh water.

⁕ **Exercise**—Moderate exercise increases the "natural killer" cells that are a key part of your immune system, killing all the nasty bugs that might otherwise infect you. Even if you want to slouch on the couch, at least try to get a good laugh in every day: Studies show that people who have the giggles tend to get sick less, because when you laugh, your stress hormones go down and your "feel-good" hormones (endorphins) go up, boosting mood, reducing pain, and increasing your immunity.

Wood

If you build your immunity out of "wood," you'll be able to withstand more of the big bad wolf, especially when combined with our "straw" elements. So try some of the following supplements:

⁕ **Arabinogalactan**—This natural plant extract from the larch tree supports immune function in impressive ways. Since it's like a fiber, it attracts water while promoting better bowel movement and removal of toxins. Unlike other fibers, which are harsh and can cause diarrhea, arabino is gentle. It also helps a sluggish lymph system flow better, so that your lymph can clear all kinds of nasty toxins and dangerous invaders from your body. Many holistic practitioners think lymph system flow is particularly helpful for children who constantly get sinus and ear infections. Some products are just called "larch." I like Thorne's Arabinex powder because it's virtually tasteless when mixed in juice. *Adults: One to three scoops daily, and for children one-third to one scoop daily.* (Of course, if your child is getting frequent infections, you might want to clear his or her diet of sugar, processed foods, and dairy products for a while.)

✳ **Mushrooms**—I'm not talking about the kind you eat for dinner, but about medicinal mushrooms that come in the form of oral supplements or teas. Some well-designed clinical trials and about four hundred studies show that some mushrooms supercharge your immune system, protecting you even against such serious challenges as cancer. These have been popular in Asia for centuries, and the Japanese Health Ministry (the equivalent of our FDA) even allows health insurance to cover the cost of them in many cases. Yet in America, you hardly ever hear about these healing mushrooms.

One of the best—and top-selling—mushrooms for your immune system is Coriolus versicolor; its extract is called PSK (Polysaccharide K). The Coriolus story started when someone successfully used it to treat stomach cancer and caught the attention of a Japanese scientist, who helped launch the research for what became known as PSK. Now people overseas spend hundreds of millions of dollars a year to get the precious extract of this mushroom—called "turkey tail" in North America—which ranges in color from brown to gray. Some studies prove clinically that PSK will enhance your own natural defenses, which protects you if some unconscious soul coughs in your space while you're standing in the movie line for a ticket.

Another magical mushroom from the Orient is maitake, sold as "Maitake D." This one grows so large that it can weigh up to 100 pounds! The extract from maitake is a powerful immune booster and has shown antiviral activity against human immunodeficiency virus (HIV) in a study confirmed by the U.S. National Cancer Institute in 1992.

I like JHS Mushroom's brand because of their careful attention to purity and the way they extract the "essence" of the mushrooms with hot water so the active ingredients are not destroyed. You can contact them at www.jhsnp.com or 888-330-4691; they sell Coriolus versicolor for about $60 for 90 capsules. There are also other terrific companies that pay attention to extraction and purity, so pick the one that feels right for you. Dosage varies according to your condition; follow the instructions that come with the product. And please don't worry about these mushrooms causing fungal infections like vaginal yeast infections or Candida...they won't do that!

Brick

* **Antioxidants**—These vital substances do offer you some protection. Without them, you're defenseless against the nasty bacteria, fungi, parasites, viruses, and cancer-causing substances that are everywhere and on everything you touch. For a few dollars a year, antioxidants vacuum these dangers out of your body and destroy them before they can destroy you. The best way to stock up on these is through colorful fruits and veggies, but juicing is also a fast and easy way to build up your immune system. Why not invest in a Juiceman or Jack La Lanne's Juicer? Or buy grape juice, pomegranate juice, and specialized juices like Noni, Goji, and Mangosteen Complete at your health-food store. You get lots of brick bang in these berry juices!

You should also take an antioxidant supplement every day throughout the year, not just when you feel a cold coming on. You can buy an all-in-one formula: Some good ones are Nature's Way Antioxidant Formula and Enzymatic Therapy's Doctor's Choice Antioxidant. In addition, I'd like you to take Coenzyme Q10 *(100 mg daily)*.

* **Probiotics**—These are the friendly bacteria (good bugs) that keep your gut working well and support your immunity—so be sure to take them regularly. Also, probiotics reduce the incidence of vaginal yeast infections. Either have several weekly servings of organic unsweetened yogurt, or take a high-quality probiotic supplement, such as Nature's Sunshine's Probiotic Eleven or Thompson's Multidophilus. GNC, The

Vitamin Shoppe, Mother Earth, and Whole Foods all carry a wide selection of terrific brands, as do many other health-food and natural-foods stores. Most probiotics are found in the refrigerator section, but it depends on the brand. Look for such key words as *Lactobacillus acidophilus*, *L. bulgaricus*, *L. plantarum*, *Bifidobacterium bifidus*, and *B. longum*. Sometimes you can find a friendly yeast called Saccharomyces boulardii (brand name is Florastor), which is terrific for reducing antibiotic-associated diarrhea—a problem that practically everyone has when they're being medicated. I know these names sound foreign and strange, but it's really easy to find these types of supplements at health-food stores, and I feel strongly that *your immune system is based on the integrity of your gastrointestinal tract.* Gut-friendly flora such as this is precisely what you need to build (or rebuild) your digestive tract and boost your immune system. You'll know if your product works because many digestive problems disappear. I'm often asked if it's okay to take an extra dose or two of probiotics. Follow the dosage on any package you buy, but it's practically impossible to take too much unless you just eat the bottle. I pop them several times a day, on an empty stomach. If you are taking an antibiotic, these are especially critical (because antibiotics are drug muggers of friendly bacteria), so take them freely, but do separate your probiotic capsules from the antibiotic by at least two hours, preferably four hours. Remember, good bugs make a happy gut.

✳ **Adaptogens**—These increase the body's defense mechanism and make the immune system work better during stress, so you are less likely to get sick. They automatically shift the balance of hormone production up or down, whatever you need to bring balance—that's why they're called "adaptogens." I really like Astragalus root, Eleuthero, Ashwagandha, and Rhodiola. You could try Thorne's Phytisone or Metagenics's Adreset.

Green Is Great!

I love my greens and drink them every day as part of my daily routine. I'm talking about a powdered supplement that you stir into some fresh water and then drink—a powdered form of every vegetable you should be eating, but don't want to! I always recommend greens because most Americans find it hard to get as many servings of fruits and vegetables as they need. So drinking greens in a pleasant-tasting beverage once a day is terrific and can boost immunity, rev up energy, help with weight loss and digestion, and also ease joint pain. I've noticed that my greens are as good as coffee at erasing fatigue—try this out for yourself and see what you think. It's a good habit to drink greens as part of your daily routine, kind of like taking a multivitamin each day. Greens are a quick, effective way to ingest some of nature's finest antioxidants, enzymes, and minerals in a single sip.

Now, even though greens offer you the nutritional benefit of about a dozen servings of fruits and vegetables, they aren't a real substitute for eating fresh fruits and veggies. But they're a good supplement if you simply don't have the time to eat *enough* veggies *every* day. Some of them even contain probiotics, like Jordan Rubin's Primal Defense made by Garden of Life.

Here's another benefit: Whenever you take greens, you are automatically getting chlorophyll, the pigment that makes plants green. Chlorophyll neutralizes the acids in our body, creating more alkalinity, which many nutritionists and alternative practitioners believe to be an important factor in promoting wellness. It also beats bad breath!

The taste of greens differs from brand to brand. So if your brand tastes like you're drinking freshly mowed grass, switch brands and try again. The better brands are mild in flavor and taste slightly minty—and surprisingly good. I like Nanogreens because they use a patented technology to make delivery of the nutrients easier in the body; plus, they post all their purity and potency tests for every batch online to provide transparent quality control. This particular brand is sold through qualified healthcare professionals, and online. You can also call 877-772-4362. Some websites and clinicians offer a free sample to try—just ask.

Some other good brands available at health-food stores include pHion Alkalive and Greens Plus (GREENS+ is what it says on the label), Berry Greens, and Greens to Go (sold through Costco and other club stores). Or visit your local health-food store and shop around. Whichever drink you choose, make sure that it's not sweetened with one of those artificial sweeteners—those chemicals don't enhance your health. Also, try to find a brand that contains "certified organic" fruits and vegetables with no sugar added.

More Zip with Zinc

Zinc is a mineral, and oysters contain the most zinc of all. Most people associate oysters with sexual appetite, since they are considered an aphrodisiac, but zinc works everywhere in your body. You can tell if you're low in this mineral because you may have a reduced sense of taste or smell, and you may not see very well at night.

Zinc is a very strong antioxidant that shortens the misery time of a cold and eases symptoms without causing drowsiness the way typical cold medications can. Using zinc boosts immune function in a natural way, as zinc is needed for hundreds of chemical reactions in the body. In one study, zinc lozenges shaved three to four days off a cold, but the trick is you have to take zinc at the first sign of your cold. It works in part by attaching to the rhinovirus and basically obliterating it. So the virus gets stopped in its tracks before it can spread. Sucking on lozenges is best because zinc is soothing to a scratchy throat and the flavor of lozenges masks the metallic taste of zinc. The better-name brands have honey or a citrus extract to improve flavor. At the onset of a cold, *take one lozenge two or three times daily,* and for prevention each year, start in August and *take one lozenge daily* so you'll be ready before cold season hits.

Silver—It's Not Just for Jewelry

Colloidal silver is a form of silver that's broken up into tiny particles and suspended in liquid. You take it with a dropper (because you don't need much), and you can also find nasal sprays (Source Naturals makes one), which are great if you're suffering from congestion, sinus trouble, or allergies.

This form of silver is a powerful weapon against hundreds of pathogens that infect humans. It used to be the main anti-infective we had until patented drugs entered the scene. Colloidal silver is a powerful germ fighter, and I think it's relatively nontoxic in normal doses, so just follow the label. I use it myself every year at the height of cough/cold season, along with the other immune-boosting supplements I've been recommending to you.

How does this miracle metal work? It suffocates bacteria—without harming human tissue. That's what sets it apart for me from the meds behind my counter (which, by the way, might harm your brain, liver, GI tract, and kidneys). Silver works for me on those rare occasions when I feel something coming on, but because I've built a house of straw, wood, and brick, I hardly ever have to take the silver.

> *It's possible that colloidal silver could interfere with the body's absorption of penicillamine quinolone antibiotics (Cipro, Levaquin), tetracyclines, and thyroid medications. So if you're taking colloidal silver with any of these drugs, you should separate the silver from the pill-popping by at least two hours.*

Suzy's Secrets from Behind the Counter
Humidifiers Rock!

A cool-mist humidifier is a terrific nondrug way to help loosen chest congestion and unstuff noses. This is particularly good for children, especially if you're as concerned as I am about how much medication children are getting these days. Humidifiers are a side-effect-free way to improve breathing, and their sound sometimes lulls an anxious toddler to sleep. I have a Vicks V3500 Cool Mist humidifier, which costs $50, but there are lots of good choices out there.

German Chamomile—Try this aromatherapy fix if you're suffering from allergies. Put some pure essential oil of chamomile on a hankie, in your bath, in a facial steam bath, in your favorite lotion, or even better, in your massage oil.

Sip Tea for Spectacular Results

If you are dealing with any kind of immune system challenge, I want you to drink some Essiac tea, which was formulated—and named—by a Canadian cancer nurse named Rene Caisse (spell her name backward and you get Essiac). The powerful combination of herbs was shared with Caisse by an Ojibway Indian man: The tea includes sheep sorrel, slippery elm bark, burdock, and rhubarb root, which provide valuable trace elements, vitamins, minerals, phytoestrogens, antioxidants, and other active substances that improve gastrointestinal problems, boost your immune system, clean up your blood, reduce inflammation, and remove free radicals. There are two great companies that produce high-quality forms of Essiac tea: Essiac Herbal Supplement Extract Formula (www.essiac-canada.com, 561-585-7111); and Flor-Essence Herbal Tea Blend (www.florahealth.com).

19

Toenail Crud and Other Really Icky, Weird Stuff

You never forget the first time someone hikes up his pants and shows you that unsightly boil or a plastic cup of phlegm. I can't exactly call it job satisfaction—but I am gratified to help you solve these icky problems so long as you don't make me closely examine the goods! We pharmacists are front-line healthcare professionals and are used to taking care of simple problems. In fact, most people come to us first, before they spring for a doctor's appointment, so I call us "drugstore doctors," offering free, on-the-spot advice and sending you off with a remedy in hand—no doctor required!

Let's go behind the counter and see what might walk in on a typical day. Keep it quiet, though—this isn't exactly dinner conversation!

Sorry, These Things Are Just Gross!

✳ **Lice**—You can show us your kid's head if you absolutely must, but most of the time, we'll believe you without seeing the bugs. Rule #1: Comb! Rule #2: Comb again! Rule #3: Comb some more. If you don't get the baby nits out—the little lice that have already hatched—it doesn't really matter what else you do. You can soften the nits' attachment and possibly kill them with coconut oil before you comb. Coconut oil is sold at health-food stores.

Because nits can survive four to ten days, you need to spray the beddng and probably your car seats, too. But most OTC lice shampoos and bedding sprays contain a pesticide (pyrethrin), to which you might not want to expose your kids. It doesn't kill the unhatched babies anyway. You've got two options: Try the tea tree oil products found in health-food stores, which have a good reputation; or do what most people do and use the conventional pharmacy products sold nationwide. Be careful with those lice sprays, though—never spray near food, eyes, or skin. Launder everything sprayed and add a second "rinse" cycle to your washer to get all the pesticides out. And if you or your child is allergic to ragweed, use pyrethrin-containing products with caution—and get your doctor's approval because these products could trigger an asthma attack.

While certain lice products (containing lindane) have come under fire in other countries and been banned, some products that are free of lindane are very popular in the United States and sold without prescription. It's easy to find brands such as Nix, Rid, and A-200, and their store-brand equivalents. These do contain a pesticide, but not lindane. I think the best one is Nix (permethrin) because it's better at killing off both the lice *and* the nits. For more holistic treatments, go to your health-food store: Some carry natural products free of toxic chemicals; these include Licefreee! and Hair Clean 1–2–3.

Suzy's Secrets from Behind the Counter

Shampoo Those Bugs Away!

To protect your children's scalps, buy a bottle of Cetaphil Gentle Skin Cleanser at your drugstore or retailer. This liquid soap is free of pesticides, but if you're willing to go through a laborious process, you can use it instead of conventional lice products. Here's the drill:

1. Massage it into every single last strand of hair.
2. After a few minutes, comb out the nits with a strong metal comb. Be very meticulous—one missed nit and you can count on reinfestation.
3. Dry your child's hair with a hair dryer. As the hair dries, it feels almost like shrink-wrap.

4. Let your child go to bed all shampooed up—the Cetaphil has to remain in place for eight hours.

5. In the morning, shampoo as normal, dry your child's hair—then comb again!

6. Repeat the process once a week for two or three weeks, and make sure to thoroughly wash bedding, pillows, pajamas, and car seats to prevent reinfestation—and of course, vacuum and empty the contents of the bag.

✳ **Wounds and cuts**—Most pharmacists don't have guts of steel, but we will have to actually look at your wounds so we can tell you whether you need to go to the emergency room. You'd be shocked how many times people come in with a piece of their finger hanging off, or a bleeding gash to the leg. Once a guy came into my pharmacy with a gunshot graze! Okay, so technically we don't run triage—but it sure feels that way sometimes.

What do we recommend? The standard pharmacist favorite is Betadine liquid to disinfect the wound, then Neosporin Plus to prevent infection. Store-brand generics of these products can save you lots of money, and they work just as well as the branded items. Of course, you'll need to cover your wound with a bandage or gauze—so for obvious reasons, get the nonstick gauze. If the gauze does stick to your wound, soak it with saline wound spray to get it to lift off easily. Another option is butterfly closures, a type of bandage that squeezes your skin back together when the wound is slightly deeper. Generally speaking, I don't recommend those spray-on bandages for wounds; they don't usually work too well on anything more serious than minor cuts and scrapes. Minor staph infections can be treated with StaphAseptic sold at many pharmacies and online at www.staphaseptic.com.

✳ **Scars**—The product Mederma—derived from onions—is sold widely at pharmacies, but taking oral nutrients could be more effective. Try natural vitamin E by mouth (*800 IU daily for six weeks*) or apply the oil to your skin *twice daily for six weeks*. You can also drink orange juice for the vitamin C. Signs that you're low in vitamin C are bleeding gums, easy bruising, and slow healing of wounds. As far back as 1969, researchers studied a handful of people in which they induced a state of vitamin C deficiency, and then cut a 5-centimeter incision into their thighs. The group then began taking various doses of vitamin C, ranging from 4 mg to 32 mg daily—not even the amount recommended by the U.S. RDA. Regardless of the dose, the study concluded that any amount of vitamin C could support improved wound healing. You can also supplement with buffered vitamin C, taking approximately *100– 250 mg three times a day for a few weeks.*

Another effective anti-scarring trick is to eat pineapple, which contains bromelain, a very useful compound in wound healing. Surgeons who are alternative-minded often recommend bromelain to patients undergoing surgery, but since the compound thins the blood, it's important to begin supplementation after the surgery, not before. Bromelain is an anti-inflammatory, but it also has the ability to break down hematomas...or, rather, to minimize bruising. We've known this for decades, when researchers conducted a study on 53 patients undergoing rhinoplasty. Each patient received either bromelain or placebo. Those patients who had received bromelain dealt with swelling and redness for only two days, compared to an entire week for those patients receiving placebos.

Elderly people who take forever to heal up their wounds, and seem more susceptible to bed sores, may be dealing with a zinc deficiency, making it harder to heal. This is very common in seniors, especially if they are being mugged by a drug that zaps zinc (see Chapter 26) or if they don't get enough zinc-rich foods such as seafood, fortified cereals, meat, poultry, dairy products, and beans. Most people eat enough zinc, but if you don't, then you can always supplement. Zinc lozenges are very popular and safe in normal doses, *around 10–15 mg daily.* Stay within these guidelines for effectiveness, and don't be tempted to take more because excessive intake of zinc (or any mineral) can tilt the delicate balance of all your minerals, especially copper and zinc. In fact, it's a good idea to supplement with about 2 mg of copper if you take about 15 mg of zinc. Keep this ratio in mind.

Finally, aloe plants are handy. Cut a leaf open and apply the gel right on your scar *two or three times a day for a few weeks.* This is particularly helpful if you can start right away.

✳ **Cold sores/fever blisters**—There are so many great products for this condition. One popular product is Abreva, and another is Zilactin, because they really get the lesion to go away quickly. Most cold sore products contain numbing ingredients to relieve pain, such as benzocaine, benzyl alcohol, lidocaine, tetracaine, camphor, or phenol.

However, the real trick to avoid suffering with cold sores is not getting them at all! Take *500 mg L-lysine every morning* to tilt your amino acids in the right direction. That's because cold sores are sometimes related to excessive arginine, a naturally occurring amino acid. An excess of arginine creates an imbalance with lysine, an amino acid. In fact, some vegetarians are more prone to cold sores because they eat lots of high-arginine foods, such as peanut butter, nuts, tahini, wheat products (including cream of wheat, whole-wheat bread, and wheat germ), oatmeal, orange juice, and grape juice. Sunlight is also thought to trigger cold sores, so lip balms that have "zinc oxide" might help reduce episodes.

If you catch the sore as soon as you first feel it tingling on your lip, one of the best and free cold sore treatments is to just hold an ice cube to it as long as you can stand it, ideally for five to ten minutes, but it's also okay to keep dabbing it. Do this every thirty minutes during the "tingly" stage and you will drop the temperature of the area, stifling a full-blown lesion. (Don't bother with the ice cube if you're past the tingly phase—it won't help.) You can also apply a moist tea bag so its tannic acid can interrupt cold sore formation, but you've still got to get there during the tingly stage.

✳ **Earwax**—This uncomfortable condition can cause you to experience a clogging sensation, ringing in your ears, or an uncomfortable itching in the canal. Most products sold over-the-counter contain peroxide to loosen the wax along with a syringe to siphon the wax out. Three popular OTC products are Debrox, Murine, and Physician's Choice, all of which are fine, but I myself prefer Similasan, a homeopathic remedy that's peroxide-free.

Be warned: *No* earwax remedy should ever be used if you have serious ear pain, dizziness, or discharge. You need a doctor for that. It's not that popular, but some holistic practitioners like ear candling, a process in which you lay on your side and one end of a special type of candle is inserted into your ear as the other end is lit. It supposedly draws out a lot of toxins, but I don't personally recommend this because I don't like flames near a person's head! At a health expo, I did have a professional candler try it on me, but I can't say it worked, although curious spectators gathered to watch the "magic" show. Whatever stuff collected on the plate did not come out of *my* head! I'd like to think it was just melted wax, rather than gray matter from my brain.

✻ **Corns and calluses**—If you're a diabetic, do *not* treat yourself for this condition—please see your physician. Everyone else, read on! When a piece of thick, hard skin forms on the bottom of your feet—usually the ball—it's called a callus; when it's on your toes, it's called a corn. Both happen from friction or pressure, perhaps from wearing a too-tight shoe.

I must admit, I've been burned, literally. I developed a callus from some high heels and tried one of those self-sticking pads with salicylic acid—and it gave me a chemical burn. In any case, I don't usually recommend OTC products for these problems because they never relieve the underlying problem, which could be a deformity or bone spur. And, of course, a medicated pad can't fix the constant pressure from your shoes; you could need orthotics, special inserts that help your shoes better fit your feet.

So donate uncomfortable shoes to the thrift shop, buy nonmedicated corn or callous pads for temporary relief, and consider comfy gel inserts for your shoes that do fit. These are sold at most pharmacies and retailers. Then get a pedicure by a gentle, licensed aesthetician, and, most importantly, see a podiatrist who can help you map out a long-term solution.

✻ **Pimples**—Resist the urge to pop them—you could wind up with a scar. Get into the habit of cleansing your face, toning it, and moisturizing it in the areas of dryness. If you must do something about a blemish, dab a bit of mud mask on the spot, and when it dries, wipe it off; it will draw toxins out of the pimple. You can also apply any one of those acne medications containing benzoyl peroxide or salicylic acid. I also like one containing 10 percent sulfur called Bye-Bye Blemish Drying Lotion—just dab it on and when it dries, wipe it off. Do this a few times in the evening, and by morning the beast should be dried out. I had a hard time finding this recently at my local pharmacies and ended up buying it from www.drugstore.com.

Pimples may result from either hormones or stress, and they do go away on their own, but if you have a serious case of acne, you may need to do a bit more. Carefully consider your choices before you take the popularly prescribed drug Accutane (isotretinoin); in my opinion, it has too many potential risks. Even suicide has been associated with it! Because the vitamin-A derived drug is known to cause birth defects, pregnant women are not allowed to take it, and women of childbearing age may take it only if they agree to adhere to strict rules and regulations stating that they will use two forms of contraception and take monthly pregnancy tests to assure dispensing pharmacists that they are not pregnant while on this medication. You can learn more about the terms of this program, which was developed in the United States and is designed to prevent fetal harm, by going to www.ipledgeprogram.com or calling 866-495-0654.

Because Accutane and its various generics are under a black cloud because of the fetal harm issue as well as potential psychiatric problems that might be associated with it, try something safer, such as zinc. Most doctors don't even realize that zinc deficiency is a culprit in acne, especially for women who take drug muggers such as estrogen drugs (birth control or HRT) or acid blockers. You need zinc for clear skin (and thyroid hormone), so if you're tired and pimpled, zinc may be the answer. Careful, though—a little zinc goes a long way; *try 10–20 mg at dinnertime.* You can buy liquid zinc when supplementing, and stop taking it when it starts to taste bitter, which means you have sufficient amounts. Or you can try it in a more palatable form with inexpensive lozenges that taste good and are sold at pharmacies and health-food stores nationwide as the brand Cold-EEZE. *Take one or two lozenges daily.* Finally, if you can, get routine facials by a qualified aesthetician.

And These Are Kind of Icky Sometimes . . .

✳ **Vaginal itching or yeast infection**—As we saw in earlier chapters, these could be the result of antibiotics, birth control pills, or leaky gut.

Turn to Chapters 11 and 18 for longer-term solutions, but you might also try to avoid perfumed, colored toilet paper; scented tampons; and any powders, sprays, or irritating lubricants that may cause vaginal irritation.

For yeast infections, I like the combination packs that come with a cream to apply to the outside, and a vaginal suppository or applicator for use inside. Popular brands include Monistat, Femstat 3, Vagistat-1, and Gyne-Lotrimin—or try a store-brand generic. If you think creams are messy, you might prefer a prescription pill like fluconazole (Diflucan), but remember that it comes with such side effects as headache, nausea, cramping, dizziness, and possible liver damage. Why go through all that when you can use the cream and wear a panty liner one night, especially since OTC creams work faster than oral medications?

Itching and soreness aren't always related to yeast—they may result from a sexually transmitted disease. So check with your doctor and don't douche, which could drive infectious organisms up through your cervix, worsening both your infection and your discomfort. In fact, I don't recommend douching as a general rule because it appears that many women who douche wind up with more vaginal irritations and infections compared to those who don't douche. I'm not alone in this: The American College of Obstetricians and Gynecologists agrees. If necessary, try an anti-itch cream (hydrocortisone or Vagisil), but see your gynecologist right away—if you have an STD, you'll need antibiotics or an antiviral drug as soon as possible. Now if you're one of those women who feels adamant about douching regardlesss of what I've said here, you can try an old folk remedy: Add about 1 tablespoon of grapefruit seed extract (buy it at your local health-food store) to a pint of water. Douche twice a day for about a week.

✳ **Urinary tract infection**—Lower pelvic pain, cramps, and burning when you pee—it happens to many women, especially as they approach menopause. Another symptom is urgency—that feeling that you have to go, not to mention that it hurts when you try. Ouch!

We can sell you something to get you through the night, but for longer-term relief, you'll need an antibiotic from your doctor. The

OTC medicine is called "phenazopyridine," and is sold under the brand name Azo-Standard or Uristat. If you take it with plenty of water, you should get pain relief within a half hour of the dose; *take up to 200 mg three times a day* if it's needed for pain. Don't freak out if it turns your pee bright orange or red—it's only a harmless dye. Remember: You can't live on this; it's only a temporary fix-me-up until you see your doctor.

If you find yourself getting UTIs frequently, especially the day after sex, it could be a sign that some *E. coli* bacteria sneaked out of your gut, where they normally live, and have taken up residence in your urinary tract or bladder. *E. coli* is the culprit in UTIs 80 to 90 percent of the time. So try to make things inhospitable for this bacteria: Acidify your urinary tract with high doses of buffered vitamin C (*500 mg three times a day with food*). And absolutely wipe front to back!

Some people claim that OTC cranberry tablets help, and they might, because they also make your urinary tract more acidic, or "slippery," so that *E. coli* can't stick to it. But cranberry is not the answer for everyone and definitely not a choice if you take blood thinners (warfarin), because it may cause hemorrhage. Although either the tablets or daily cranberry juice (100 percent juice, not sugary "cocktails") might help you reduce the frequency of infection, they won't resolve an established UTI.

I can recommend two natural products: D-Mannose is a natural substance that keeps *E. coli* from sticking to your urinary tract; and Thorne's Uristatin will help build healthy normal flora down there. What will also help with any type of infection, including pelvic ones, is drinking plenty of water to flush your kidneys and taking probiotics regularly. And one more really good trick is to urinate right after sexual intercourse (get out of bed first of course!), then take an immediate shower to cleanse. I've had women tell me repeatedly how well this prevents infection.

✳ **Warts**—Common warts have that "cauliflower" look to them, and they match the color of your skin. Plantar warts usually appear only on the bottom of the feet, and they're smooth in appearance. OTC products now available use the same technology that your dermatologist does to "freeze" the little devils right off. The treated wart falls off on its own within two weeks.

Pharmacists often recommend two wart-removal products: Compound W Freeze Off or Wartner. Either of these will cost about $25–$30. I prefer these brands because you don't spray them on, you dab the chemical on with a swab. You don't want to spray because if you miss, you will burn otherwise healthy skin! Older, traditional formulas containing salicylic acid are much cheaper (about $5), but they don't work as well.

You can also try nail polish. Apply a dab of clear polish to a wart, morning and night, to starve them of oxygen. They might fall off in a week or two.

✳ **Phlegm**—This is the stuff that comes out when you cough. I promise you, we don't need to see it—you can just tell us what color it is. Clear, white, or pale might mean you're suffering from a virus, such as a cold or flu, which means in turn that antibiotics shouldn't be necessary, because they only work against bacterial infections. However, doctors tell me that yellowish-green phlegm generally indicates bacterial infection, in which case your physician may want to prescribe an antibiotic or some other medication to help cure the infection.

Either way, the key to healing is getting that phlegm up and out of you, not drying it up. It may be wise to avoid cold and cough products that contain antihistamines, because they dry you up. You may also want to stay away from cough syrups that contain dextromethorphan or "DM" because this will suppress your cough when you are trying to cough the phlegm out. Feel free to ask your local "drugstore doctor" what is best for your particular cough.

Diet plays a role too. I would suggest that you avoid dairy products if you are coughing or dealing with sinus congestion. Some experts feel that milk (even rice milk and soy milk) creates more mucus in the body, which could make you spit up still more phlegm.

Now before I go on, I need to warn you that coughing is a symptom, not a disease in itself. You don't know how many people come in and say to us, "I've had this cough for a few months now and..." A few months? Stop right there, that's your ticket to the doctor! Another ticket is coughing up blood—we can't help you with that! Long-standing coughs could be a sign of something serious like allergies, bronchitis, pneumonia, emphysema, or worse. See your doctor for any cough that persists beyond a week.

Of course, if you have a garden-variety cold, just drink fluids, rest, and lay a microwavable hot pack on your chest for some soothing relief. Try a steam shower to loosen the phlegm, or run a steam vaporizer or a humidifier.

For the cough itself, try Mucinex DM, Robitussin DM, or Delsym liquid. Or try marshmallow tea for coughs, colds, sore throats, and asthma. And then check out Chapter 18 on colds, flu, and immunity—you'll find lots of soothing ideas.

Bear in mind that prescribed heart meds called Angiotensin Converting Enzyme or ACE inhibitor drugs have a side effect of coughing—without phlegm. If you take any of the following medications and you have a bothersome cough that is nonproductive, ask your doctor to switch you to something else: captopril (Capoten), benazepril (Lotensin), enalapril (Vasotec), lisinopril (Prinivil, Zestril), fosinopril (Monopril), ramipril (Altace), perindopril (Aceon), quinapril (Accupril), moexipril (Univasc), and trandolapril (Mavik).

✳ **Dandruff**—In the 1990s, the FDA banned a bunch of ingredients found in dandruff shampoos, but nowadays, the products on the shelves are relatively safe. Today you can choose from many products like XSeb, Head & Shoulders, Sebulon, and DHS Zinc, with such active ingredients as selenium sulfide, zinc pyrithione, or coal tar. If you want a non-medicinal route, get some grapefruit seed extract from the health-food store. Mix ten drops into whatever shampoo you use and massage it in for two minutes before rinsing; it acts as an antifungal. Or buy some apple-cider vinegar and apply 2 or 3 tablespoons—enough to cover your head. Leave it on for about thirty minutes, then shampoo it out and condition lightly.

Whatever you choose, your best weapon against dandruff is to cut out sugars and starches, and start taking either fish oils or evening primrose oil. That's because all that itching and flaking may be the result of excess yeast, or maybe overactive oil glands. So clean up your diet, and the flakes will fade away. And add a few drops of rosemary essential oil to your shampoo to promote scalp health.

And Don't Even Show Me These!

✳ **Nasal discharge**—If you have anything dripping out of your nose, the pharmacist will hand you a Kleenex and then sell you an antihistamine to dry you up. Runny noses are often accompanied by sneezing and itchy eyes and throat—and pure misery. So if these are chronic for you, I recommend herbs and dietary changes to boost your immune system.

Alas, most "drugstore doctors" will just send you to aisle 4 for a box of Claritin or Alavert, both of which contain the active ingredient loratadine—and then quickly run back behind the counter! Most pharmacists like loratadine because you only have to take it once a day, and it doesn't make you drowsy. Older antihistamines like Tavist (clemestine) and Benadryl (diphenhydramine) work just as well, but they zonk you. If your runny nose comes with stuffy sinuses, you might need an antihistamine/decongestant combination drug. Fine if you want to take it at night only, but it's *very* dangerous to take sedating antihistamines during the day when you have to work, drive the kids around, or operate machinery like a lawn mower, power tool, or espresso machine!

✳ **Toenail fungus**—This icky condition can be the result of many things. It grows in moist areas, perhaps because of an internal overgrowth of yeast. Some women who take estrogen drugs (birth control or HRT) may experience this. You can clean up your diet, but you'll still need medicine. Try OTC creams and solutions like Lamisil or Lotrimin, or pick up a bottle of tea tree oil at the health-food store.

Many customers use another trick to get rid of toenail crud: They buy Vicks cold formula rub and apply it three times daily to their toes. The menthol penetrates the area and kills the fungus, and within six to nine months, you have pretty nails again. Here's another folk remedy: Gently buff the shiny topcoat of your nail and then apply tea tree oil three times a day. It might take several months, but it's safer than liver-damaging oral antifungals.

✳ **Pinworm**—These little worms are very common among 5- to 10-year-old kids; the worms live in your child's intestine and occasionally crawl out his or her rear end. Some ambitious parents who need to *see* the worms to believe will literally sneak up on their sleeping children, pull off the covers, and shine a flashlight deep into said orifice—and then stick a piece of tape in there to snag a worm when it leaves the anus. If your child wakes up while you're applying the tape, he or she will most certainly require psychological intervention for years to come! Seriously, these worms are freaky, but not all that dangerous. Still, they're uncomfortable, and you do want to treat them.

Symptoms always include an itchy butt, among other things. Give your child a good shower just to make sure the itchiness isn't related to hygiene—but if you still hear complaints, it's probably pinworms. You can use anti-itch cream (hydrocortisone) to get through the night of discomfort, but this isn't a cure—it just buys a few hours' time.

Pinworms look like whitish-yellow thread, and you can see them if you peek in the potty and look at a bowel movement. Parents, I speak for all the pharmacists in the nation, *don't bring us samples in Ziploc baggies*—we promise to take your word for it!

We'll probably recommend Pronto Plus or Pin-X sold OTC, giving the dosage according to your child's weight. Transmission is "hand to mouth," so your child may have picked up this unwelcome guest from a sandbox (where animals have pooped), those giant ball pits that kids play in, clothing, bedding, or toys. Keep their little hands *clean* and out of worm zones, and though it's impossible, I have to tell you, *keep their hands out of their mouths*!

✳ **Hemorrhoids**—These are caused by veins in or around the anus that swell up to create pain, itching, bleeding, and swelling, especially while you're passing bowel movements. They're pretty common in pregnant women and people over 50, and they may get worse if you have chronic constipation, diarrhea, or anal intercourse. They're uncomfortable but hardly life-threatening; however, *please* check out any blood in your stool, because that could be a sign of something serious. To soothe hemorrhoidal tissue, try Cellfood Essential Silica. *Dosage: 15 drops twice daily.*

To ease straining, your pharmacist will probably suggest a fiber supplement like Metamucil or Citrucel. My advice is also to cut back on constipating foods like starches and meats, and to eat more fibrous vegetables and fruits, especially broccoli, cabbage, carrots, apples, pears, and berries.

A stool softener eases passage of fecal matter, while hydrocortisone ointment—1 percent—can relieve the pain. Tucks hemhorrhoidal pads (which are drenched in witch hazel) are great, too. Store them in the fridge to cool them down so when you apply them rectally, they feel really cool and refreshing. Or try a sitz bath: Sprinkle some Epsom salts in lukewarm water, and soak for fifteen minutes.

✳ **Boils**—They start out as red spots, then fill with pus and get tender. Most boils come to a head on their own, and often rupture and drain by themselves within a week or two. They tend to pop up where you sweat or feel friction, especially on your neck, armpits, bottom, thighs, or sometimes on your forehead or face. You're most likely to get them if you have a suppressed immune system or diabetes, or if you're simply run down.

Your pharmacy sells Boil Ease to numb the pain and promote healing. Or get some tea tree oil at the health-food store, or perhaps a natural ointment containing slippery elm. My readers tell me that rubbing some oil of oregano onto their boils right at the onset keeps them from fully developing and lessens their duration. Another folk remedy has you eating lots of fresh garlic and turmeric spice, and applying the juices of garlic and onion to the boil to bring it to a head. Finally, there's an old-time pharmacy remedy called ichthammol, a thick black ointment that draws out the toxins. Most drugstores still sell it under the brand name Draw Out Salve.

✳ **Flatulence**—If your gas occurs mainly with certain foods, such as cabbage, broccoli, onions, and green beans, buy Beano (or maybe skip those foods at business luncheons and before your massage!). You can also soak dried beans (kidney, black, red, pinto, white, and garbanzos) for twelve hours in plain filtered water before cooking. It takes the pressure out of them and subsequently out of you! Taking digestive enzymes such as Enzymedica's Digest can help you break down food and improve digestion. Probiotics are also important to combating yeast and cutting down on gas production.

If you find that dairy products give you gas, you may be lactose-intolerant—unable to digest milk products. Some people buy a remedy called Lactaid to help them digest the dairy, but why not just avoid the problem foods? "F" = Flatulence! Fatty foods and those with fiber (beans, broccoli, bran) are combustible!

If your gas is a more general problem, the number-one thing you can do is buy enzymes from your local health-food store to help you break down the foods you eat. (See Chapter 4.) You can also buy activated charcoal, an internal detoxifier that absorbs odors in the digestive tract. I like CharcoCaps, which are sold at most pharmacies. Other popular remedies include Gas-X, Phazyme, and Mylanta Gas. Just remember that gas is generally a symptom of poor digestion, so the key is to improve your gut integrity and clean up your diet. Frequent and regular gas may indicate leaky gut, candida, or irritable bowel syndrome, so check out Chapter 3 for more information.

part V

Think Outside the Pill

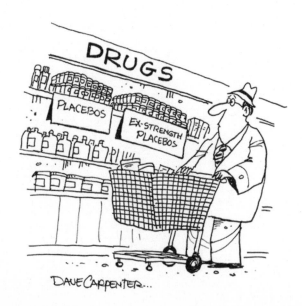

20

Plant Extracts and Vitamins

Plant Extracts That Give Stellar Drugs a Run for Their Money

⊕ *Saw Palmetto (Serenoa repens) vs. Finasteride (Proscar) for Prostate Problems*

It's been proven with good solid clinical trials—saw palmetto extract is more effective than placebo at easing problems with urination, and when compared with our stellar drug, it worked equally well. Because finasteride can change PSA levels (a cancer marker) and saw palmetto is less likely to interfere with PSA, I think those stubby little palm trees give finasteride a run for its money!

⊕ *St.-John's-Wort (Hypericum perforatum) vs. Fluoxetine (Prozac) for Depression*

This popular plant extract generates millions of dollars of sales in the U.S. because people know that it promotes better sleep and a happier mood. Some clinical trials show that St.-John's-wort is significantly more effective than fluoxetine—a blockbuster antidepressant—and seems to have fewer side effects. Plus, St.-John's-wort is widely used and trusted in Europe for depression, infection, insomnia, and low sex drive.

✿ *Black Cohosh (*Cimicifuga racemosa*) vs. Conjugated Estrogen (Premarin) for Hot Flashes*

Again, proven: Women with surge problems get cooling relief from black cohosh extract—and in some studies, even more relief than from conjugated estrogens. And a 2002 study found that the plant extract had favorable effects on bone health and cholesterol levels—all without increasing endometrial tissue (a harmful side effect of many estrogen drugs).

Is Your Vitamin Pill Worth It or Worthless?
Six Rules to Guarantee Quality

The debate gets heated when people talk about vitamins because some people really believe they work, while others really believe they just make expensive urine. But a recent study published in the *Journal of the American Medical Association* looked over thirty years of supplement studies and decided that multivitamins really can help us prevent many serious diseases, including cancer, heart disease, and osteoporosis.

Wow, did we need to spend all that money on a study to learn that nutrients improve wellness? Of course, eating well is the best way to get your nutrients, because lab-created supplements do not capture the essence of what nature made—although some companies do a better job than others. Supplementing with vitamins is not a substitute for eating well—but it is still a good idea.

Though I didn't mention it in every chapter, I think a multivitamin should be your first daily supplement. Make sure that you select the highest-quality brands that you can afford. Also, there are certain things on the label that may help you decide if these products are right for you. Here are some guidelines that can streamline your decision-making:

✿ *Rule #1: Don't buy a thousand tablets of anything for $6.99.*
What exactly do you think you'll get for that price? I hate to say it, but sometimes you do get what you pay for.

✿ *Rule #2: Choose capsules over tablets whenever you can.*
Capsules are easier for your body to absorb.

⚙ *Rule #3: If you have any chronic medical conditions, take a lot of medications, or have gastrointestinal difficulties, choose liquids or powdered supplements.*

Again, these are more easily absorbed. Of the two—liquids and powders— I think powders are better because many liquids contain preservatives.

⚙ *Rule #4: Don't buy anything that promises to cure seventeen conditions.*

Unless you're also interested in this bridge I'd like to sell you . . .

⚙ *Rule #5: When it comes to multivitamins, taking something is better than nothing—but multiple doses are better than one.*

That's why the best multivitamins tell you on the label to take them two or three times a day. If you take a multivitamin just once a day, the effect washes out after a few hours. This is frustrating for some people, who like to just take multivitamins once in the morning—but your cells are constantly regenerating, so your body really will benefit from multiple doses.

⚙ *Rule #6: It's great to buy supplements that have certification.*

You can be sure that a nutraceutical company is better than the competition if they have GMP certification—that's Good Manufacturing Practices—or even better, full certification by a governmental agency such as the Australian TGA (Therapeutic Goods Administration).

GMP is something that quality companies will pay for, but TGA certification is independent of the manufacturer and you can't just buy it.

What adds to the confusion is USP certification. USP stands for U.S. Pharmacopeia, and USP certification is fine, as are other certifying organizations, but they have a limited number of validated quality-assurance tests. In other words, testing is not necessarily comprehensive, so a USP-certified company may only have a few of their products actually tested. Some companies paste pretty labels onto their bottles—but the tablets inside come up short. A GMP logo or a TGA certification means a superior company by most standards.

21

Placebos and
Healing Treats

Take Two Sugar Pills and E-mail Me in the Morning:
Understanding the Placebo Effect

A placebo is an inert pill—usually a sugar pill—that people get in clinical trials so that researchers can compare the beneficial effects of the real drug compared to that of the inert pill. Typically, neither the person receiving the drug nor the researcher administering it knows who got the real medication and who got the placebo. When all the results are in, a new drug has to perform better than a placebo to get a thumbs up from the FDA.

However, after years of using placebos in medical research, scientists discovered something astonishing: The placebos themselves work fairly frequently! According to some research, a plain old sugar pill—nothing medicinal about it—will make people better about one-third of the time, *just because they believe it will.*

Think about that for a minute. One-third of the time, taking a sugar pill that you *think* is some terrific new wonder drug does just as much for you as the wonder drug itself. Never underestimate the power of placebo!

Between you and me, this is something most pharmacists know, even if we don't all like to admit it. For example, many drugs on the market today work just slightly better than placebos—certainly nothing to brag about—yet advertisements make them out to be some kind of wonder drug. And some prescription drugs have been "grandfathered" into the pharmacy without even a single clinical trial to back up their efficacy. In other words, they're sold today only because they have been used for decades, not because they are proven to work. I personally am deeply respectful of all methods of healing and keenly aware that we are more than our physical bodies—especially on a molecular level, where we are composed of energy. In fact, it may very well be that our belief in placebos works on that molecular level, which is why I feel that placebos play an important role in healthcare. Understanding how and why placebos work can help scientists to discover all sorts of treatments that may one day lead to healing our entire energy field on a molecular level, rather than focusing on a particular compromised organ. As a pharmacist, I know that many medications have unpleasant side effects and that some are downright deadly. So I've become very open and flexible in my practice—always careful to consider many different methods of healing, including those that are less tested.

In the end, I think people will heal faster if they believe in what they are taking. This is exactly why placebos work, because they put your mind at ease and you believe that you will heal. This isn't just my opinion; it's a commonly accepted scientific phenomenon: People who take placebos in clinical trials think they are getting the real drug—and they show a clinical response.

Many people will agree that a number of factors can affect your response to a drug: the drug itself, of course, but also touch, words, gestures, and the genuinely good intentions of your practitioner. For example, we know that patients who receive more empathy, counseling, and attention during surgery will fare better than those who get less compassion.

And what about medicine? How much medicine is, in truth, placebo? We know that the brain is capable of releasing strong opiates—feel-good chemicals, or "endorphins," that are more powerful than a prescription painkiller. Some studies suggest that as soon as we anticipate relief, we release endorphins and feel better—even if we're given a placebo rather than an actual pain medication.

I've seen this work in my own pharmacy repeatedly. Sometimes a person comes to my counter in a great deal of pain. If they have someone to drive them home, I'll usually advance them a tablet of the prescribed painkiller immediately while I go and process their prescription, which could easily take forty-five minutes in a busy store. Now here's the placebo effect: Within five minutes, most of these people are suddenly chitchatting, joking around with the staff, color back in their cheeks—even though, pharmacologically, the painkiller won't begin to work for another hour! I have noticed this effect time and time again—and I was recently fascinated to see that my observations were supported by several studies cited in the books *The Anatomy of Hope* and *How a Doctor Thinks* by Jerome Groopman, MD, professor of medicine at Harvard Medical School.

Or consider the billions of consumer dollars that have been spent on antidepressants like Prozac, Paxil, and Zoloft—and then remember that in one study published in the *Journal of the American Medical Association*, the sugar pill did a better job of alleviating symptoms of depression. Other studies have shown similar effects. For example, one team of researchers compared people who took an antidepressant such as Effexor or Prozac with those who took placebos. Brain scans for both groups showed definite improvements in the prefrontal cortex—a part of the brain that controls mood. But while 52 percent of those taking medications showed improvement, an impressively high 38 percent of those taking placebo also showed improvement.

Another study compared people suffering from depression who took St.-John's-wort (an herb) with those who took Zoloft (a medication), and those who took a placebo. The med and the herb were equally effective, helping some 25 percent of the people who took them—but the placebo helped 32 percent! (Now, don't suddenly stop taking your antidepressants on this account. ***Never suddenly stop taking antidepressants without a doctor's care,*** or you could make yourself extremely sick.) Psychologists also notice effects with antidepressants like the one I observed with painkillers—patients start to feel better as soon as they start taking the meds, even though pharmacologically, results aren't supposed to appear for at least two or three weeks. Studies show that surgery may have a placebo effect as well. In 1950, a small study on patients who underwent arterial ligation surgery to treat chest pain (angina pectoris) revealed that 76 percent of those who received the surgery improved—while 100 percent of those who *believed* they had surgery—but had only a chest incision—improved. Or consider the one hundred men in an English study who were told that they were receiving chemotherapy while they were actually given only an inactive saline solution. Some 20 percent of these men believed in the treatment so much they even lost their hair! Dr. Groopman cites other "surgical placebos" in his book, too.

I want you to remember that the power of the mind is spectacular! We can convince ourselves of pretty much anything. So please be open to the possibility of getting help without any active ingredients. Why not? Since my husband and I both dabble in energy work and hands-on healing, it is not a stretch for me to believe that we can bring healing to the body by unblocking trapped energy in core centers of our physical bodies. Healing with energetic touch has worked on me, and I've used it to help other people, too. Be creative and imagine beautiful visualizations of healing. For example, if you have cancer, imagine that the chemotherapy is like Pac Man eating up all the bad cells. If you have heart problems, imagine someone you love hugging you and filling your heart up with warm energy. See it beating in perfect rhythm. If you are prone to blood clots, close your eyes and see them dissolving and surround yourself in violet light. Sound delusional? Not if it works, and it does for some people. One of the most famous healers is Adam, author of *The Path of the Dreamhealer* and other books. He has a DVD available that helps those with less imagination do healing visualizations on their bodies. Adam is in his early twenties and believes that people can harness their own healing power and cure disease through visualizations; check out www.dreamhealer.com. I agree that this is possible; we already accept that stress induces physical illness, so the opposite must hold true. Relaxation and joy (and positive thinking) should induce wellness and healing, and with visualizations, there are no side effects. Plus it's free. Laughing is another proven way to reduce pain and improve healing outcomes. Rent hilarious movies, hang around funny people, and find witty cartoons and humorous books.

Now, don't abandon your current medical treatments and drugs, but start thinking positively. This will break the cycle of negativity and help you shake off that feeling of being victimized and trapped by your illness. Thinking positively and acting "as if" you are healthy will start attracting wellness into your cells and tissues. I have to tell you, all that mental berating takes a toll on your body. I believe every time you think or declare a negative self-concept—"I'm worthless, I'm so stupid, I hate my body, This sickens me"—your body releases chemicals that reinforce your condition and pain.

Take notice that even during times of what should be joy, some of you will still talk about the pain you felt earlier that day or the misery in your life. If you imagine that your words and thoughts instantly translate into harmful substances in your cells, then you will be more choosy about what you say and think. Your goal should be to think and talk in ways that create feel-good endorphins in your body, not destructive chemicals. Finding something (anything) to be grateful for is part of the healing pie.

Attitude is another key factor. A famous study showed that women who took control of their lives after being diagnosed with breast cancer showed stronger immune responses than those who were resigned to the diagnosis. Mind over matter—it's not just a slogan!

So do yourself a favor and think more flexibly. Listen to that quiet voice inside—your intuition—which sometimes helps you figure out what's going wrong in your body when blood tests can't. Realize that your body believes what you think and what you say—one more reason to think and speak positively.

Finally, be open to the possibility that healing comes in various forms. As the placebo effect suggests, we can alter our physical response to healing by changing our perceptions, using prayer, or relying upon various alternative methods of healing. Even if you're taking prescription meds, you can still use your mind to take advantage of and harness the power of your soul and spirit to heal.

Sinful Pleasures That Help You Heal: Good News for Java Junkies and Chocoholics!

Chocolate is good for you because it . . .

* contains magnesium, which is good for circulation and mood

* helps relax our blood vessels

* slightly thins the blood (that's nothing to worry about, so don't freak if you take blood thinners)

* improves the balance of compounds called "eicosanoids," which help the heart

* contains antioxidants, which vacuum up nasty free radicals that want to hurt you

* activates the same receptors in our brains that marijuana does (and chocolate is legal!)

And here's some more good news: Chocolate is not as fattening as people think!

I know your mind is racing with thoughts of some gooey, caramel-swirled chocolate bar—but messing up a perfectly nice cocoa bean with additives, extra fat, sugar, and grease is not exactly what I had in mind. No, I'm thinking real, dark chocolate, the kind that's pure and unadulterated, at least 70 percent cocoa. Milk chocolate is primarily fat and nonnutritive. Dark chocolate is the one that is studied in trials. It's more natural and it has exponentially more nutrients, so that's the type of chocolate that is good for the soul. It will help your heart and soothe your brain—and best of all, it's not fattening!

So find one of the many delicious organically grown forms of chocolate that they sell at health-food stores. This isn't a license to eat a bar every day, but do have a few guilt-free squares of fine chocolate now and then. I've always thought that behind every successful woman, there's a box of chocolates in her desk, just in case of emergency. In fact, I'm eating some right now!

Coffee is good for you because it . . .

* temporarily boosts your energy

* improves your focus and alertness

* creates a temporary sense of well-being

* might lower your risk of liver damage

* may protect against colon cancer

* seems to ease memory disorders (like dementia or Alzheimer's)

* can help you lose weight

* may help diabetes, according to some studies

* makes most people move their bowels (which could help with constipation)

* can ease pain such as a headache (which is why many pain relievers contain caffeine)

Now, moderation in all things! After all, coffee is a drug—it contains a powerful mood- and body-altering substance that speaks to your body, so treat it with respect. Next time you're standing in line at Starbucks—which serves as a human gas station!—remember that caffeine also has a number of less pleasant effects, including the jitters, diarrhea, anxiety, nausea, racing heart, and, in some people, depression. If you're used to drinking coffee, a caffeine shortage can trigger a headache. And if you rely on coffee as your primary source of energy, you probably have adrenal burnout and long-term problems with fatigue (see Chapter 1).

So enjoy that hazelnut soy latte every once in a while—maybe even two or three times a week. Just make sure that you drink plenty of water, green tea, and other healthy beverages the rest of the time. And by healthy beverages, no, I do not mean soda pop! Hey, I'm not an ogre—I've let you have coffee and chocolate! Please quit while you're ahead!

22

The Most Misunderstood Drugs in America

⚙ *Xanax and other benzodiazepine sleeping pills*
Misunderstood because people think that sleeping pills help them sleep better—which is not necessarily true. In the long run, this class of prescribed sleepers won't allow for restful, refreshing sleep because they cut out deeper stages of restorative REM sleep. Read Chapter 9.

⚙ *Premarin, PremPro, and other synthetic estrogen/progestin drugs*
Misunderstood because people think the pharmacy version of these hormones is a copy of their own naturally produced hormone. Not true. Both Premarin and PremPro contain ingredients from horse urine. These and other manmade hormones mimic a few of the beneficial actions of our own hormones—but they also pose many risks. Read Chapters 11–13.

⚙ *Lipitor, Zocor, and other cholesterol-reducing drugs*
Misunderstood because people think that these drugs will lower cholesterol and protect them from a heart attack. False. They do a good job of lowering cholesterol, but some people still get heart attacks while taking these drugs. They don't get to the heart of *why* someone makes all that cholesterol, and *why* the blood vessels in the body are so clogged up to begin with. Statin drugs are

drug muggers that deplete our Coenzyme Q10, which we need for optimal heart health. Read Chapter 2.

✿ *Viagra and other sexual enhancers*

Misunderstood for two reasons: 1) People think that sex pills create erections, but they don't—they only prolong and harden them (and sometimes not even that). So if that spark isn't there, these drugs won't start a fire. 2) Sex pills carry big risks for people with heart problems and vision trouble. Read Chapter 10.

✿ *Marijuana*

Misunderstood because people assume pot is for getting high: They associate it with hippies, drug addicts, wayward teens, and people with bad morals. But according to clinical data, this botanical extract has authentic medicinal value. It's even FDA-sanctioned and sold as the drug Marinol to help overcome nausea and vomiting in cancer patients receiving chemotherapy and restore appetite in AIDS/HIV patients.

✿ *Ibuprofen, naproxen, and other over-the-counter arthritis drugs (nonsteroidal anti-inflammatory drugs, or NSAIDs)*

Misunderstood because people think these drugs cure their arthritis when they only mask the pain. Plus, they all pose such risks as GI upset, excessive bleeding, high blood pressure, and potential heart problems. The real cure for arthritis is in adding shock-absorbing quality to your joints rather than masking the pain. Read Chapter 17.

✿ *Warfarin (coumadin)*

Misunderstood because people fear that if they eat green vegetables while taking this blood thinner, it makes the drug stop working. Actually, it's okay to eat greens and salads—but you have to do so *consistently*. That way, the doctor can fine-tune your drug dosage based on your daily vegetable intake.

✿ *Oxycontin and other enteric-coated painkillers*

Misunderstood because people hear news stories of overdosing and deaths and think this is a harmful drug. Fact is, it's very effective and has given people back some quality of life. Only take recommended doses and don't crush it, chew it, or combine it with alcohol—and that's no different than any other painkiller in this class. The people you heard about on TV may have abused it, misused it, combined it with alcohol or other narcotics, or crushed it, releasing a large dose of medication that should have been released slowly over 24 hours.

Commonly Prescribed Drugs in America

Their Side Effects, and Natural Remedies for Side Effects

DRUG NAME	SIDE EFFECT	NATURAL REMEDY
Advair discus	Upper respiratory infection	Vitamin C, glutathione
Amoxicillin	Diarrhea, yeast infections	Probiotics, saccharomyces
Anticonvulsants	Liver damage	SAMe
Antidepressants	Low sex drive, inability to climax	Ginkgo biloba
Celebrex	Edema, elevated blood pressure	Fish oils, folic acid
Nexium	Mouth sores and fatigue	B vitamins
Prevacid	Mouth sores and fatigue	B vitamins
Procrit	Leg swelling, high BP, heart attack	Coenzyme Q10
Statins (Lipitor, Zocor)	Muscle weakness and fatigue	Coenzyme Q10
Zyprexa	Zombielike mood	Quercetin, rhodiola

23

Aromatherapy—The Nose Knows What's Nice

Aromatherapy: Essential Oils Are Good Medicine, Too

I love plants. They give us powerful remedies—remedies that have been used for centuries and by many cultures. Essential oils are extracts from aromatic plants. Their therapeutic value was discovered in the 1930s by R.M. Gatte-fossé, a French chemist and perfumer. When he had a laboratory accident that burned his hand, he plunged it into the only liquid nearby—a vat of lavender essential oil. He noticed the pain of the burn subsided quickly, and it healed much sooner than expected. Gattefossé spent the rest of his life studying the therapeutic properties of essential oils.

Aromatherapy is defined as the art and science of using essential oils to promote health and well-being. It is valued for its effectiveness and holistic nature in a variety of situations where it can be used for self-care. Essential oils are manufactured within the plant for various uses, such as to protect the plant from disease, repel bugs, or attract bees for pollination. Essential oils are extracted from many different plant parts, such as flowers, seeds, leaves, and grasses, and they can come from many different geographical locations. We need essential oils for the Earth to flourish, but humans can also benefit from their healing properties.

Essential oils are unique. They are highly concentrated—one hundred times stronger than the dried herb of the same plant. They exist in a variety of colors and viscosities and are soluble in alcohol and vegetable oils. (They are not soluble in water.) They will last for many years when stored properly in dark-colored glass bottles with tight-fitting caps away from heat and light. Essential oils do not become rancid because they do not contain fatty acids.

The price of an essential oil depends on the quality and the availability. It can vary greatly from oil to oil. For example, rose essential oil is expensive because it takes about 2,000 pounds of rose petals to produce one pound of essential oil. One ounce of pure rose essential oil may cost $800. In contrast, one ounce of peppermint essential oil may cost $40. However, because these are nature-produced products, if the peppermint supply was depleted or destroyed, the price would go up dramatically.

Essential oils are versatile in their physical applications. They can relieve pain, soothe irritations, reduce inflammation, relax muscles, stimulate circulation, and fight a broad spectrum of infections. In 1988, scientists tested three specific essential oils (armoise, oregano, and eucalyptus) against hospital-pathogenic bacteria. The study found that they had an effect comparable to standard antibiotics.

Psychologically, aromatherapy is used to promote positive mental and emotional states, such as mental clarity or optimism, and to reduce negative mental and emotional states, such as mental fatigue or anxiety. This is achieved in two different ways: first, by choosing an essential oil with the appropriate properties, such as rosemary or peppermint for mental clarity, and second, by using memory and association with an aroma to re-create positive feelings. The psychological effects of aromas were first tested in 1966 by R. Moncrieff. He tested a variety of essential oils and found that some produced beta patterns (attention and alertness) and some produced delta patterns (euphoria and calmness).

Spiritually, aromatherapy is used to assist a variety of transformative techniques, such as meditation, affirmation, prayer, and visualization. In this subtle realm, the essential oil is chosen for its energetic or vibrational properties. Joni Keim, an essential oil specialist and co-author of *Aromatherapy and Subtle Energy Techniques*, says, "The aromatic qualities of plants have been used for religious ritual, meditation, and prayer for thousands of years. Fragrances were chosen for their ability to promote feelings of oneness with the universe, and a closeness with God." In an excerpt from her book, Joni goes on to say:

These spiritual connections have been passed down through the ages from ancient Egypt, Arabia, Greece, and Asia, as well as other cultures such as Native Americans. Dried herbs were burned as incense, and the rising smoke was believed to communicate with the deities. As it rose to the heavens, prayers were offered. Frankincense was the most common aromatic used, and is mentioned several times in the Bible, most notably as a gift to baby Jesus. Sage was traditionally used by Native Americans in ceremony.

People have long held on to the idea that we need mushrooms, LSD, or Ayahuasca to access other realms or have a spiritual experience. It appears that certain essential oils allow you to tune in better to God, your spiritual guides, or Angels…if not as potently as the drugs mentioned above! Frankincense is fabulous for this purpose, but if this scent doesn't appeal to you, consider sandalwood, cedarwood, or rosewood. By now, you're probably wondering how to use the oil for this purpose. Simply inhale a drop of the essential oil from a tissue. Or you can put one drop in the palm of your hands (if your skin is not too sensitive), rub your hands together, and breathe in the aroma. Pause and inhale again. If you're taking a bath, put a few drops right into the bathwater. Essential oils can heighten any meditative experience that you're having. You can also wear it in a little glass bottle around your neck; these are found in many health-food stores or metaphysical book shops.

When you use essential oils, their effects cannot be completely separated or isolated into one realm or the other of body, mind, or spirit. For example, when you apply lavender to your skin to soothe a sunburn, you also inhale the aroma, which will have a soothing effect on your psyche. In *Daily Aromatherapy: Transforming the Seasons of Your Life with Essential Oils*, Joni Keim states, "This demonstrates the true wholistic nature of essential oils, which aligns so beautifully with the wholistic nature of human beings."

Essential oils are used to promote health and well-being by application to the skin and by inhaling the aroma. (They are not taken internally unless under the supervision of a qualified aromatherapist.) The most common methods of use are massage, bath, compress, steam inhalation, and diffusion. When applied to the skin, essential oils' small molecular structure and attraction-to-oil (*lipophylic*) characteristics allow certain constituents to be absorbed. When the aroma of an essential oil is inhaled through the nose, some molecules enter the lungs and others contact the olfactory bulb. Those connecting with the olfactory bulb travel to the limbic part of the brain and produce a variety of responses related to emotions and memories.

Essential oils must be of high quality in order to achieve the desired results. Two essential oil lines that are excellent are Oshadhi (707-763-0662, www.oshadhiusa.com) and Primavera (www.primaveralife.com). If aromatherapy appeals to you, there are many books available to teach you how to incorporate these incredible gifts from nature into your life. Here are some ideas to get you started:

✴ Put a few drops of neroli (*Citrus aurantium*) essential oil on a tissue and put it in a baggie in your purse for easy access to help relieve anxiety. Open the baggie and simply inhale the aroma. Pause and inhale again.

✴ If you have trouble sleeping, try putting a few drops of lavender (*Lavandula angustifolia*) on a cotton pad and place it inside a corner of your pillowcase. Lavender helps many people to go to sleep.

✴ To ease congestion, make a chest rub by combining 10–20 drops of eucalyptus (*Eucalyptus globulus or radiata*) with 1 ounce of fragrance-free lotion. Apply to your upper chest and upper back.

✴ To make a personalized lotion, put 20–30 drops of your favorite skin-pampering essential oil, such as geranium, lavender, or rose, in 8 ounces of fragrance-free lotion.

Where "massage" is mentioned in the following table, you may use oil or lotion. This is a matter of personal preference. Most people prefer adding the drops of oil to a fragrance-free lotion because it doesn't leave the skin feeling "greasy" and won't stain clothes like an oil. But, of course, oil is certainly acceptable and may be preferred by those with dry skin, or by massage therapists who wish to heighten the relaxation experience for their clients. You might choose to use hazelnut oil, apricot kernel oil, sweet almond oil, or avocado oil. These all penetrate the skin well; however, some are heavier than others, so experiment with them to see which feels the best and provides the right amount of massage "slip."

Essential Oils and Their Uses

CONDITION	ESSENTIAL OIL THAT MAY HELP	HOW TO USE
Allergies	German chamomile	Steam inhalation
Anxiety	Neroli	Massage, inhalation
Arthritis	Lemongrass	Massage, compress
Athlete's foot	Tea tree	Massage, compress, foot bath
Blemishes	Lavender, tea tree	Spot application
Colds/flu	Eucalyptus	Steam inhalation, chest rub
Dandruff	Rosemary	Scalp tonic
Depression	Ylang ylang	Bath, massage, inhalation
Fatigue	Rosemary	Inhalation
Grief	Rose, frankincense	Inhalation
Headache	Peppermint, spearmint	Massage (temples, back of neck)
Immune support	Eucalyptus, frankincense	Massage, inhalation
Insect bites	Lavender, tea tree	Spot application (1 drop)
Insomnia	Lavender, clary sage	Bath, massage, inhalation
Muscle cramp	Roman chamomile	Massage
Nerve pain	Lavender, eucalyptus	Gentle massage

CONDITION	ESSENTIAL OIL THAT MAY HELP	HOW TO USE
PMS	Geranium, clary sage	Massage, bath, inhalation
Sex drive	Jasmine, sandalwood	Massage, bath, inhalation
Sinusitis	Ravintsara	Steam inhalation
Skin beautification	Lavender, rose	Massage, compress
Sore throat	Sandalwood	Steam inhalation
Stretch marks	Immortelle, rosa rubiginosa	Massage
Warts	Tea tree, palmarosa	Spot application

Note: Essential oils are for external use and must be diluted if they are used on the skin. The percent of dilution, the method of use, and the duration of use depend on the oil used, the purpose of its use, the location of its use, and the condition of the person it is used on.

24

Finding Your
Dream Doctor

He listens for more than five minutes and can figure out the root cause for all seven of your weird symptoms that don't even feel remotely connected. His staff promptly returns your calls and phones in refills for your prescription. If something he tries doesn't work on you, he doesn't give you a higher dose of it—he tries something new. He reads the articles you bring in from the paper or the Internet—and his medical knowledge keeps growing and changing. He doesn't find it strange at all that you think Coenzyme Q10 is good for you, or that you want to try ginseng. In fact, he just recommended some herbs to another patient. Hello, Dr. McDreamy!

Does that sound like *your* dream doctor too? Someone who's open to both conventional and alternative medicine, someone who knows how to think outside the pillbox, and understands that amazing cures don't always come from the pharmacy?

Now, let's be reasonable. Once we leave the world of television, doctors aren't superhuman, and they're going to make mistakes, become confused, or just plain miss something they should have caught. They can't possibly know everything; every day, dozens of studies come across the wire, and each month, hundreds are printed in various journals and periodicals. No doctor—hey, no *human*—could possibly keep up with all that literature. But your doctor *can* be open-minded, flexible, sensitive to the importance of nutrition, and willing to consider alternative techniques like acupuncture, massage, and homeopathy. In fact, some doctors are so committed to integrating alternative and conventional medicine that they've joined organizations dedicated to that purpose.

Your dream doctor may not even be a medical doctor. These organizations will train all sorts of practitioners, including nurses, dentists, physical therapists, chiropractors, acupuncturists, and pharmacists—yes, I am a member too, but of course you could tell that if you read my book! So if you'd like to find *your* dream doctor somewhere outside a TV medical show, read on.

Institute of Functional Medicine (IFM)

This is a nonprofit international organization of practitioners who think outside the pillbox. Their mission is to improve health and well-being through preventive means. Their goal is to identify the underlying cause of your condition, and they believe that the best way to do that is by integrating lifestyle changes, diet, and nutraceuticals, along with other practitioners and other complementary healers. Their priority is to care for the whole patient, not to treat one symptom at a time, adding drug after drug.

Call them or look on their website to find a doctor near you. Or if your current MD is interested, invite him or her to use the group as a resource.

Institute of Functional Medicine
4411 Point Fosdick Drive NW, Suite 305
P.O. Box 1697
Gig Harbor, WA 98335
800-228-0622
www.functionalmedicine.org

American College for Advancement of Medicine (ACAM)

This is another nonprofit medical society that educates physicians and other healthcare professionals on the latest findings in preventive and nutritional medicine. The group is committed to integrating complementary and alternative medicine with conventional medicine through research, practice, and education. ("Complementary medicine" is the term for treatments that complement, o rt, conventional procedures.)

Celebrating more than a quarter century of service, ACAM represents physicians in more than 30 countries. It's the largest and oldest organization of its kind anywhere in the world, and you can also use their website to locate a doctor near you.

American College for Advancement of Medicine
24411 Ridge Route
Suite 115
Laguna Hilla, CA 92653
949-309-3520
www.acam.org

Health-Food Stores

Visit your local health-food store or natural supermarket and ask the staff. They are a terrific source of information and know which doctors and holistic healers practice in your area. Many stores have an information board with pamphlets and business cards to help you find the dream doctor for your needs.

The Phone Book

You can also look in your yellow pages under "physicians" to find doctors who practice alternative medicine. They often advertise themselves as "holistic," "complementary," or "integrative" physicians. Today, with the demand for safer, natural treatments exploding, more and more traditional doctors are opening their minds and educating themselves in the "naturopathic" methods of healing. Conventional doctors often know who the holistic practitioners are and may give you a lead if you ask.

American Academy of Anti-Aging Medicine (A4M)

This nonprofit organization has worldwide membership representing doctors and scientists from about 65 countries. Their mission is to detect, prevent, and treat aging-related disease and promote research into slowing down the aging process. I've been to their international seminars, and if you're a healthcare professional, it's really nothing short of fascinating. I'd encourage all doctors to participate at least once!

773-528-1000
www.worldhealth.net
E-mail: info@worldhealth.net

American Association of Naturopathic Physicians (AANP)

This organization can help you find a naturopathic physician in your area. Naturopathic doctors think of the body as a whole system, and use natural and safer methods of treatment to help one heal. Oftentimes, naturopathic care is covered by insurance and can be used alongside conventional medicine. They are not licensed in every state, so visit the website or call to find out if a naturopathic doctor is near you.

877-969-2267
www.naturopathic.org

American Chiropractic Association (ACA)

Many chiropractors have a strong nutritional background and can offer recommendations for herbals and vitamins. Some carry physician-only formulas (like Thorne, Metagenics, and Xymogen) as well as other certified supplements. Chiropractors will also know which doctors in town practice alternative medicine.

703-276-8800
www.acatoday.com

American Holistic Medical Association (AHMA)

505-292-7788
Fax: 505-293-7582
www.holisticmedicine.org

American Holistic Health Association (AHHA)

This nonprofit organization provides free and impartial health information to help you help yourself and gives you the power of choice. AHHA's mission is unique and unbiased, and they will help you find the right organization, health professional, or research article to suit your individual needs. They believe that you should be a participant in your own health, rather than a spectator. AHHA has a free and extensive list of resources and referrals so that anyone, sick or healthy, can connect to the resources they need in order to improve health or maintain well-being.

714-779-6152

www.ahha.org

E-mail: mail@ahha.org

American Osteopathic Association (AOA)

800-621-1773

www.osteopathic.org

Council for Responsible Nutrition (CRN)

202-776-7929

www.crnusa.org

E-mail: webmaster@crnusa.org

Professional Referral Network

www.healthreferral.com

Alternative Medicine Network

A free service listing healthcare professionals who use natural hormones, by state.

www.altmednetwork.net

The Health Resource

This internationally acclaimed information service will provide you with individualized bound reports on your specific medical condition. The nice thing is that the research is tailored to fit your customized needs, and provides all treatment options, addresses for specific questions and concerns, and practitioners who could help. They will provide cutting-edge, comprehensive research. I think this service is indispensable, especially if you have a rare or serious condition. There may be a charge, but it's well worth it.

933 Faulkner Street
Conway, AR 72034
800-949-0090 or 501-329-5272
www.thehealthresource.com
E-mail: moreinfo@thehealthresource.com

Stanford Health Library Research Services

This is a free information service offered by Stanford University to help you locate answers to your health questions, including treatment options for health conditions. Information packets include journal articles and excerpts from books and special databases. If you have any medical condition, and you are not satisfied with your treatment, this is a terrific resource.

800-295-5177
http://healthlibrary.stanford.edu
E-mail: healthlibrary@stanfordmed.org

For information on progesterone in the United Kingdom and Europe:

The Natural Progesterone Information Service provides information on all aspects of the use of natural progesterone to women, doctors, and other health-care providers. NPIS also makes available many books, tapes, videos, and scientific papers related to natural progesterone.

The Natural Progesterone Information Service
PO Box 24, Buxton, SK17 9FB
Phone: 07000 784849
FAX: 01298 70979
www.npis.info
E-mail: news@npis.info

Finding a Doctor to Prescribe Bioidentical Hormones

If you want to find a doctor who can prescribe bioidentical hormones, ask your local compounding pharmacist—any pharmacist who compounds medicines right there in the pharmacy. The doctors who most frequently prescribe natural hormones are medical doctors (MDs), naturopathic doctors (NDs), and osteopathic doctors (DOs). In some states, naturopaths do not have prescribing privileges, so you may need to ask your medical doctor to prescribe what the naturopath suggests.

If you can't find a compounding pharmacy in your yellow pages, you can also contact any of these three organizations:

The International Academy of Compounding Pharmacists (IACP)
P.O. Box 1365
Sugarland, TX 77487
800-927-4227
www.iacprx.org
E-mail: iacpinfo@iacprx.org

Professional Compounding Centers of America, Inc. (PCCA)
9901 S. Wilcrest
Houston, TX 77099
800-331-2498
www.pccarx.com

National Association of Compounding Pharmacies (NACP)
4015 River Road
Amarillo, TX 79108
800-687-7850

25

Issues with Estrogen and Progesterone

Coping with Environmental Estrogens: Identifying and Responding to Xenobiotics

Common xenobiotics—substances that mimic estrogen:

* Dry-cleaning chemicals

* Fresh paint

* Gasoline

* Household cleaners with solvents

* Cigarette smoke

* Nonylphenol (a by-product of spermicide nonoxynol-9)

* Bisphenol-A (found in polycarbonate plastic water bottles and in many canned foods)

* Pesticides

* Ant killer

* Herbicides

* Weed killer

✳ DDT

✳ PVC, or polyvinyl chloride, found in shrink wrap and plastic bottles and food containers. Don't freeze it or microwave it because it can release the poison dioxin.

✳ Benzene (a gasoline additive)

✳ Parabens and phthalates, found in many cosmetics

✳ Dioxins (found frequently in contaminated meats and fatty fish)

✳ PCBs

✳ Some shampoos that contain placenta, hormones, estrogen, oestradiol, or oestragen, usually marketed to black women who want to deep-condition their hair

A Dartmouth University study found that plastic wrap heated in a microwave oven with vegetable oil had 500,000 times the minimum amount of xenoestrogens needed to stimulate breast cancer cells to grow in the test tube.

✳ Plastics that contain phthalates, which are added to make them flexible. Don't microwave your plastic containers, which might release phthalates from the container into the food you are heating. Buy the thicker, heavier-grade plastics rather than the superthin flexible kinds.

What you can do to counteract these chemicals:

✳ Get a HEPA filter or another type of indoor air purifier, like an ionizer.

✳ Avoid heating or freezing plastics whenever possible.

✳ Take NAC (N-acetylcysteine), which can help break down pesticides in your body. Follow the dosage on the bottle or try *500 mg twice daily.*

✳ Take a chlorophyll supplement, eat greens (kale, broccoli, chard, turnip greens), or supplement with drinkable greens—these powdered mixed "green drinks" are sold at health-food stores.

✳ Take curcumin—it's found as a supplement, and in the spice turmeric. Curcumin can block the doorways to your cells that might otherwise allow in xenobiotics.

❋ Consider Thorne Research's Pesticide Protector, available at www. thorne.com or 800-228-1966. Cost: $25.

Direct and Indirect Causes of Estrogen Dominance

❋ trans fatty acids (found in mass-produced pastries and processed foods)

❋ working nights/sleeping in the daytime

❋ lack of antioxidants

❋ sedentary lifestyle

❋ obesity

❋ chronic stress (excess cortisol)

❋ sleep deprivation

❋ insulin resistance (brought about from excessive starches and sugar)

❋ fluoridated water and toothpaste

❋ cigarette smoking

❋ progesterone deficiency

❋ zinc deficiency

❋ magnesium deficiency

❋ environmental xenobiotics (industrial chemicals)

❋ lack of sulfur-containing amino acids (for example, SAMe or S-adenosylmethionine)

❋ lack of the nutrient L-glutamine

❋ using drugs that impair liver function

Using Progesterone Creams

Progesterone cream is sold OTC, but the creams don't always come in the same dose. Generally ¼ teaspoon contains 20 mg USP progesterone, but read the label.

I want you to pick a good brand that feels right for you. Find one that is free of the methyl or propyl parabens (a harmful preservative in some creams), because parabens are xenobiotics, with an estrogen-like behavior in the body.

Work with a physician to determine your dosage, because balance is critical. Using unopposed progesterone for too long can raise your risk for cancer. Likewise, deficiencies may increase risk for cancer, so progesterone should be limited to those who prove to need it. Progesterone (like any bioidentical or prescribed hormone) must have its risks weighed to its benefits. Because progesterone is sold without a prescription, I realize that some of you will begin self-treatment despite my repeated warnings. You should start on the low end of the dosage guidelines I've suggested and use the lowest effective dose to improve symptoms. If your condition worsens, or you develop any new symptoms, see your physician. If you have fibroids or cervical dysplasia, there are some guidelines I suggest in Chapter 12; however, these are serious conditions, so you should get your doctor's approval before starting any new supplements or herbs.

> *If you experience sleepiness, weight gain, bloating, an increase in triglycerides, a decrease in HDL cholesterol, or a decrease in thyroid hormone, this is a sign to lower your progesterone dosage, either by applying less cream, or applying the cream less often.*

How to Apply Progesterone Cream:

Squeeze out the proper amount and apply directly to your breasts, chest, inner arms, inner thighs, hands, or neck. Pick one site each time, and then rotate so you're applying to a range of places on your body. The cream feels like a moisturizer, and you don't have to wash your hands afterward—but you can if you want to.

If you're in your reproductive years:

With Day 1 as your first day of bleeding:

* ✳ Use no cream on Days 1–14.

* ✳ On Days 15–21, apply *¼ teaspoonful (20 mg) twice daily.*

✳ On Days 22–28, apply ¼–½ *teaspoonful (20–40 mg) twice daily.*

✳ Stop the progesterone cream as soon as you start bleeding.

If you're perimenopausal:
With Day 1 as your first day of bleeding:

✳ Do not use on Days 1–7.

✳ On Days 8–21, apply ¼ *teaspoonful (20 mg) twice daily.*

✳ On Days 22–28, apply ¼–½ *teaspoonful (20–40 mg) twice daily.*

*If you're menopausal, postmenopausal, or have had your uterus
or ovaries removed:*
With Day 1 as the first day of each month:

✳ Do not use on Days 1–13.

✳ On Days 14–30/31, apply ¼–½ *teaspoonful (20–40 mg) twice
daily.*

You can also try it this way:
Use throughout the month, taking five days off each month.

✳ Apply ¼–½ *teaspoonful (20–40 mg) once or twice daily.*

> *Some women who are perimenopausal or menopausal have
> insulin swings or diabetes. Be aware that doctors can test you
> very easily with blood tests. And if you're prone to insulin swings, use less
> progesterone than I've suggested—work with your doctor to find the
> best dosage.*

Drug Muggers

Install a Nutrient Security System

Nutrients You Need If You Take These Drugs

DRUG	WHAT'S MUGGED, AMONG OTHER THINGS . . .
Acetaminophen	Glutathione
Acid blockers	Zinc and B vitamins
Antacids	Calcium and vitamin D
Antibiotics	B vitamins and probiotics
Aspirin	Folic acid and vitamin C
Benazepril	Zinc and vitamin D
Betoptic eye drops	Coenzyme Q10
Bisacodyl (Dulcolax)	Potassium
Boniva	Calcium and vitamin D
Butalbital	Biotin, calcium, and folic acid

DRUG	WHAT'S MUGGED, AMONG OTHER THINGS . . .
Carbamazepine	Biotin, calcium, folic acid, and vitamin D
Celebrex	Folic acid
Chlorpropamide	Coenzyme Q10
Chlorthalidone	Zinc
Conjugated estrogen (Premarin/Prempro)	Magnesium and B_6
Cyclosporine	Magnesium and potassium
Diclofenac	Folic acid
Didanosine	Carnitine, B_{12}, copper, and zinc
Digoxin	Calcium, magnesium, thiamine, and phosphorus
Doxepin	Coenzyme Q10 and riboflavin
Enalapril	Zinc
Estrogens	B vitamins
Fluticasone nasal spray	Selenium
Fosamax	Calcium and vitamin D
Furosemide	Calcium
Gemfibrozil	Vitamin E
Glipizide	Coenzyme Q10
Glyburide	Coenzyme Q10
Haloperidol	Coenzyme Q10
Hydrochlorothiazide	Coenzyme Q10, magnesium, potassium, zinc, and phosphorus

DRUG	WHAT'S MUGGED, AMONG OTHER THINGS...
Hydrocodone and acetaminophen	Glutathione
Ibuprofen	Folic acid
Indapamide	Coenzyme Q10, magnesium, potassium, zinc, and phosphorus
Isoniazid (INH)	B_6, vitamin D, and niacin
Lansoprazole (Prevacid)	B_{12}
Levodopa/Carbidopa	Potassium and SAMe
Levonorgestrel	Folic acid, magnesium, B_2, B_6, B_{12}, vitamin C, and zinc
Lisinopril	Zinc
Lithium	Inositol
Meloxicam	Folic acid
Metformin	Coenzyme Q10, folic acid, and B_{12}
Methotrexate	Folic acid
Metoprolol	Coenzyme Q10
Mineral oil	Beta-carotene
Moexipril (Univasc)	Zinc
Nadolol	Coenzyme Q10
Nicotine patches and gums	Vitamin C
Nortriptyline	Coenzyme Q10 and riboflavin
Omeprazole (Prilosec)	B_{12}
Orlistat (Xenical and Alli)	Beta-carotene and vitamins D and E

DRUG	WHAT'S MUGGED, AMONG OTHER THINGS . . .
Oxcarbazepine (Trileptal)	Biotin, calcium, folic acid, and vitamin D
Oxycodone	Melatonin
Pantoprazole (Protonix)	B_{12}
Phenobarbital	Calcium, folic acid, and vitamins D and K
Pravastatin	Coenzyme Q10
Prednisone	Calcium, magnesium, folic acid, potassium, selenium, zinc, and vitamins C and D
Propafenone (Rythmol)	Coenzyme Q10
Propranolol	Coenyzme Q10
Questran	Vitamins A, B_6, and D
Quinapril (Accupril)	Zinc
Raloxifene	Magnesium and B_6
Ramipril (Altace)	Zinc
Repaglinide	Coenzyme Q10
Sildenafil (Viagra)	Not known at this time
Simvastatin (Zocor)	Coenzyme Q10
Statin cholesterol drugs	Coenzyme Q10
Steroids	Calcium, potassium, and vitamins C and D
Sulindac (Clinoril)	Folic acid
Trandolapril/Verapamil (Tarka)	Zinc

DRUG	WHAT'S MUGGED, AMONG OTHER THINGS . . .
Triamterene	Calcium, folic acid, and zinc
Valproic acid (Depakote)	Carnitine and folic acid
Xenical	Vitamins A, D, and E
Zidovudine (Retrovir)	B_{12}, carnitine, copper, and zinc
Zonisamide (Zonegran)	Biotin, calcium, folic acid, inositol, B_1

Drug Muggers That Mug Vitamin B_6 (Pyridoxine)

Vitamin B_6 is important for mood, sleep, and the nervous system. If you become deficient, you could experience depression, insomnia, PMS, fatigue, anemia, seborrheic dermatitis, and elevated homocysteine (an inflammatory chemical that has been tied to heart disease). Some common meds that "mug" vitamin B_6 include:

* Amoxicillin

* Azithromycin

* Bumetanide

* Cephalosporin antibiotics

* Clarithromycin

* Dicloxacillin

* Doxycycline

* Enalapril and HCTZ

* Erythromycin

* Estrogen-containing drugs (hormone replacement therapy and birth control)

* Fluoroquinolone antibiotics (ciprofloxacin, levofloxacin, lomefloxacin, moxifloxacin)

* Furosemide

* Hydralazine

* Isoniazid

* Levonorgestrel

* Minocycline

* Penicillin

* Raloxifene

* Tetracycline

* Trimethoprim

Drug Muggers That Mug Vitamin B₉ (Folic Acid or Folate)

You need folic acid to make healthy red blood cells, which carry oxygen throughout your body. You also need it to make healthy DNA—your genetic structure. Without folic acid, every cell potentially suffers. Deficiencies of folic acid may ultimately result in the development of cancer, cervical dysplasia, atherosclerosis, birth defects, and depression. So if you're taking one of the following meds, you may need to supplement with some extra folic acid or an active body-ready form like 5-MTHF.

* Acid blockers (most, but not all)

* Anti-inflammatory drugs (most, but not all)

* Aspirin

* Carisoprodol

* Celecoxib

✳ Cholestyramine

✳ Estrogen-containing drugs (hormone replacement therapy and birth control)

✳ Glyburide and Metformin

✳ Ibuprofen

✳ Indomethacin

✳ Levonorgstrel

✳ Metformin

✳ Naproxen

✳ Nizatidine

✳ Oxycodone aspirin (percodan)

✳ Seizure meds (carbamazepine, ethosuximide, phenobarbital, phenytoin)

✳ Steroids (betamethasone, dexamethasone, methylprednisone, prednisone)

✳ Sulindac

✳ Triamterene/HCTZ (Dyazide, Maxzide)

✳ Valproic Acid

Drug Muggers That Mug B_{12} (Cyanocobalamin)

Vitamin B_{12} is important for energy and for your nervous system. When you run low on B_{12}, you feel tired and forgetful. You may become depressed, and you could develop tongue and mouth sores as well as low appetite, confusion, and memory loss. B_{12} shortages may lead you to experience easy bruising and peripheral neuropathy, that pins and needles sensation in your hands and feet. B_{12} drug muggers include:

* Acid blockers (nizatidine, omeprazole, ranitidine)

* Amoxicillin

* Azithromycin

* Cephalosporin antibiotics

* Colchicine

* Colestipol

* Dicloxacillin

* Estrogen-containing drugs (hormone replacement therapy and birth control)

* Famotidine

* Levofloxacin

* Metformin

* Norethindrone

* Phenytoin

* Sulfamethoxazole

* Tetracyline

* Trimethoprim

* Zidovudine

Drug Muggers That Mug Biotin

Biotin belongs to the B complex group of vitamins. It is produced in the intestines, so having a natural healthy camp of friendly bacteria is important in order for you to make biotin. Its most important role is to help us break down carbohydrates, fats, and proteins. People who have brittle nails or slow-growing, dull hair often utilize biotin supplements. Symptoms of deficiency could include balding, premature graying, depression, abnormal sensations on the skin, muscle aches, and inflammation of skin or membranes. You can find biotin in foods such as brewer's yeast, whole grains, strawberries, watermelon, grapefruit, legumes, egg yolks, bananas, and cauliflower. Dosage for supplementation ranges widely: *100–5,000 mcg daily.* The following are muggers of biotin:

✳ Alcohol

✳ Antibiotics—all of them are muggers; a few popular ones include: Amoxicillin, Cephalexin, Ciprofloxacin, Clarithromycin, Doxycycline, Levaquin, SMZ/TMP, Tetracycline, Z-packs

✳ Butalbital-containing drugs (Fioricet, Fiorinal)

✳ Seizure meds: carbamazepine (Tegretol), phenobarbital, phenytoin (Dilantin), zonisamide (Zonegran)

Drug Muggers That Mug Vitamin C (Ascorbic Acid)

Vitamin C is crucial for warding off infections and protecting your arteries. That's because C helps keep your capillaries strong, so that your entire cardiovascular system benefits from it. And because C concentrates in your adrenal glands, it's crucial for your energy levels. People who become deficient in C (a condition known as "scurvy") may develop bleeding gums, anemia, slow wound healing, muscle weakness, swollen and tender joints, constant infections, and even cancer. Here are some of C's most common muggers:

✳ Aspirin

✳ Bumetanide

✳ Carisoprodol with aspirin

✳ Dexamethasone

✳ Estrogen-containing drugs (hormone replacement therapy and birth control)

✳ Fluocinonide

✳ Fluticasone

✳ Furosemide

* Levonorgestrel

* Oxycodone/aspirin (Percodan)

* Steroids (methylprednisolone, prednisolone)

* Torsemide

* Triamcinolone

Drug Muggers That Mug Calcium

You need calcium to form strong bones and teeth, and to maintain blood pressure. Also, calcium helps make your muscles work properly and comfortably. Calcium deficiency could put you at greater risk for osteoporosis, muscle cramping, tooth decay, high blood pressure, heart disease, cancer, insomnia, and digestion problems. Take calcium supplements if your body's supply is being mugged by any of these meds:

* Acid reducers (famotidine, nizatidine)

* Butalbital-containing drugs

* Carbamazepine (Tegretol)

* Colchicine

* Digoxin

* Diuretics (bumetanide, furosemide)

* Laxatives

* Mineral oil

* Seizure meds (ethosuximide, methsuximide, phenobarbital, phenytoin, primidone)

* Steroids (dexamethasone, fluticasone, hydrocortisone, prednisone, triamcinolone)

* Triamterene/HCTZ (Dyazide, Maxzide)

Drug Muggers That Mug Coenzyme Q10

Coenzyme Q10 is a powerful antioxidant that is crucial to every cell of the human body because it makes ATP, the energy molecule required for normal blood sugar, proper heart function, muscle contraction, immune function, and brain health. Without adequate amounts, we would literally die. And as we age, the amount we make diminishes. Studies show that coenzyme Q10 improves angina pectoris, arrhythmias, high blood pressure, cholesterol issues, and energy levels. Food sources of coenzyme Q10 are not so appetizing to me, but include organ meats such as kidney, heart, and liver. Today there are many high-quality brands of coenzyme Q10 sold in health-food stores. It can reduce your risk for congestive heart failure, so it's ironic that meds used to lower cholesterol and blood pressure are on this list! Coenzyme Q10 can dramatically reduce the side effects you may get from beta blockers and statin cholesterol drugs. Here are the drug muggers for coenzyme Q10:

* Acebutolol

* Anti-psychotics (haloperidol, thioridazine)

* Atenolol

* Bisoprolol (Zebeta)

* Candesartan/HCTZ (Atacand HCT)

* Carvedilol (Coreg)

* Chlorpropamide

* Clomipramine (Anafranil)

* Clonidine

* Fenofibrate (Tricor)

* Gemfibrozil (Lopid)

* Glimepiride (Amaryl)

* Glipizide (Glucotrol)

* Glyburide (Diabeta, Glynase, Micronase)

* Glyburide/Metformin (Glucovance)

* Hydrochlorothiazide (HCTZ) and any drug containing HCTZ (Avapro HCT, Dyazide, Hyzaar, Maxzide, Micardis HCT)

* Indapamide (Lozol)

* Labetalol

* Methyldopa

* Metoprolol (Lopressor, Toprol XL)

* Nadolol (Corgard)

* Propafenone (Rhythmol)

* Propranolol

* Repaglinide (Prandin)

* Sotalol (Betapace)

* Statin cholesterol drugs (Advicor, Lescol, Lipitor, Mevacor, Pravastatin, Zocor)

* Tri-cyclic antidepressants (Amitriptyline, Desipramine, Doxepin, Imipramine, Nortriptyline)

Drug Muggers That Mug Vitamin D (Calciferol)

Most people get enough D from the sun because the sun's ultraviolet rays help our bodies make this hormone naturally. But some people don't get enough of the "sunshine" vitamin, so they need to supplement. Vitamin D is needed to make strong bones and teeth and to ward off cancer. In children, a deficiency could result in knock knees, bowed legs, spinal curvature, or dental problems. In adults, a deficiency could show up as osteoporosis, SAD (seasonal affective disorder), depression, rheumatic pains, muscle weakness, hip fracture, gradual loss of hearing, and even a higher risk of cancer, particularly prostate and breast cancer, according to some cutting-edge research. These OTC and prescription drugs can "mug" your D:

* Acid-reducing drugs (cimetidine, famotidine, ranitidine)

* Antacids

* Cholestyramine

* Colestipol

* Laxatives containing aluminum hydroxide or magnesium hydroxide

* Mineral oil

* Orlistat

* Seizure medication (carbamazepine, ethosuximide, phenytoin, primidone)

* Steroids (dexamethasone, fluticasone, hydrocortisone, methylprednisolone, prednisone)

Drug Muggers That Mug Magnesium

Magnesium contributes to better moods, higher energy levels, and a healthy heart. A deficiency of this vital mineral could result in more frequent headaches, muscle pain and tenderness, poor cardiovascular function, thicker blood, high blood pressure, asthma, osteoporosis, and PMS symptoms. Don't let these meds mug your magnesium:

* Blood pressure drugs containing hydrochlorothiazide (HCTZ)

* Cholestyramine

* Cyclosporine

* Digoxin

* Doxycycline

* Enalapril

* Estrogen-containing drugs (hormone replacement therapy and birth control)

* Furosemide

* Metolazone

* Minocycline

* Raloxifene

* Steroids (dexamethasone, fluticasone, methylprednisolone, prednisone)

* Tetracycline

Drug Muggers That Mug Potassium

Potassium is an electrolyte because it is "charged" and it helps with water balance and electrical circuitry in the body. When you run out (and it's easy to do if you have severe diarrhea, for example) or if you get mugged by a drug, you could develop problems all over your body. Potassium deficiency could result in heart rhythm abnormalities, high blood pressure, inadequate reflexes, muscle weakness, fatigue, confusion, constipation, osteoporosis, constant thirst, and ultimately heart disease. You can find it in many foods such as fresh fruits and vegetables, nuts, and dairy. Cantaloupes, spinach, and bananas are very high in potassium. Supplementation is okay; just get approval from your doctor. It's ironic, but many medications that are taken to reduce blood pressure are drug muggers of potassium! The following are drug muggers of potassium:

* Alcohol

* Aspirin

* Bisacodyl (Dulcolax)

* Bumetanide (Bumex)

* Butalbital compound/aspirin (Fiorinal)

* Caffeine

* Carisoprodal/aspirin (Soma compound)

* Colchicine

* Cyclosporine

* Dexamethasone

* Dicloxacillin

* Docusate/Casanthranol (Peri-Colace)

* Excessive salt intake

* Fluticasone (Flonase)

* Furosemide

* Hydralazine

* Hydrochlorothiazide (HCTZ) and any drug that contains HCTZ (Dyazide, Maxzide, etc.)

* Levodopa/Carbidopa

* Methyclothiazide

* Oxycodone/aspirin (Percodan)

* Steroids (methylprednisolone, prednisolone, prednisone)

* Valsartan and HCTZ (Diovan HCT)

Drug Muggers That Mug Selenium

Selenium is a trace mineral needed to help us make thyroid hormone and keep our immune systems working properly. Because it is often depleted from soil, it's possible to run out even if you don't take a drug mugger on the list below. Also, people with digestive or bowel problems will run out of this mineral. Deficiencies can lead to heart disease, exhaustion, hypothyroidism, and poor immune function. Some studies indicate that death rates from cancer (lung, colon, rectal, and prostate cancers) are lower among people with higher selenium intake. Food sources include nuts, tuna, turkey, beef, oatmeal, and vegetables. All steroids are drug muggers of selenium, including:

* Betamethasone

* Cortisone

✳ Dexamethasone

✳ Fluocinolone (Synalar cream)

✳ Fluticasone (Flonase)

✳ Fluticasone/Salmeterol (Advair)

✳ Methylprednisolone

✳ Prednisolone

Drug Muggers That Mug Zinc

Levels of this trace mineral decline as we age, plus our soils have become depleted of zinc in many parts of the world. Zinc deficiency is quite common; in fact, elderly people are usually deficient, as are alcoholics, vegetarians, and those with kidney or liver disease. Because zinc works in tandem with vitamin A, a deficiency could cause macular degeneration and blindness. Zinc is needed to make both insulin and thyroid hormone, so a deficiency could lead to diabetes and hypothyroidism, respectively. Zinc is a well-known immune protector, boosting activity of our T-lymphocytes, natural killer cells, and interleukin. Without enough zinc, we will get frequent colds or infections. And its final perk: Zinc boosts sex drive. See if you take any of the following drug muggers of zinc:

✳ Ace inhibitors: Benazepril (Lotensin), Enalapril (Vasotec), Lisinopril (Prinivil, Zestril), Ramipril (Altace)

✳ Acid blockers

✳ Alcohol

✳ Antacids

✳ Calcium supplementation, when done excessively

✳ Cholestyramine (Questran)

✳ Coffee

* Conjugated estrogens (Premarin or Prempro)

* Diuretics—some (but not all) are muggers, including Bumetanide and Furosemide

* Oral contraceptives and hormone replacement therapy (HRT)

* Raloxifene (Evista)

* Steroids

Drugs That Can Cause or Worsen Arthritis and Joint Pain

* Erectile dysfunction drugs

* Many stimulant drugs for attention deficit disorder

* Most vaccinations

* Osteoporosis drugs

* Some acid blockers

* Some antibiotics and antivirals

* Some blood pressure pills

* Statin cholesterol drugs

* Steroids (methylprednisolone, prednisone)

Drugs That Can Cause Hair Thinning or Loss

* Acid blockers (famotidine, omeprazole, ranitidine)

* Antidepressants (doxepin, fluoxetine)

* Any blood pressure drug containing hydrochlorothiazide (HCTZ)

* Benazepril

* Blood pressure (atenolol, betaxolol, metoprolol, nadolol, pindolol)

* Carbamazepine

* Chemotherapy drugs

* Colchicine

* Conjugated estrogens with medroxyprogesterone (Prempro)

* Diethylpropion

* Estrogen-containing drugs (hormone replacement therapy or birth control)

* Isotretinoin

* Medroxyprogesterone (Provera)

* Methyltestosterone

* Statin cholesterol drugs (atorvastatin, lovastatin, pravastatin, simvastatin)

* Tamoxifen

* Valproic acid, Divalproex sodium

* Valsartan

* Warfarin

Drugs That Can Cause Muscle Pain

* Acyclovir

* Antidepressants (buspirone, citalopram, fluoxetine, paroxetine, sertraline)

* Azathioprine

* Fibrate cholesterol drugs (fenofibrate, gemfibrozil)

* Interferon

* Isotretinoin

* Losartan

* Mefloquine

* Metformin

* Moexipril

* Norfloxacin

* Orlistat

* Osteoporosis drugs (bisphosphonates and calcitonin)

* Quinolone antibiotics (ciprofloxacin, ofloxacin)

* Raloxifene

* Salmeterol

* Sex pills (sildenafil, tadalafil, vardenafil)

* Some blood pressure pills (pindolol, propranolol)

* Some sleeping medications (zaleplon)

* Statin cholesterol drugs (atorvastatin, lovastatin, pravastatin, simvastatin)

* Steroids (betamethasone, dexamethasone, methylprednisone, prednisone)

* Zafirlukast

* Zolmitriptan

Drugs That Can Interfere with Sex Drive

* All headache medications containing butalbital

* Appetite suppressants (diethylpropion, phentermine)

* Diuretics (anything containing HCTZ or spironolactone)

* HIV drugs

✳ H2 acid blockers (cimetidine, ranitidine, etc.)

✳ Most antidepressants (duloxetine, escitalopram, fluoxetine, imipramine, nortriptyline, paroxetine, sertraline, venlafaxine, etc.)

✳ Most anti-epileptic drugs (carbamazepine, gabapentin, phenytoin, etc.)

✳ Most antipsychotics (olanzapine, promethazine, risperidone, etc.)

✳ Most cholesterol drugs (atorvastatin, fenofibrate, lovastatin, simvastatin, etc.)

✳ Most heart or blood pressure pills (atenolol, bisoprolol, clonidine, digoxin, diltiazem, doxazosin, metoprolol, verapamil)

✳ Most oral antifungal drugs (ketoconazole)

. . . and these popular drugs (brand name is in parentheses):

✳ Diazepam (Valium)

✳ Finasteride (Proscar)

✳ Fluvoxamine (Luvox)

✳ Medroxyprogesterone (Provera)

✳ Scopolamine patches (for seasickness) (Transderm-Scop)

✳ Tamoxifen (Nolvadex)

Drugs That Can Cause Weight Gain

✳ Acid-blocking drugs

✳ Birth control pills and shots

✳ Hormone replacement therapy

✳ Ibuprofen

* Insulin

* Lithium

* Mirtazapine

* Prednisone

* Psychiatric drugs (olanzapine, risperidone)

* Raloxifene

27

Food–Drug Interactions

* **Alcohol**—Any alcoholic beverage, including beer, interacts badly with certain types of medications.

    * *Antibiotics, especially metronidazole:* Avoid all alcoholic beverages as well as cough syrups; otherwise, you could face prolonged, repeated, and violent vomiting.

    * *Drugs that affect your brain, including antidepressants, antianxiety meds, antihistamines, antipsychotics, muscle relaxants, painkiller tablets and patches, seizure meds, sleeping pills, and tranquilizers:* These drugs slow down your nervous system, and so does alcohol. The combination can be dangerous or even deadly because it slows down heartbeat and breathing.

* **Caffeinated beverages, including coffee, soda, black tea, and energy drinks such as Red Bull**—Caffeine is a stimulant that speeds up your nervous system—and so do some drugs.

    * *Asthma medicines, inhaled bronchodilators, SSRI antidepressants, and stimulant drugs for attention deficit disorder:* All of these interact badly with caffeine, giving your nervous system a dangerous and potentially deadly jolt.

✳ **Cheese**—For some people, the tyramine in aged cheeses can interact with MAO inhibitors to cause a potentially fatal rise in blood pressure. Be aware that you risk this effect with Parmesan, Brie, Cheddar, Camembert, and Roquefort.

> ✳ *MAO inhibitors, including Parnate, Marplan, Nardil, and Emsam.* Note: MAO inhibitors should also not be taken with red wine, beer, fava beans, sauerkraut, and pepperoni.

✳ **Dairy products**—These are high in calcium, which can interfere with your body's ability to take up certain antibiotics.

> ✳ *Some antibiotics, including ciprofloxacin (Cipro), levofloxacin (Levaquin), and tetracycline:* Avoid dairy while on these antibiotics, or you may not get well. At the very least, separate your meds and your consumption of dairy by two hours.

✳ **Grapefruit and grapefruit juice**—The enzyme in grapefruit (naringen) prevents you from effectively breaking down some medications.

> ✳ *Statin cholesterol drugs, including simvastatin (Zocor) or felodipine (Plendil), nifedipine (Procardia), nisoldipine (Sular), cyclosporine (Sandimmune and Neoral):* Avoid grapefruit and its juice.

> ✳ *Other medications:* If you want to consume grapefruit and grapefruit juice, make sure you do so consistently, so your body gets used to it.

✳ **High-fiber foods**—High-fiber foods include apples, pears, carrots, berries, cabbage, and whole grains, including breads and cereals. Generally, they can blunt the effects of some medications, so if you're used to eating a lot of fiber, *don't* stop suddenly, or your medication may begin to work more intensely than you're used to. Taper off slowly or follow the suggestions below.

> ✳ *Acetaminophen:* High-fiber food can flatten the effects of this pain reliever, so eat your oatmeal a couple of hours away from taking your acetaminophen (Tylenol).

> ✳ *Antibiotics:* High-fiber foods could lessen the effect of your antibiotic by binding the medication, keeping it from your gut; or they might slow

down your absorption of it. Consume high-fiber foods at least four hours after your antibiotic dose.

✳ *Digoxin:* Bran cereals can slow down the absorption of this heart drug.

✳ **Vitamin K–rich foods**—Foods that are rich in K include green leafy vegetables, such as broccoli, spinach, kale, turnip greens, chard, asparagus, and red leaf lettuce. These foods promote blood clotting, which counters a blood-thinning drug's effect.

✳ *Blood-thinning drugs, including aspirin, Coumadin (warfarin), Plavix (clopidogrel), Lovenox, and Heparin:* Be consistent. A regular daily intake of green vegetables is so good for your health, most experts *don't* advise giving up greens entirely. Instead, keep your intake consistent, so that your doctor can adjust your drug dosage based on your vegetable intake.

Acknowledgments

I could not have completed this book without the patience and understanding of my loving family. Thank you for slipping food under the door to my office! Sam, you are my constant inspiration and my better half. My sweet Michael, can you even fall asleep without the clicking of keystrokes at night? Samara, you are my champion editor—making crunch time fun with your brilliant eyes. Rachel, you are one terrific researcher! Mom, Dad—thanks for everything. You all have given me more joy than I ever thought possible. I love you all so much!

Thank you David Brown, for giving me my start—I hope that I have made you proud. Steve Doyle at the *Orlando Sentinel*—I am eternally grateful: Because of you, the *Tribune* took an interest in me, syndicating my column for so many years.

Kim Pearson, you are simply the best! Just knowing that your skillful eyes are watching over my company is a deep sigh of relief. The world needs more people like you.

Thank you Susan Berg and Nancy Hancock for publishing this body of work, and for making my original book so much better. We share the same dreams, and I am grateful to you for recognizing my true intentions and spirit. I also want to thank Joe Tessitore, Mary Ellen O'Neill, and Laura Dozier for making my dreams come to life in the pages of the original version of *The 24-Hour Pharmacist*. You believed in me and took a chance, and for this I will be eternally grateful. My agent, Janis Vallely, you have hauled me all around New York in crazy taxi cabs (Oy!). What can I say, you are still an Angel for me and a huge blessing. Of course, Rachel Kranz, this book would not exist without your industrious writing skills, sensible input, and magic editorial eye. You are wonderful, and by now, I hope you have gotten some sleep.

I'd like to also thank some brilliant friends and technical geniuses whose pioneering work has eased the suffering of so many. You've freely given me your time and knowledge, and this gift will be paid forward to all who read my book. Doug Kaufmann from *Know The Cause* TV show, you are such a wonderful and kind man, your work has saved so many people from suffering. Thank you for lighting a fire under me and giving me such grand opportunities to spread the healing word alongside you. Michael Dresser, your 'solutions' will live long in me and I adore you. I am so honored to have a weekly voice on your radio show, *The Michael Dresser Show*. And Health Ranger Mike Adams: Mission accomplished! Because of NaturalNews.com, the world is healthier and people are wiser. You inspire me to do more, and I feel lucky to call you friend. Bless you always, all ways. The following unsung heroes and heroines don't have glitz or glamour, but in my book, you are the real celebrities:

Adam, Dr. Frederick Behringer, Dr. John F. Berg, Dr. Jeffrey Bland, Dr. Stanislaw Burzynski, Dr. Tsu-Tsair Chi, Dr. Martin Cohn, Al Czap, Sheila Dean, MS, RD, Dr. Robert Erickson, Dr. Edwin Ernest, Dr. Kenneth Fine, Marita Graves, Dr. Douglas Hall, Dr. Patrick Hanaway, Dr. Kathi Head, Virginia Hopkins, Dr. David Klein, Dr. Peter and Alena Langjsoen, Dr. Jay Lombard, Dr. Alison McAllister, Dr. Alan Miller, Lorraine Mobley, R.Ph., Dr. Richard Nesmith, James Paoletti, R.Ph., Dr. David and Leize Perlmutter, Azad Rastegar, Dr. Ray Sahelian, Barbara Brandon Schwartz, A.P., Dr. Dean Silver, Janet W. Slimak, LMT, Dr. Gregg Stern, Caroline Sutherland, Dr. Bear and Susan Walker, Dr. Brian Weiss, Dr. Julian and Connie Whitaker, Dr. James Wilson, Dr. Jonathan Wright, Dr. David Zava, and Phyllis Zermeno.

Crystal Wright, you are *my* Superstar. Your professional nudging and friendship have changed my life for the best. Craig Fuller, Gale Bensussan, and Kurt Proctor, your belief in me and support has meant so much. Also, Dean William Riffee and Art Wharton from the University of Florida. Go Gators!

Joni Keim, you took my aromatherapy chapter to another realm with your expertise and artful writing. It now shines with vibrant energy and allows us all to access our inner strength through aromas.

You all know what good deeds you did to make my life easier and this project better. I am thankful to have you in my life: Susan Anton, LMT, Bob Brewster, Linda Cirulli-Burton, Carol Colman, Christine Gallick, Sandy

Long, Daryl Collier, Sandy Ezell, Peggy Dace, Paul Franck, Bob Gruber, Susan Hussey, Dr. Jeffrey and Linda Pitts, Marta Aman, Barbara Close, Dr. George Graves, Danny Gurvich, Bill Cheek, Ed Oberhaus, Ryoichi Ojima, Sarah Hill, Gail Murphy, Jan and George Specht, Laurie Johnson, Mark Marinovich, Sherry McCullough, Sheila Still, Peter Awad, Sam at Elite, Joy Hannon, Terry May, Cindy Turner, Brooke Patillo, Mike Rose, Larry Whitler, the late Tony Rodriguez, Tyrone Russell, Carrie Scharf, and Rebecca Walker.

Resources

Recommended Reading

Abramson, John, MD. *Overdosed America: The Broken Promise of American Medicine.* (HarperCollins, 2004)

Adam. *The Path of the Dream Healer.* (Penguin, 2006) www.dreamhealer.com

Arem, Ridha MD., *The Thyroid Solution: A Mind-Body Program for Beating Depression and Regaining Your Emotional and Physical Health.* (Ballantine Books, August 2000)

Balch, Phyllis A., CNC. *Prescription for Nutritional Healing,* 4th Ed. (Avery, 2006)

Bland, Jeffrey, PhD. *The 20-Day Rejuvenation Diet Program.* (Keats, 1997)

Braverman, Eric. R., MD. *The Edge Effect.* (Sterling, 2004)

Brennan, Barbara Ann. *Hands of Light.* (Bantam, 1987)

Brownstein, David. *Iodine, Why You Need It, Why You Can't Live Without It,* 2nd Ed. (Medical Alternative Press, 2006)

Campbell, T. Colin, PhD, and Thomas M. Campbell II. *The China Study.* (BenBella Books, 2006)

Challem, Jack, Burton Berkson, MD, and Melissa Diane Smith. *Syndrome X–The Complete Nutritional Program to Prevent and Reverse Insulin Resistance.* (Wiley & Sons, 2000)

Crook, William G., MD, Hyla Cass, MD, Elizabeth B. Crook, and Carolyn Dean. *The Yeast Connection and Women's Health.* (Professional Books/Future Health, 2005)

Duke, James A., PhD. *The Green Pharmacy.* (St. Martin's Press, 1997)

Eden, Donna and David Feinstein. *Energy Medicine.* (Tarcher, 1998)

Fuller, DicQie, PhD, DSc. *The Healing Power of Enzymes.* (Forbes, 1998)

Gottschall, Elaine. *Breaking the Vicious Cycle—Intestinal Health Through Diet.* (Kirkton Press, 1994)

Groopman, Jerome, MD. *The Anatomy of Hope: How Some People Prevail in the Face of Illness.* (Random House, 2005)

Hyde, Stephen S. *Prescription Drugs for Half Price or Less.* (Bantam Books, 2005)

Janse, Allison and Charles Gerba, PhD. *The Germ Freak's Guide to Outwitting Colds and Flu.* (Health Communications, 2005)

Lawless, Julia. *The Illustrated Encyclopedia of Essential Oils.* (Element Books, 1995)

Lee, John R., MD, and Virginia Hopkins. *What Your Doctor May Not Tell You About Menopause.* (Warner Books, 1996)

Lee, John R., MD, David Zava, PhD, and Virginia Hopkins. *What Your Doctor May Not Tell You About Breast Cancer.* (Warner Books, 2003)

Lee, John R., MD, Jesse Hanley, MD, and Virginia Hopkins. *What Your Doctor May Not Tell You About Premenopause.* (Warner Books, 1999)

Levine, Barbara Hoberman. *Your Body Believes Every Word You Say.* (Words Work Press, 2000)

Lowell, Jax Peters. *Against the Grain.* (Henry Holt and Company, 1995)

Mitchell, Deborah R. and David Charles Dodson, MD. *The Diet Pill Guide.* (St. Martin's Press, 2002)

Murray, Michael, MD. *The Healing Power of Foods.* (Prima Publishing, 1993)

Myss, Caroline, PhD. *Anatomy of the Spirit.* (Crown Publishers, 1996)

Myss, Caroline, PhD. *Why People Don't Heal and How They Can.* (Harmony Books, 1997)

Northrup, Christiane, MD. *The Wisdom of Menopause.* (Bantam, 2003)

Northrup, Christiane, MD. *Women's Bodies, Women's Wisdom.* (Hay House, 2006)

O'Neill, Brian E. *The Testosterone Edge.* (Healthy Living Books, 2005)

Perlmutter, David, MD, and Carol Colman. *Raise a Smarter Child by Kindergarten.* (Bantam Dell, 2006)

Perlmutter, David, MD, and Carol Colman. *The Better Brain Book.* (Riverhead Books, 2004)

Pert, Candice B., and Deepak Chopra. *Molecules of Emotion: Why You Feel the Way You Feel.* (Scribner, 1997)

Pierce, Tanya Harter. *Outsmart Your Cancer: Alternative Non-Toxic Treatments That Work.* (Thoughtworks Publishing, Stateline, NV, 2004)

Rath, Matthias, MD. *Why Animals Don't Get Heart Attacks but People Do.* (MR Publishing, 2003)

Ravnskov, Uffe, MD, PhD. *The Cholesterol Myths: Exposing the Fallacy That Saturated Fat and Cholesterol Cause Heart Disease.* (New Trends Publishing, 2000)

Redmond, Geoffrey, MD. *The Hormonally Vulnerable Woman.* (HarperCollins, 2005)

Robbins, John. *The Food Revolution: How Diet Can Help Save Your Life and Our World.* (Conari Press, 2001)

Rogers, Sherry A., MD. *No More Heartburn.* (Kensington, 2000)

Roizen, Michael F., MD, and Mehmet C. Oz, MD. *You: The Owner's Manual.* (HarperCollins, 2005)

Rubin, Jordan S., N.MD, and Joseph Brasco, MD. *Restoring Your Digestive Health.* (Kensington, 2003)

Rubin, Jordan S., N.MD, PhD. *The Maker's Diet.* (Siloam, 2004)

Sapolsky, Robert M. *Why Zebras Don't Get Ulcers.* (W. H. Freeman and Company, 1994)

Seidman, Michael D., MD, FACS, and Marie Moneysmith. *Save Your Hearing Now.* (Warner Books, 2006)

Shames, Richard, MD, and Karilee Shames, PhD, RN. *Feeling Fat, Fuzzy or Frazzled?* (Penguin, 2005)

Shealy, C. Norman, MD, PhD. *The Illustrated Encyclopedia of Healing Remedies.* (Element Books, 1998)

Shippen, Eugene, MD, and William Fryer. *The Testosterone Syndrome.* (M. Evans and Co., 2001)

Somers, Suzanne. *Ageless: The Naked Truth About Bioidentical Hormones.* (Crown Publishers, 2006)

Sutherland, Caroline M. *The Body "Knows"—How to Tune into Your Body and Improve Your Health.* (Hay House, 2001)

Talbott, Shawn, PhD. *The Cortisol Connection.* (Hunter House Inc., 2002)

Teitelbaum, Jacob, MD. *From Fatigued to Fantastic.* (Avery, 2001)

Tolle, Eckhart. *A New Earth.* (Penguin, 2005)

Tolle, Eckhart. *The Power of Now.* (Namaste Publishing, 1997)

Weil, Andrew. *Eight Weeks to Optimum Health, Rev. Ed.: A Proven Program for Taking Full Advantage of Your Body's Natural Healing Power.* (Knopf, 2006)

Weil, Andrew. *Healthy Aging: A Lifelong Guide to Your Physical and Spiritual Well-Being.* (Knopf, 2005)

Weiss, Brian L., MD. *Mirrors of Time.* (Hay House, 2002)

Weiss, Brian L., MD. *Through Time into Healing.* (Simon & Schuster, 1992)

Whitaker, Julian, MD. *Dr. Whitaker's Guide to Natural Healing: America's Leading Wellness Doctor Shares His Secrets for Lifelong Health!* (Three Rivers Press, 1996)

Whitaker, Julian, MD. *The Whitaker Wellness Weight Loss Program.* (Rutledge Hill Press, 2006)

Williamson, Marianne. *A Return to Love: Reflections on the Principles of a Course in Miracles.* (HarperCollins, 1992)

Wilson, James L., ND, DC, PhD. *Adrenal Fatigue: The 21st Century Stress Syndrome.* (Smart Publications, 2001)

Wright, Jonathan. *Natural Hormone Replacement for Women Over Forty-Five.* (Smart Publications, 1995)

Young, Robert O., PhD, and Shelley Redford Young. *The pH Miracle.* (Warner Books, 2002)

CDs and DVDs

Adam. Dream Healer: Visualizations for Self-Empowerment.

www.dreamhealer.com This is a DVD narrated by Adam, and it outlines fourteen powerful visualizations. I really like this DVD, and you can play it anytime. It teaches you how to "see" yourself heal through creative imagery.

Byrne, Rhonda. The Secret DVD. *(Beyond Words, 2006)*

Positive thinking helps you feel better. This interesting movie teaches you how to stay in the positive and learn about Laws of Attraction.

Dyer, Wayne W. The Power of Intention. *Audio CDs. (Hay House, 2004)*

www.drwaynedyer.com

Franco, Lisa Lynne, and George Tortorelli. Love and Peace. *(*Lavender Sky Records, 1997)

Halpern, Steven.
www.innerpeacemusic.com Halpern's music helps you relax, reduce stress, sleep better, and connect with your spiritual essence. His music is designed to reorganize your brain waves in a positive manner.

Thompson, Dr. Jeffrey. Brainwave Suite.
www.unwind.com or call 888-4-UNWIND. $28.
This is a set of four CDs that uses inaudible pulses of sound, based on brain maps, to trigger your brain to produce the alpha, theta, delta, or alpha-theta brain states. Choose your CD based on whether you want to feel relaxed, intuitive, sleepy, or fully awake.

Tolle, Eckhart. The Power of Now, Stillness Speaks, *and* A New Earth: Awakening Your Life's Purpose.
www.eckharttolle.com These are audio versions of his books—try them if you live on the go!

Virtue, Doreen. Chakra Clearing.
www.angeltherapy.com A CD designed to manipulate energy patterns, giving you a sense of vitality and wellness.

Weiss, Brian, MD. Mirrors of Time.
www.brianweiss.com
The CD contains the actual regression techniques Dr. Weiss uses with his patients. Now you can go back through time and recall past events that may have led to symptoms or difficulties in the present time.

Aromatherapy

Oshadhi USA
www.oshadhiusa.com 707-763-0662 This company harvests their plants from all over the world with a commitment to organic and sustainable harvesting. Their oils are authentic, unlike those of many companies who dilute them. Oshadhi offers fantastic synergistic blends of oils for all types of purposes. You can get lost in their website for hours.

Primavera Life
www.primaveralife.com Offers worldwide distribution and sales off their website with headquarters based in Germany. This company is committed to purity and quality and cultivates their plants from the purest soils in the world. You can email them at info@primavera-life.de.

Cosmetics and Skin Care Resources

Aminocare Lotion and Cream
www.aminocare.com 800-856-8006 Formulated by an internationally known researcher and holistic cancer specialist, Dr. Stanislaw Burzynski, this beauty breakthrough alters your genes and switches off the ones that age you. For more information on his cancer clinic, visit www.cancermed.com or call 713-335-5697.

Aubrey Organics
www.aubrey-organics.com 800-282-7394 They make a complete line of skin care essentials, soaps, and shampoos sold widely at most health-food stores and online.

Blue Lagoon Iceland
www.bluelagoon.com Yes, Iceland! I recommend you go there at least once in your life. Their incredible Blue Lagoon geothermal water, a hot spring, contains healing silica mud, minerals, and algae, which are soothing and helpful for all kinds of skin problems, even psoriasis. If you can't fly there, go online and see their silica-infused beauty products.

The Body Shop
www.bodyshop.com You'll see this store in lots of malls and shopping districts—their bath, body, and makeup line is very natural.

Botox Injection
www.botoxcosmetic.com You can go on their website to learn more about Botulinum toxin, the "pretty" poison that people use to erase wrinkles and frown lines.

Bremenn Research Labs
www.hylexin.com 800-621-9553 They make Hylexin—the undereye cream that removes dark circles.

Dermalogica
www.dermalogica.com 310-900-4000 They sell to fine salons where you can buy their products (not direct to consumer). They make a nice acne mask, the Anti-Bac Cooling Masque, among other wonderful products.

Enzymedica
www.enzymedica.com E-mail: request@enzymedica.com 888-918-1118 They make terrific high-quality enzymes. A basic one is called Digest, but they have a full range of enzymes for all sorts of conditions.

HairMax
www.lasercomb.net This is a "laser" hair brush that thickens hair. It used to be offered only in salons.

Ideal Image Laser Hair Removal
www.idealimage.com They specialize in permanently removing unwanted hair using laser technology.

Jan Marini Skin Research
www.janmarini.com 800-347-2223 She makes a supercool eyelash builder and other innovative products that utilize alpha hydroxy acids and a skin-loving form of vitamin C.

Kinerase

www.kinerase.com E-mail: kinerasesupport@kinerase.com 800-321-4576

Klein-Becker

www.strivectin.com 800-919-9715 They make the cream StriVectin-SD, which they advertise as being "better than Botox."

Naturopathica

www.naturopathica.com E-mail: service@naturopathica.com 800-592-7995 They are committed to using only the highest-quality botanicals from around the world in their complete line of skin and body care products. They make unique eye creams that reduce puffiness and dark circles (Coneflower Eye Recovery Gel and Vitamin K Eye Cream), and my readers tell me that their Arnica Muscle and Joint Bath and Body Oil helps ease sore muscles and minor arthritic pain.

Purist Company

www.purist.com Australian based: + 61 2 9420 7400 They use natural botanical extract for their makeup and skin care line, "certified organic" where possible.

Restylane

www.restylane.com An injectable "filler" that some women use in their lips, laugh lines, and under eyes.

Safe Cosmetic Organization

www.safecosmetics.org This website can tell you if a beauty company has signed a document promising not to use harmful chemicals.

Sephora

www.sephora.com 877-SEPHORA (or 877-737-4672) Picture a *huge* cosmetic and skin care store that you can get lost in for six hours straight! They are found in many cities in the U.S., but if there's not one in yours, go online.

Skin Deep

www.ewg.org/reports/skindeep This website allows you to assess the safety of personal care items and cosmetics. It is a project of the Environmental Working Group, and they provide in-depth information on more than 7,000 ingredients that are found in our bathroom drawers. You can find out how safe your favorite products are, like shampoos, lip balms, sunscreens, deodorants, lotion, cleansers, and nail polish. This website actually lists products of highest concern to lowest concern.

SkinMedica

www.skinmedica.com They sell Retinol Complex, a vitamin A–derived formula (similar to prescription Retin-A) that helps to ease fine lines and improve the overall architecture of your skin. Go to their home page and click on "find a physician" to find a doctor you can buy it from.

Vaniqa

www.vaniqa.com This prescription cream slows the growth of unwanted facial hair after about six months of use.

Zia Natural Skincare

www.zianatural.com 800-334-SKIN

Foods

Gluten Free Mall

www.glutenfreemall.com 800-986-2705

Lucy's Kitchen Shop

lucyskitchen.com or scdkitchen.com E-mail: lucy@lucyskitchenshop.com 888-484-2126 This is where you order almond flour and get recipes for the Specific Carbohydrate diet mentioned in Chapter 14. Great for diabetics and people with neurological or gastrointestinal problems.

Madhava

www.madhavahoney.com A source for agave syrup.

Sweet Cactus Farms

www.sweetcactusfarms.com A source for agave syrup.

Whole Foods Market

www.wholefoodsmarket.com This unique health supermarket offers meats, fish, and poultry that are free of hormones and antibiotics. They have aisles of specialty natural and organic foods/produce and other personal care items/cosmetics that promise to be free of harmful additives, colorants, sweeteners, dyes, and other toxic chemicals. Their website lists all the chemicals that you will NOT find in their store. Shop with confidence at Whole Foods. If there isn't one close to home, you can shop securely online at their website. Whole Foods supports local growers.

Labs and Testing

Billings Ovulation Method

www.billings-ovulation-method.org

Doctor's Data, Inc.

www.doctorsdata.com E-mail: inquiries@doctorsdata.com 3755 Illinois Avenue, St. Charles, IL 60174-2420 800-323-2784 FAX: 630-587-7860

Dr. John Lee

www.johnleemd.com E-mail: info@johnleemd.com 16612 Burke Lane, Huntington Beach, CA 92647 877-375-3363 FAX: 714-848-8311 Right up to the moment of his death in 2003, John R. Lee, MD, dedicated his life to helping people overcome health issues related to hormone imbalances. He worked tirelessly to bring awareness to millions of women that there are safe, natural alternatives to synthetic hormones and their disturbing side effects. Men and women can order hormonal test kits from this site to help determine their levels of DHEA, cortisol, estrogen, testosterone, and much more. No doctor required; they sell directly to consumer.

EnteroLab.com
www.enterolab.com 10875 Plano Road, Suite 123, Dallas, TX 75238 972-686-6869 Specialized stool testing for gluten and other food sensitivities and gastrointestinal disorders. Dr. Kenneth Fine, founder and director of EnteroLab.com and the non-profit Intestinal Health Institute (www.intestinalhealth.org), is a leading expert in GI health. You don't need to have a doctor order these specialized tests. EnteroLab.com is willing to sell their test kits directly to the public.

Genova Diagnostics
www.gdx.net 63 Zillicoa Street, Asheville, NC 28801 800-522-4762 FAX: 828-252-9303

Hemex Laboratories
www.hemex.com 800-999-CLOT (2568) They specialize in a wide variety of blood testing and can find out how "thick" your blood is and how well it coagulates. They offer other exciting blood panels.

Meridian Valley Laboratory
www.meridianvalleylab.com E-mail: info@meridianvalleylab.com 801 SW 16th, Suite 126, Renton, WA 98055 425-271-8689 FAX: 425-271-8674 They offer a broad range of labs, including saliva, blood, and 24-hour urine panels. They are also willing to sell their hormone kits directly to consumers. Call for pricing.

Metametrix Clinical Laboratory
www.metametrix.com E-mail: inquiries@metametrix.com 4855 Peachtree Industrial Blvd., Suite 201, Norcross, GA 30092 800-221-4640 FAX: 770-441-2237

Tahoma Clinic
www.tahomaclinic.com Founded by international lecturer and author Dr. Jonathan Wright, the Tahoma Clinic focuses on disease prevention and treatment by natural biochemical and bioenergetic means. Dr. Wright has developed the use of bioidentical estrogens and the proper use of DHEA, and I consider him one of the best physicians of our time.

ZRT Laboratory
www.zrtlab.com E-mail: info@zrtlab.com 8605 SW Creekside Place, Beaverton, OR 97008 866-600-1636 FAX: 503-466-1636 This is a great lab for at-home saliva and

blood-spot tests that you can order yourself without a doctor. Their Comprehensive Hormone Profile test measures your levels of estrogen, testosterone, cortisol, DHEA, and thyroid, among others. Their report is easy to read, and you can take it to any doctor for evaluation.

Organizations

American Association of Retired Persons (AARP)
www.aarp.org 888-OUR-AARP (888-687-2277)

American Board of Hypnotherapy
www.abh-abnlp.com 888-823-4823

American Board of Medical Specialties
www.abms.org 866-275-2267 (866-ASK-ABMS) This website can tell you whether your doctor is board certified.

American College for the Advancement of Medicine (ACAM)
24411 Ridge Route, Suite 115, Laguna Hills, CA 92653 949-309-3520
www.acam.org

American College of Obstetricians and Gynecologists
www.acog.org

American Council of Hypnotist Examiners
www.hypnotistexaminers.org E-mail: hypnotismla@earthlink.net 818-242-1159

American Sleep Apnea Association (ASAA)
www.sleepapnea.org

The Broda O. Barnes, MD, Research Foundation Inc.
www.brodabarnes.org Great resource for thyroid information.

Centers for Disease Control
www.cdc.gov You can find out what drugs have been approved, including generics.

Clinical Pharmacology
www.clinicalpharmacology.com A great reference for clinicians on medications and herbals.

Federation of State Medical Boards
www.docinfo.org This is the website mentioned in Chapter 15 that sells reports outlining any disciplinary actions against a physician.

Hospice Foundation of America
www.hospicefoundation.org 800-854-3402

Institute of Functional Medicine (IFM)
www.functionalmedicine.org 800-228-0622
4411 Point Fosdick Drive NW, Suite 305, P.O. Box 1697, Gig Harbor, WA 98335

National Guild of Hypnotists
www.ngh.net E-mail: ngh@ngh.net 603-429-9438

National Institutes of Health
www.nih.gov Bethesda, Maryland

National Sleep Foundation
www.sleepfoundation.org

Natural Products Association
www.naturalproductsassoc.org

Sleepcenters.org
They'll help you find a sleep center close to your home.

Plan B

www.go2planB.com
Information on Plan B birth control.

Products

AntiSnore Therapeutic Ring
www.antisnore.com

Aubrey Organics
www.aubrey-organics.com 800-282-7394 A very natural beauty product line widely available at natural health-food stores and online.

Aveda
www.aveda.com 866-823-1425 They make a line of environmentally friendly skin-care and bath products sold at fine salons and online.

Bath and Body Works
www.bathandbodyworks.com They make a nice Energizing Body Wash and lots of special "me time" pampering bath and body products.

CPAP machines
www.cpap.com 800-356-5221

emWave
www.emwave.com 800-450-9111 The antistress toy: a small handheld biofeedback device that helps you train yourself to balance your heart rhythm by feeling positive emotions, mentioned in Chapter 2.

Head Spa Massager
www.gadgetuniverse.com 800-429-1139 Gadget Universe sells an innovative product called the Head Spa Massager that fits over your head and vibrates to relieve headache pain. The site also offers a bunch of other very neat, unique gadgets.

Juvent 1000
www.juvent.com They sell the Juvent 1000, a device for people who have osteoporosis.

MIGRA-CAP International
www.migracap.com E-mail: sales@migracap.com This South Wales company produces a unique headcover that combines pressure, coldness, and darkness to relieve your head pain. It costs about $75 (U.S.) when you buy it online.

Myself Bladder Trainer
www.deschutesmed.com www.dependonmyself.com E-mail: info@dependonmyself.com 800-323-1363 This biofeedback training device helps you with those embarrassing leaks by training your bladder to stay shut. You can buy "Myself" at Walgreens, The Medicine Shoppe, Drug Emporium, and other pharmacies as well as online.

Noiselezz
www.nosnorezone.com

Pillar Procedure
www.pillarprocedure.com Helps with snoring and is described in Chapter 8.

Snore Free nose clip
Sold online through various websites, but I found the best prices on Ebay.com.

Snoreclipse
www.snoreclipse.com 877-662-9500

Somnoguard
www.nosnorezone.com

Spa Petite

www.therabath.com A paraffin wax bath mentioned in Chapter 17 that offers drug-free
   pain relief for joint pain in your hands and feet.

Vigorelle

www.vigorelle.com A topical sex cream for women.

Wise Woman Herbals

www.wisewomanherbals.com 541-895-5172 This website offers a vitamin E suppository
   that helps with vaginal dryness and other high-quality nutritionals using very pure ingredients and essential oils.

Zestra

www.zestraforwomen.com A topical sex cream for women, sold at chain pharmacies and
   most major retailers.

Salt

Gourmet Salts

www.seasalt.com E-mail: info@seasalt.com 800-353-7258 SaltWorks has all sorts of exotic and delicious salts from around the world. I think their Bamboo Salt Sampler by
   Artisan is supercool! It comes with twenty-four exotic and uniquely colored natural
   salts extracted from seas all over the world, including the Himalayas, Peru, France, the
   Mediterranean, and Hawaii. Cost: $115.

Redmond RealSalt

www.realsalt.com E-mail: mail@realsalt.com 800-367-7258

Supplements

Alkalol

www.alkalolcompany.com E-mail: info@alkalolcompany.com 800-967-4904

Allergy Research Group

www.allergyresearchgroup.com E-mail: info@allergyresearchgroup.com 800-545-9960

Canada RNA Biochemical Inc.

www.canadarna.com 866-287-4986 FAX: 866-287-8671 They make the Boluoke brand of
   Lumbrokinase—used in clinical trials and sold through physicians' offices. Lumbrokinase is an over-the-counter clot buster.

Country Life

www.country-life.com They have an extensive product line of all sorts of nutraceuticals sold
   at natural health-food stores.

Desert Burn
www.desertburn.com E-mail: help@desertburn.com 919-783-4049
They sell the weight-loss supplement hoodia.

Dr. Chi's Products
www.chi-health.com E-mail: veinlite@mindspring.com 800-457-5708 Dr. Tsu-Tsair Chi,
　N.D., Ph.D., makes Eastern-blend herbal products like Myomin and Super X.

Emerita's Response Cream
www.emerita.com 800-648-8211 Emerita makes a soothing progesterone cream that is free
　of parabens (an additive that mimics the effects of estrogen).

Enzymatic Therapy
www.enzy.com 800-783-2286

Enzymedica
www.enzymedica.com E-mail: info@enzymedica.com 888-918-1118 These people are en-
　zyme experts who offer a complete and innovative line of quality enzymes sold at health-
　food stores and online. Their products are 100 percent vegan.

Florastor
www.florastor.com This is a terrific probiotic supplement (Saccharomyces boullardii)
　that helps prevent antibiotic-induced diarrhea (mentioned in Chapter 18).

Future Formulations, LLC
www.futureformulations.com 800-357-5027 This is Dr. James Wilson's line of adrenal fa-
　tigue and other nutritional supplements.

Garden of Life
www.gardenoflife.com 561-748-2477 Dr. Jordan Rubin makes Primal Defense and other
　premium whole-food supplements.

Green Health
www.greenhealth.co.nz E-mail: enquiries@greenhealth.co.nz This is your New Zealand
　source for GMP-certified green-lipped mussel extract.

Healthy Origins
www.healthyorigins.com Extensive product line—I like their Coenzyme Q10, but they
　have other good products as well.

Hoodia Gordonii Plus
www.hoodiagordoniiplus.com 800-238-1413 HoodiSpray www.hoodispray.com 800-941-
　4171 HoodiSpray is a form of hoodia gordonii, an herb for weight management, manufac-
　tured by Prime Life Nutriceuticals. Certified to be authentic.

HoodiThin

www.hoodithin.com 800-310-6013 Another quality form of hoodia gordonii, an herb for weight management. Manufactured by Prime Life Nutriceuticals. Certificate of authenticity is on the website.

Illness Is Optional

www.illnessisoptional.com 888-794-4325 This is one source to buy Iodoral, a tablet form of iodine that provides iodine-iodide complex, 12.5 mg per tablet.

iNutritionals

www.inutritionals.com E-mail: info@inutritionals.com 800-530-1982 They sell Dr. Perlmutter's Brain Sustain, which supports overall brain health and memory.

Jarrow

www.jarrow.com They have an extensive product line of all sorts of nutraceuticals sold at natural health-food stores. They also make a nice brand of coconut oil.

JHS Natural Products

www.jhsnp.com E-mail: jhsinfo@jhsnp.com 888-330-4691 They make Reishi Gano 161 and VPS Coriolus versicolor mushroom extract. Mushrooms are powerful immune boosters.

Kaneka Texas Corporation

www.kanekatexas.com 800-526-3223 One of the world's leading sources of Coenzyme Q10.

Life Enhancement

www.life-enhancement.com 800-543-3873 They make PropeL, a sexual enhancement supplement formulated by Dr. Jonathan Wright.

Life Extension Foundation

www.lef.org 800-544-4440 Life Extension has offered a generous gift valued at $30. Call toll-free anytime or e-mail and ask for the free six-month subscription to *Life Extension* magazine. Be sure to include your mailing address in your e-mail. You will love it! Mention *The 24-Hour Pharmacist* coupon code CMX01X to receive this gift.

Life Line Foods

www.lifelinefoods.com 800-216-3231 They make Mangosteen Complete, a whole-foods berry juice that also contains noni and goji juices. Very comprehensive.

Liv Kit

www.liv.com/home.html Olivia Newton-John's Liv Kit is a breast self-examination tool sold at most pharmacies and online. The product is really nothing more than two thin sheets of soft, latex-free polyurethane filled with liquid lubricant. During a self-exam, you get better sensitivity because it's easier to feel. This improves your ability to detect potential trouble spots. Sells for about $20.

Metabolic Maintenance
www.metabolicmaintenance.com 800-772-7873 As a reader bonus, they will give you 20 percent off your total purchase price if you buy directly from them. Just mention my name, or tell them you've read *The 24-Hour Pharmacist*.

Metagenics
www.metagenics.com 800-692-9400 Metagenics products are available through healthcare professionals. You have to call them or go online to their website to find a practitioner in your area. You can also ask your doctor to fax them his or her license and order supplements for you.

Morningstar Minerals
www.msminerals.com They make Energy Boost Plus: D-Ribose with Fulvic Minerals, mentioned in Chapter 2 and also fabulous for chronic fatigue and fibromyalgia.

Nanogreens
www.biopharmasci.com E-mail: support@biopharmasci.com 877-772-4362

Natrol
www.natrol.com Extensive product line. I like their glucomannan.

Natural Factors
www.naturalfactors.com E-mail: us_custservice@naturalfactors.com 800-322-8704

Nature Made
www.naturemade.com 800-276-2878 They produce a complete line of nutraceuticals. I especially like their SAMe.

Nature's Way
www.naturesway.com I mentioned their Calcium Complex Bone Formula in Chapter 3, their glucomannan in Chapter 14, and their Antioxidant Formula in Chapter 18.

Nordic Naturals
www.nordicnaturals.com E-mail: info@nordicnaturals.com 800-662-2544 They specialize in pure fish oils, cod-liver oil, and other essential fatty acids.

Orange Peel Enterprises, Inc.
www.greensplus.com 800-643-1210 They make GREENS+, mentioned in Chapter 18.

Physician Formulas

www.physicianformulas.com 877-225-2466 They make Serrapeptase, Lyprinol, and other innovative products formulated by Dr. Ray Sahelian, MD.

Rath Vitamins

www.drrathvitamins.com www.drrathresearch.org E-mail: contact@drrath.com 800-624-2442 This is the cardiologist who makes Epican Forte, mentioned in Chapter 2.

Solgar

www.solgar.com E-mail: productinformation@solgar.com 877-SOLGAR-4

Sound Nutrition

www.soundnutrition.com 800-437-6863 A division of Thorne Research, this company sells direct to consumer and makes a high-quality, pure, hypo-allergenic dietary supplement line sold at Whole Foods markets and other health-food stores. They make high-quality 5-MTHF.

Swanson Health Products

www.swansonvitamins.com 800-824-4491 They have a huge selection of supplements that you can buy, including interesting formulations like Ultimate Stress Pills, which are helpful if you have anxiety or insomnia, and MSR-3, which is a potent immune booster containing arabinogalactin combined with mushroom extracts. This is a terrific website for information and articles, too.

Thompson Nutrition

www.thompsons.co.nz A New Zealand–based company that makes high-quality supplements, including Multidophilus, a probiotic.

Thorne Research, Inc.

www.thorne.com E-mail: info@thorne.com 800-228-1966 This premier nutraceutical company sells their supplements internationally. They are TGA-certified and GMP-certified—this means very high quality. I like that they don't make tablets; rather, they make capsules, powders, and liquids, which are so much easier to absorb. You have to call them with a practitioner's name. You can ask your doctor to fax them his or her license so your doctor can order supplements for you.

Triple Whammy

www.triplewhammycure.com This is where you can buy the hot-flash supplement called Menopause Transition with black cohosh mentioned in Chapter 13 on hot flashes. Dr. David Edelberg and Heidi Hough wrote an interesting book entitled *The Triple Whammy Cure* (Free Press, December 2005), and there is more information on this website.

Valen Labs, Inc.
www.corvalenm.com 866-267-8253 They make another brand of D-Ribose sold under the
  brand of CORvalenM, which is very helpful for the heart and for fatigue.

Vitamin Research Products
www.vrp.com E-mail: customerservice@vrp.com 800-877-2447

Vitamin World
www.vitaminworld.com E-mail: info@vitaminworld.com 800-228-4533

Xymogen
www.xymogen.com E-mail: info@xymogen.com 800-647-6100

Tea

Essiac
www.essiac-canada.com 561-585-7111 You can buy Essiac Herbal Supplement Extract Formula from them and learn how the powerful botanicals in this tea support good health
  and possibly prevent cancer.

Flora's Natural Health Products
www.florahealth.com 800-446-2110 Here's the website for Flor-Essence Herbal Tea Blend,
  an Essiac tea blend.

The Republic of Tea
www.republicoftea.com

Revolution
www.revolutiontea.com

Water

Essentia
www.essentiawater.com

Evamor
www.liveacidfree.com

Fiji
www.fijiwater.com

Zephyrhills
www.zephyrhillswater.com

Websites

Cohen, Suzy

www.DearPharmacist.com My website devoted to helping you get on the right track to health. You can sign up to receive my free syndicated column delivered to your e-mail once a week, discussing matters of health that could be important to you. The latest-breaking news health stories are on the home page.

Consumer Labs

www.consumerlab.com 914-722-9149 They evaluate supplements for quality, and you can view this published information right off their website if you subscribe for about $27 a year. I like that they do independent testing because it helps consumers and healthcare professionals evaluate nutritional products.

Emoto, Masaru

www.masaru-emoto.net and www.hado.net A cool website and book by the author of *Messages from Water*, showing that our words and thoughts affect molecules of water.

Gottschall, Elaine

www.breakingtheviciouscycle.com The late Elaine Gottschall, author of *Breaking the Vicious Cycle*, created this great resource for the Specific Carbohydrate diet mentioned in Chapter 14, a diet for people who suffer from Crohn's, colitis, celiac, and other inflammatory bowel diseases.

Hopkins, Virginia

www.virginiahopkinshealthwatch.com She is the coauthor of *What Your Doctor May Not Tell You About Premenopause*. She has terrific information for your hormonal health and much more.

Lee, John R., MD

www.johnleemd.com The late Dr. Lee wrote many books in the *What Your Doctor May Not Tell You* series about all sorts of women's issues. He coined the term "estrogen-dominance" and utilized progesterone in his practice.

Perlmuter, David

www.brainrecovery.com Dr. Perlmutter wrote *The Better Brain Book* and *Raise a Smarter Child by Kindergarten*. He's a brilliant neurologist, pioneering new and complementary ways to improve brain health, memory disorders, and other debilitating neurological disorders.

Schlesinger, David, L.Ac.

www.modernherbalist.com/betaine.html This is a terrific, easy-to-understand resource for herbals and other nutrients. I particularly like the discussion on acid and its beneficial role in the gut.

United States Food and Drug Administration
www.fda.gov

U.S. Pharmacopeia
www.usp.org

Whitaker, Julian, MD
www.whitakerwellness.com 800-488-1500 He is a fantastic resource for alternative health advice, along with sensible conventional advice—the best of both worlds. Dr. Whitaker runs the Wellness Institute and offers a *Health & Healing* newsletter subscription ($50 a year) that you can receive by e-mail, which gives you health advice. His website is packed with free health solutions as well as health products and his eye-opening books.

Wilson, James, DC, ND, PhD
www.adrenalfatigue.org 888-ADRENAL (888-237-3625) He is the author of *Adrenal Fatigue: The 21st Century Stress Syndrome*, a fabulous resource for people who are tired and dealing with multiple symptoms. He is dedicated to providing solutions to today's health problems of stress, poor nutrition, and lowered immunity.

Wright, Jonathan, MD
www.tahomaclinic.com One of the world's leading experts on bioidentical hormone replacement, founder of the Tahoma Clinic (which offers natural preventive therapies), and author of many books including *Natural Hormone Replacement for Women Over Forty-Five*.

The Yeast Connection
www.yeastconnection.com Dr. William Crook's website; he's a leading expert on candida.

Zava, David, PhD
www.zrtlab.com Zava, another leading expert in hormone therapy, is the founder of ZRT Laboratory. He is also coauthor of *What Your Doctor May Not Tell You About Breast Cancer*.

Buying Prescriptions and Personal Care Products Without Leaving the House

1. You can send a friend or family member in to purchase your medication, but they will be asked a few personal questions at the register before your medicine is handed over.
2. Shop with your local community pharmacy or compounding pharmacy. They often deliver right to your home, and they offer personalized service. If you need home medical supplies (like a cane tip, crutch, or new walker), independent pharmacies are ideal because they specialize in home medical equipment and cater to consumers who need extra attention. To find one, visit **www.irxplus.com** and then click on "Find an independent pharmacy." You can also call the Professional Compounding Centers of America and ask, at (800) 331-2498.

3. Buy online. I know many of you are nervous about this, and with all the bogus pharmacies and counterfeit pills sold off the Internet, who could blame you? But trust me; there are respectable pharmacies that offer safe and secure shopping. Big-name retailers would not risk your security, and they all encrypt credit card information. Buying online reduces stress—you don't have to wait in long pharmacy lines, breathe in germs during cough and cold season, or risk embarrassment when the cashier hollers out, "Price check, aisle 6, Preparation H" or "Manager, is Vagisil still buy one, get one?"

Here are some tips to help you shop online securely:

Only buy from online pharmacies that have VIPPS certification, another level of authenticity. The VIPPS emblem will be clearly visible on the home page. You can get your medications with just a few clicks of a button. Most pharmacies will deliver everything to your door for a small shipping fee, including prescriptions, unless they are Class II narcotics or other non-shippable drugs.

If you are concerned about keying in a credit card number on the Internet, don't worry. If you call your bank (or go to its website), they can issue a temporary credit card number (a fake one) that you can use on the computer. Banks offer this service for free so consumers can shop online safely without ever revealing their true credit card number.

There are others, but here are a few reputable, big-name pharmacies that you can trust:

www.albertsons.com

www.costco.com

www.cvs.com

www.drugstore.com

www.duanereade.com

www.kerrdrug.com

www.kmart.com

www.kroger.com

www.medicineshoppe.com

www.riteaid.com

www.samsclub.com

www.target.com

www.walgreens.com

www.walmart.com

www.winn-dixie.com

References

Part I: Above the Waist
Chapter 1: Overcoming Fatigue:
From Stupor Woman to Super Woman

Agarwal, R., Diwanay, S., Patki, P. et al. Studies on Immunomodulatory Activity of Witha-nia somnifera (Ashwagandha). *J Ethnopharmacol.* Oct 1999;67(1):27–35.

Blumenthal et al. *The Complete German Commission E Monographs.* Integrative Medicine Communications; Boston, MA; 1998.

Boone, K. Withania—Indian Ginseng. *Nutrition and Healing.* Jun 1998;5(6):5–7.

Challem, Jack, Burton Berkson, MD, and Melissa Diane Smith. *Syndrome X.* (John Wiley & Sons, 2000)

Ellis, J.M., Reddy, P. Effects of Panax ginseng on Quality of Life. *Ann Pharmacother.* Mar 2002;36(3):375–79.

Gebhart, B., Jorgenson, J. Benefit of ribose in a patient with fibromyalgia. *Pharm* 2004;24(11):1646–1648.

The Journal of Clinical Endocrinology & Metabolism; Vol. 87, No. 4, 1687–91.

Lamperti, C. et al. Muscle coenzyme Q10 level in statin-related myopathy. *Arch Neurol.* 2005 Nov;62(11):1709–12.

Langsjoen, P.H., Langsjoen, A.M. The clinical use of HMG CoA-reductase inhibitors and depletion of CoQ10. *Biofactors.* 2003;18(1–4):101–11.

Mishra, L.C. et al. Scientific Basis for the Therapeutic Use of Withania somnifera (Ashwa-gandha). *Alternative Medicine Review.* Aug 2000;5(4):334–46.

Morales, A.J., Nolan, J.J., Nelson, J.C., Yen, S.S.C. Effects of replacement dose of DHEA in men and women of advancing age. *J Clin Endocrionol Metab.* 1994;78:1360.

Panda, S., Kar, A. Withania somnifera and Bauhinia purpurea in the Reg of Circulating Thy Hor Conc in Mice. *J Ethnopharmacol.* Nov 1999;67(2):233–39.

Patton, B.M. Beneficial effect of D-ribose in patient with myoadenylate deaminase defi-ciency. *Lancet.* 1982 May8;1(8280):1701.

Rai, D. et al. Anti-stress effects of Ginkgo biloba and Panax ginseng: Central Drug Re-search Institute, Lucknow, India. *J Pharmacol Sci.* Dec 2003;93(4):458–64.

Shevtsov, V.A., Zholus, B.I., Shervarly, V.I., Vol'skij, V.B., Korovin, Y.P., Khristich, M.P., Roslyakova, N.A., Wikman, G. A randomized trial of two different doses of a SHR-5 Rhodiola rosea extract versus placebo and control of capacity for mental work. *Phytomedicine* 2003;10(2-3):95–105.

Thampan, P.K. 1994. *Facts and Fallacies about Coconut Oil.* Asian and Pacific Coconut Community. P9.

Tiano, L., Belardinelli, R., Carnevali, P., Principi, F., Seddaiu, G., Littarru, G.P. Effect of Coenzyme Q10 administration on endothelial function and extracellular superoxide dismutase in patients with ischaemic heart disease: a double-blind, randomized controlled study. *Eur Heart J.* 2007 Sep;28(18):2249–55. Epub 2007 Jul 19.

Torjeson, P.A., Birkeland, K.I., Anderssen, S.A. et al. "Lifestyle changes may reverse development of the insulin resistance syndrome." *Diabetes Care*, 1997;20:26–31.

Wilson, James L., N.D., D.C., PhD. *Adrenal Fatigue: The 21ˢᵗ Century Stress Syndrome.* (Smart Publications, 2001)

Chapter 2: Straight from the Heart: Don't Let Your Ticker Become a Time Bomb

Auer, J., Berent, R., Lassnig, E., Eber, B. C-reactive protein and coronary artery disease. *Jpn Heart J.* 2002 Nov;43(6):607–19.

Chang, Y.C., Riby, J., Chang, G.H. et al. Cytostatic and antiestrogenic effects of indole–3-carbinol. *Biochem Pharmacol.* 1999;58:825–34.

Circulation: Journal American Heart Association. www.circ.ahajournals.org.

Dodd, S.L. et al. The role of ribose in human skeletal muscle metabolism. *Med Hypotheses.* 2004;62(5):819–24.

Jacobs, D. et al. Report of the conference on low blood cholesterol: Mortality associations. *Circulation* 86, 1046–60, 1992.

Krumholz, H.M. et al. Lack of association between cholesterol and coronary heart disease. *JAMA* 272, 1335–40, 1990.

Langsjoen, Peter et al. Usefulness of CoQ10 in Clinical Cardiology. *Molecular Aspects of Medicine*, 1994, 15 Suppl: 165–75.

Miller, E.R., Paster-Barriuso, R., Dalal, D. Riemersma, R.A., Appel, L.J., Guallar, E. Meta-analysis: high-dosage vitamin E supplementation may increase all-cause mortality. *Ann Intern Med.* 2005 Jan 4;142(1):I40.

Omran, H., Illien, S., MacCarter, D., St. Cyr, J.A., Luderitz, B. D-Ribose improves diastolic function and quality of life in congestive heart failure patients: a prospective feasibility study. *The European Journal of Heart Failure* 2003;5:615–19.

Omran, H., Illien, S., MacCarter, D., St. Cyr, J.A. Ribose improves myocardial function and quality of life in CHF. *J Mol Cell Cardiol,* 2001;33(6):A173.

Packard, C.J. et al. Lipoprotein-associated phospholipase A2 as an independent predictor of CHD. *NEJM.* 2000 Oct 19;343(16):1148–55.

Pauly, D.F., Pepine, C.J. Ischemic heart disease: Metabolic approaches to management. *Clin Cardiol.* 2004;27(8):439–41.

Ravnskov, Uffe. *The Cholesterol Myths—Exposing the Fallacy That Saturated Fat and Cholesterol Cause Heart Disease.* (New Trends Publishing, October 2000).

Shechter, M. et al. Effects of oral magnesium on exercise tolerance, chest pain, and quality of life in patients with CAD. *Am J Cardiol.* 2003 Mar 1;91(5):517–21.

Wolfgang, Pliml et al. Effects of ribose on exercise-induced ischemia in stable coronary artery disease. *Lancet.* Aug.1992; Vol 340, No. 8818. p507–10.

The Writing Group for the WHI Investigators. Risks and benefits of estrogen plus progestin: *JAMA* 2002;288(3):321–33.

www.americanheart.org American Heart Association

Chapter 3: Strong Bones and Straight Bodies: Ways to Keep Things Healthy Under the Skin

Agnusdei, D., Buffalino, L. Efficacy of Ipriflavone in established osteoporosis and long-term safety. *Calcif Tissue Int* 1997;61 Suppl 1:S23–7.

Bonjour, J.P. et al. 1997. Protein intake, IGF–1 and osteoporosis. *Osteoporosis International* 7:S36.

Carmona, Richard H. Bone Health and Osteoporosis: A Report of the Surgeon General, 10/14/04. www.surgeongeneral.gov/library/bonehealth/

Cooper, C. et al. Water fluoridation & hip fracture, *JAMA* 7 1991, 19(32):513–14.

Cramer, D.W. Lactase persistence and milk consumption as determinants of ovarian cancer risk. *Am J Epidemiol* 1980; 130:904–10.

Exposure to Natural Fluoride in Well Water and Hip Fracture: A Cohort Analysis in Finland. *American Journal of Epidemiology.* 150(8):817–24, October 15, 1999.

Feskanich, D. et al. Milk, dietary Ca, and bone fractures in women. 12-yr prospective study. *Am J Public Health* 1997; 87:992–97.

Hannan, M.T. et al. 2000. Effect of dietary protein on bone loss in elderly men and women: The Framingham Study. *JBMR* 15(December):2504.

Head, Kathleen. Ipriflavone: An Important Bone-Building Isoflavone. *Alternative Medicine Review.* Vol 4, No. 1, 1999.

Heaney, R.P. 2001. Protein intake and bone health: The Influence of belief systems on the conduct of nutritional science. *AJCN.* 73(Jan):5.

Kurttio, Paivi et al. Dietary calcium and phosphorus ratio regulates bone mineralization & turnover in vit D. *JBMR* 2003 Jul;18(7):1217–26.

McGartland, C.P. et al. Fruit and vegetable consumption and bone mineral density: North Ireland Young Hearts Proj. *Am J Clin Nutr* 2004;80(4):1019–23.

Melton, L.J. et al. Bone density & fracture risk men. *JBMR.* 1998; 13:No 12:1915.

Meunier, Pierre J., et al. The effects of strontium ranelate on the risk of vertebral fracture in women with postmenopausal osteoporosis. *NEJM* 350 (2004):459–68.

Munger, R.G. et al. Prospective Study on dietary protein intake and the risk of hip fracture in postmenopausal women. *Am J Clin Nutr* 1999; 69(January):147.

New, S.A., Millward, D.J. Calcium, protein, and fruit and vegetables as dietary determinants of bone health. *Am J Clin Nutr* 2003;77(5):1340–41.

Orwoll, E., Ettinger, M., Weiss., S. et al. Alendronate for the treatment of Osteoporosis in Men. *NEJM* 2000; 343:604–10.

Reginster, Jean-Yves, et al. Strontium ranelate reduces the risk of nonvertebral fractures in postmenopausal women with osteoporosis: Treatment of Peripheral Osteoporosis (TROPOS) study. *Journal of Clinical Endocrinology and Metabolism* 90 (2005): 2816–22.

Robbins, John. *The Food Revolution.* (Conari Press, 2001)

Seaborn, C.D., Nielsen, F.H. Silicon: a nutritional beneficence for bones, brains and blood vessels. *Nutr Today* 1993;28:13–18.

Sebastian, A. et al. Improved mineral balance and skeletal metabolism in postmenopausal women treated with potassium. *NEJM* 1994;330(25):1776–81.

Sellmeyer, D.E. et al. 2001. A high ratio of dietary animal to vegetable protein increases the rate of bone loss and the risk of fracture. *AJCN.* 73(Jan):118.

Sellmeyer, D.E., Schloetter, M., Sebastian, A. Potassium citrate prevents increased urine calcium excretion and bone resorption induced by a high sodium chloride diet. *J Clin Endocrinol Metab* 2002;87(5):2008–12.

Tucker, K.L. et al. 2000. Diet pattern groups are related to BMD among adults: The Framingham study. *JBMR* 15(September):S222.

Tucker, K.L. et al. "Colas, but not other carbonated beverages, are associated with low bone mineral density in older women: The Framingham Osteoporosis Study." *AJCN.* 2006; 84: 936–42.

Weaver, C.M. et al. "Dietary Calcium: Adequacy of a Vegetarian Diet." *AJCN.* 59 (Sup) 1994:1238S–41S.

www.nih.gov, The National Institutes of Health

www.nof.org/men/index.htm, The National Osteoporosis Foundation

Yiamouyiannis, John. *Fluoride, The Aging Factor.* (Health Action Press, 1986)

Chapter 4: Do You Have the Guts to Throw Away Your Antacids?

Abele, M., Schols, L., Schwartz, S., and Klockgether, T. Prevalence of antigliadin antibodies in ataxia patients. *Neurology* May 27, 2003; 60(10):1674–75.

Akcay, M.N., Akcay, G. The presence of the antigliadin antibodies in autoimmune thyroid diseases. *Hepatogastroenterology.* 2003 Dec;50 Suppl 2:cclxxix–cclxxx.

American Journal of Cardiology 8:43, 1963 Lipase Improves Fat Absorption.

Bell, S.J., Grochoski, G.T., Clarke, A.J. Health implications of milk containing beta-casein with the A2 genetic variant. *Crit Rev Food Sci Nutr.* 2006;46(1):93–100.

Bohager, Tom, Enzymes: What the Experts Know (One World Press August 2006)

Buysschaert, M. Acta. Coeliac disease in patients with type 1 diabetes mellitus and autoimmune thyroid disorders. *Gastroenterol* Belg. 2003 Jul-Sep;66(3):237–40.

Campbell, T. Colin, PhD, and Thomas M. Campbell II. *The China Study.* (BenBella Books, 2006)

Carlsson, A. et al. Prevalence of IgA-antigliadin ATB and IgA-anti-endomysium ATB related to celiac in Downs syndrome. *Pediatrics* 1998;101:272–75.

Elitsur, Y., Luk, G.D. Beta-casomorphin (BCM) and human colonic lamina propria lymphocyte proliferation. *Clin Exp Immunol.* 1991 Sep;85(3):493–7.

Elliot, R.B. Diabetes—a man made disease. *Med Hypotheses.* 2006;67(2):388–91.

Green, Bryan T. and J. Barry O'Connor. Most GERD Symptoms are not Due to Acid Reflux in Patients with very low 24-hour acid contact times. Duke University. *Digestive Diseases and Sciences.* 2004;49:1084–87.

Hadjivassiliou, M., Davies-Jones, G.A.B., Sanders, D.S., and Grunewald, R.A. Dietary treatment of gluten ataxia. *J. Neurol. Neurosurg. Psychiatry* September 1, 2003; 74(9): 1221–24.

Hadjivassiliou, M., Sanders, D.S., Grunewald, R.A., and Akil, M. Gluten sensitivity masquerading as systemic lupus erythematosus. *Ann Rheum Dis* November 1, 2004; 63(11): 1501–03.

Howell, Edward. *Food Enzymes for Health Longevity.* (Lotus Press, 1994)

Kelly, G.S. Hydrochloric Acid: Physiological Functions and Clinical Implications. *Alternative Medicine Review.* 2;2;1997.

Martorell, A., Plaza, A.M., Boné, J. et al. Cow's milk protein allergy. A multi-centre study: clinical and epidemiological aspects. *Allergol Immunopathol* (Madr). 2006 Mar-Apr;34(2):46-53

Peng, H.J. et al. Effect of cow's milk protein hydrolysate formulas on alpha-casein-specific IgE and G1 antibody responses. *J Ped Gastr Nutr* 2005 Oct;41(4):438–44.

Rogers, Sherry A., MD. *No More Heartburn.* (Kensington, 2000)

www.breakingtheviciouscycle.com

Part II: Above the Neck
Chapter 5: Antidepressants: Do You Need One to Be Happy?

Adams, P.W., Wynn, V., Rose, D.P. et al. Effect of pyridoxine hydrochloride (Vitamin B_6) upon depression associated with oral contraception. *Lancet* 1973;1:897–904.

De Vanna, M., Rigamonti, R. SAMe in depression. *Curr Ther Res* 1992;52:478–85.

Eby, George A., Eby, Karen L. Rapid Recovery from Major depression using Magnesium treatment. *Elsevier: Medical Hypotheses* 2006.

Ellis, F.R., Nasser, S. Vitamin B_{12} in the treatment of tiredness. *Br J Nutr* 1973;30:277–83.

Gelenberg, A.J. et al. Tyrosine for depression: a double-blind trial. *J Affect Disord* 1990; 19:125–32.

Gelenberg, A.J. et al. Tyrosine for depression. *Am J Psych* 1980;137:622–23.

Headache Classification Committee of the International Headache Society. Classification and diagnostic criteria for headache disorders, cranial neuralgias and facial pain. *Cephalagia* 1998;8(Suppl 7):1–96.

Holmes, J.M. Cerebral manifestations of vitamin B_{12} deficiency. *J Nutr Med* 1991;2:89–90.

Hoppe, J., Bergner, P. St. John's Wort and Major Depression: a critique of the JAMA trial. *Medical Herbalism* 12(2): 18–21.

Howard, J.S., III. Folate deficiency in psychiatric practice. *Psychosomatics* 1975;16: 112–15.

Kagan, B.L. et al. Oral SAMe in depression: A randomized, double-blind, placebo-controlled trial. *Am J Psychiatry* 1990;147:591–95.

Linde, K. et al. St. John's wort for depression—an overview and meta-analysis of randomized clinical trials. *British Medical Journal*, 313:53–58, 1996.

Littlefield, N.A. and B.S. Hass. Is the RDA for Magnesium Too Low? *NCTR, FDA,* Jefferson, AR, 72079.

Maes, M., Smith, R., Christophe, A. et al. Fatty acid composition in major depression. *J Affect Disord* 1996;38:35–46.

Martinsen, E.W., Medhus, A., Sandivik, L. Effects of aerobic exercise on depression: a controlled study. *BMJ* 1985;291:109.

Meyers, S. Neurotrans precursors for depression. *Altern Med Rev* 5(1), 64–71, Feb 2000.

Noble, S., Moore, K. Drug treatment of migraine: part II. Preventive therapy. *Am Fam Physician* 1997;56(9):2279–86.

Peet, M., Horrobin, D.F. A dose-ranging study of the effects of EPA in patients with ongoing depression. *Arch Gen Psychiatry* 2002;59:913–19.

Philipp, M., Kohnen, R., Hiller, K. Hypericum extract versus imipramine or placebo in patients with moderate depression. *BMJ* 319:1534–39, 1999.

Piscitelli, S.C., Burstein, A.H., Chaitt, D., Alfaro, R.M., Falloon J. Indinavir concentrations and St John's wort. *Lancet* 2001 Apr 14;357(9263):1210.

Reynolds, E., Preece, J.M., Bailey, J., Coppen, A. Folate deficiency in depressive illness. *Br J Psychiatry* 1970;117:287–92.

Sabelli, H. C. et al. Clinical studies on the phenylethylamine hypothesis of affective disorder. *J Clin Psychiat* 47(2):66–70, 1986.

Sandor, P.S., Afra, J., Ambrosini, A., Schoenen, J. Prophylactic treatment of migraine with beta-blockers and riboflavin: differential effects on the intensity dependence of auditory evoked cortical potentials. *Headache* 2000;40(1):30–35.

Schoenen, J., Lenaerts, M., Bastings, E. High-dose riboflavin as a prophylactic treatment of migraine: results of an open pilot study. *Cephalalgia* 1994;14(5):328–29.

Schrader D. Equivalence of St. John's wort extract (ZE 117) and fluoxetine: a randomized, controlled study. *Int Clin Psychopharm* 2000;15:61–68.

Shelton, C. Keller et al. Effectiveness of St John's Wort in Major Depression: A Randomized Controlled Trial. *JAMA* 285(15):1978–86, 2001.

Spasov, A., Wikman, G., Mandrikov, V. et al. The stimulating and adaptogenic effect of Rhodiola rosea. *Phytomedicine* 2000;7(2):85–89.

Stancheva, S., Mosharrof, A. Effect of the extract of Rhodiola rosea L. on the content of the brain biogenic monamines. *Med Physiol* 1987;40:85–87.

Tiihonen, J., Lönnqvist, J., Wahlbeck, K., Klaukka, T., Tanskanen, A., Haukka, J. *Arch Gen Psychiatry* 2006;63:1358–67.

Turner, E.H. et al. Serotonin a la carte. *Pharmocological Theraputics*, 2005 Jul. 13.

Chapter 6: Frazzled, Frustrated, and Freaked Out: Coping with Anxiety and Stress

Ahles, T.A., Tope, D.M., Pinkson, B. Massage therapy for patients undergoing autologous bone marrow transplantation. *J Pain Symptom Massage* 1999; 18: 157–63.

Blaylock, Russell L., MD. *Excitotoxins: The Taste That Kills.* (Health Press, 1996)

Cherniske, Stephen, M.S. *Caffeine Blues.* (Warner Books, 1998)

Deberry, S., Davis, S., Reinhard, K.E. A comparison of meditation-relaxation and cognitive-behavioral techniques for reducing anxiety and depression. *Journal of Geriatric Psychiatry* 1989;22:231–47.

Dhondt, W., Willaeys, T., Verbruggen, L.A., Oostendorp, R.A.B., Duquet, W. Pain threshold in patients with rheumatoid arthritis and effect of manual oscillations. *Scand J Rheumatol* 1999; 28: 88–93.

Eisenberg, D.M., Davis, R.B., Ettner, S.L., et al. Trends in alternative medicine use in the United States, 1990–1997: results of a follow-up national survey. *JAMA* 1998;280(18): 1569–75.

Field, T. et al. Chronic fatigue syndrome: Massage therapy effects on depression and somatic symptoms. *Journal of Chronic Fatigue Syndrome, 3,* 43–51.

Gaffney, C. Armed Forces Institute of Pathology. "Aspartame in Aviation." Paper presented at the 57th Annual Scientific Meeting of The Aerospace Medical Association. (April 1986)

Goats, G.C. Massage—the scientific basis of an ancient art. Physiological and therapeutic effects. *Br J Sports Med* 1994; 28: 153–56.

Greden, J.F. et al. Anxiety and depression associated with caffeinism among psychiatric inpatients. *Am J Psychiatry* 1978;135:963–66.

John, D.R. "Migraine Provoked by Aspartame." *NEJM* (October 14, 1986); p.456.

Juneja, L.R., Chu, D.-C., Okubo, T. et al. L-theanine a unique amino acid of green tea and its relaxation effect in humans. *Trends Food Sci Tech* 1999;10:199–204.

Kakuda, T., Nozawa, A., Unno, T., et al. Inhibiting effects of theanine on caffeine stimulation evaluated by EEG in the rat. *Biosci Biotechno Biochem* 2000; 64:287–93.

Kleijnen, J., Riet, G.T., Knipschild, P. Vitamin B_6 in the treatment of the premenstrual syndrome—a review. *Br J Obstet Gynaecol* 1990;97:847–52.

Maher, T.J., Wurtman, R.J. "Possible Neurologic Effects of Aspartame, a Widely Used Food Additive." *Environmental Health Perspectives* 75: 53–57 (1987).

Mason, R. 200mg of Zen; L-theanine boosts alpha waves promotes alert relaxation. *Alternative & Complementary Therapies* 2001, April; 7:91–95.

Mullarkey, Barbara. "How Safe is Your Artificial Sweetener," September/October 1994 issue of *Informed Consent* Magazine. *Psychosomatics* (March 1986).

Wiesinger, G.F., Quittan, M., Ebenbichler, G., Kaider, A., Fialka, V. Benefit and costs of passive modalities in back pain outpatients: a descriptive study. *Eur J Phys Med Rehab* 1997; 7: 182–86.

Chapter 8: Snoring and Other Things That Go "Boom" in The Night

Bailey, D.R. Sleep disorders. *Dent Clin North Am.* 1997;41:189–209.

Ballard, R.D. Sleep and medical disorders. *Prim Care.* 2005 Jun;32(2):511–33.

Breus, Michael, PhD. *Good Night's—The Sleep Doctor's 4-Week Program to Better Sleep and Better Health.* (Dutton Adult, 2006)

Deviated septum. The Centers for Chronic Nasal and Sinus Dysfunction website. www.nasal.net/otolaryngology/deviated.htm.

Hu, Frank B. et al. Prospective Study of Snoring and Risk of Hypertension in Women. *American Journal of Epidemiology.* 150(8):806–16, October 15, 1999.

Kahn, A. et al. Sleep characteristics in milk-intolerant infants. *Sleep.* 1988 Jun;11(3): 291–97.

Partinen, M., Guilleminault, C. Daytime sleepiness and vascular morbidity at seven-year follow-up in obstructive sleep apnea patients. *Chest* 1990;97:27–32.

Pritchard, A.J., *Phytother. Res.* 18, 696–99 (2004), Shrewsbury.

Resta, O. et al. Influence of subclinical hypothyroidism and T4 treatment on sleep apnea. *J Endocrinol Invest.* 2005 Nov;28(10):893–98.

Sleep Research Online 2(1): 7–10, 1999 Stanford University Sleep Disorders Clinic and Research Center, Stanford, California.

Snoring: not funny, not hopeless. American Academy of Otolaryngology—Head and Neck Surgery website. www.entnet.org

Staevska, M.T., Mandajieva, M.A., Dimitrov, V.D. Rhinitis and sleep apnea. *Curr Allergy Asthma Rep.* 2004 May;4(3):193–99.

www.sleepfoundation.org, The National Sleep Foundation

Chapter 9: A Nation of Insomniacs: Do You Really Need a Pill to Get a Good Night's Sleep?

Boato, F., Wortley, G.M., Liu, R.H., Glahn, R.P. Red grape juice inhibits iron availability: application of an in vitro digestion/caco-2 cell model. *J Agric Food Chem* 2002 Nov 6;50(23):6935–38.

Davis, W., Ziady, F. University of Pretoria, S. Africa—presented at the Second International Symposium on Magnesium, Montreal, 1976.

Hornyak, M. et al. Magnesium for periodic leg movements-related insomnia and restless legs syndrome. *Sleep.* 1998 Aug 1;21(5):501–5.

Kamm-Kohl, A.V., Jansen, W., Brockmann, P. Modern valerian therapy for nervous disorders in old age [translated from German]. *Med Welt.* 1984;35:1450–54.

Kelly, G.S. Folates: supplemental forms and therapeutic applications. *Altern Med Rev.* 1998 Jun;3(3):208–20.

National Jewish Medical and Research Center. Asthma patients cautioned about melatonin. *ScienceDaily* 2003, September 8.

Part III: Below the Waist
Chapter 10: When He Wants Viagra and You Want a Valium

Al-Ali, M. et al. Tribulus terrestris: preliminary study of diuretic and contractile effects and comparison with Zea mays. *J Ethnopharmacol.* 2003 Apr;85(2–3):257–60.

Ang, H.H., Lee, K.L. Effect of Eurycoma longifolia Jack (Tongkat Ali) on libido in middle-aged male rats. *J Basic Clin Physiol Pharmacol.* 2002;13(3):249–54.

Ang, H.H., Sim, M.K. Eurycoma longifolia (tongkat ali) increases sexual motivation in sexually naive male rats. *Arch Pharm Res.* 1998 Dec;21(6):779–81.

Arthritis Rheum. (1994) 37:1305–10 as cited in Skolnick, A.A., "Medical News and Perspectives: Scientific Verdict Still Out on DHEA," *JAMA* (Nov. 6, 1996) Vol. 276, No. 17, pages 1365–67.

Balch, James F., and Phyllis A. Balch. *Prescription for Nutritional Healing Second Edition* (Garden City Park, NY: Avery Publishing Group, 1997), page 545

Boehm, S. et al. "Estrogen suppression as a pharmacotherapeutic strategy in BPH. 1998, 110: 817–23. *British Journal of Cancer*, vol. 78 in 1998.

Bradlow, H. L., Sepkovic, D.W., Telang, N.T., Osborne, M.P. Multi-functional aspects of the action of indole–3-carbinol as an antitumor agent. *Ann NY Acad Sci* 1999;889: 204–13.

Cover, C.M., Hsieh, S.J., Cram, E.J. et al. Indole–3-carbinol and tamoxifen cooperate to arrest the cell cycle of MCF–7 human breast cancer cells. *Cancer Res* 1999;59:1244–51.

Davis, Susan. Testosterone Deficiency in Women. *Journal of Reproductive Medicine* 2001;46:291–96.

deLarminat, M. and Blaquier, J. "Effect of in vivo administration of 5 alpha reductase inhibitors on epididymal function." *Acta Physiol Lat Am* 1979, 29:1–6.

Farnsworth, W. "Estrogen in the etiopathogenesis of BPH." *J Basic Clin Physiol Pharmacol.* 2003;14(3):301–8. *Prostate.* 1999, 41: 263–74.

Farnsworth, W.E. Roles of estrogen and SHBG in prostate physiology. *Prostate* (1996 Jan) 28(1):17–23.

Farthing, M. et al. "Progesterone, prolactin, and gynecomastia in men with liver disease." Gut 1982, 23: 276–79.

Fitzpatrick, L.A. University of Pennsylvania School of Medicine. Libido and Perimenopausal Women. *Menopause.* 2004 Mar-Apr;11(2):136–37.

Ge, X., Yannai, S., Rennert, G. et al. 3,3'-diindolylmethane induces apoptosis in human cancer cells. *Biochem Biophys Res Commun* 1996; 228:153–58.

Hetts, S. "To die or not to die: an overview of apoptosis and its role in disease." *JAMA* 1998, 279: 300–7.

Klatz, Ronald, with Carol Kahn. *Grow Young with HGH* (New York: HarperCollins Publishers, 1997), pages 10, 186–89, 191

Krieg, M. et al. "Effect of aging on endogenous level of 5 DHT, estradiol, and estrone in human prostate." *J Clin Endocrinol Metab.* 1993, 77: 375–81.

Lee, J. "Prostate disease and hormones." The John R. Lee, MD Medical Letter Feb. 2002.

Lin, LW. Anti-nociceptive and anti-inflammatory activity caused by Cistanche deserticola in rodents. China Medical College, 91 Hsieh Shih Road, Taichung, Taiwan, ROC. *J Ethnopharmacol.* 2002 Dec;83(3):177–82.

Maida, Taylor. Psychological Consequences of Surgical Menopause. *Journal of Reproductive Medicine* 2001;46:317–24.

McPherson, S.J. et al. Transient Neonatal Estrogen Exposure to Estrogen-Deficient Mice (Aromatase Knockout) Reduces Prostate Weight and Induces Inflammation in Late Life. *American Journal of Pathology.* 2006;168:1869–78.

Mercola, J. "Progesterone cream can help prostate cancer." 1998. www.mercola.com/fcgi/ pf/1998/ archive/natural_progesterone2.htm.

Moynihan, R. The making of a disease: female sexual dysfunction. *British Medical Journal.* 2003;326:45–47.

Nakhla, A. et al. "Estradiol causes the rapid accumulation of cAMP in human prostate." *Proc Natl Acad Sci* USA 1994, 91: 5402–5.

Peat, R. "The Progesterone Deception," Townsend Letter for Doctors, Nov. 1987

Peat, R. Progesterone in Orthomolecular Medicine Eugene, OR, 1993: 4–6.

Petrow, V. "Endocrine dependence of prostatic cancer upon dihydrotestosterone and not upon testosterone." *J Pharmacol* 1984, 36: 352–53.

Regelson, William, and Carol Colman. *The Super-Hormone Promise* (New York: Simon & Schuster, 1996)

Scarano, W.R. et al. Intraepithelial alterations in the guinea pig prostate after estradiol treatment. *J Submicrosc Cytol Pathol.* 2004 Apr;36(2):141–48.

Simpson, E.R., Risbridger, G.P. Elevated androgens and prolactin in aromatase- deficient mice cause enlargement prostate gland. *Endocrinology.* 2001 Jun;142 (6):2458–67.

Sokeland, J. Urological Clinic of Dortmund, Training Hospital of the University of Munster, Germany. *BJU* Int. 2000 Sep;86(4):439–42.

Thompson, I.M., Pauler, D.K., Goodman, P.J. et al. Prevalence of prostate cancer among men with a PSA ≤4.0 ng per ml. *NEJM* 2004; 350(22):2239–46.

www.johnleemd.com Dr. John R. Lee Information Source for Hormone Balance

Chapter 11: The Condom Broke: Birth Control Before, During, and the Morning After

Austin, H., Louv, W.C., and Alexander, W.J. A case-control study of spermicides and gonorrhea. *JAMA* 251, no. 21 (December 6, 1985).

Bradfield, C.A., Bjeldanes, L.F. Structure-activity relationship of dietary indoles: a proposed mechanism of action as modifiers of xenobiotic mechanism. *J Toxicol Environ Health* 1987;21:311–23.

Briggs, M. and Briggs, M. Vitamin C requirements and oral contraceptives. *Nature* 238: 277, 1972.

Larsson-Cohn, U. Oral contraceptives and vitamins: a review. *Am J Obstet Gynecol* 121: 84–90, 1975.

Martinez, O. and Roe, D.A. Effect of oral contraceptives on blood folate levels in pregnancy. *Am J Obstet Gynecol* 128: 255–61, 1977.

Meng, Q. et al. Inhibitory effects of I3C on invasion and migration in human breast cancer cells. *Breast Cancer Res Treat* 2000;63:147–52.

Pfrunder, A., Schiesser, M., Gerber, S. et al. Interaction of St John's wort with oral contraceptives. *Br J Clin Pharmacol.* 2003;56:683–90.

Public Health Agency of Canada: HIV/AIDS Epi Update. Nonoxynol-9 and the Risk of HIV transmission, April 2003.

Rivers, J.M. and Devine, M. Plasma ascorbic acid concentrations and oral contraceptives. *Am J Clin Nutr* 25: 684–89, 1972.

Seelig, MS. Increased need for magnesium with the use of combined oestrogen and calcium for osteoporosis treatment. *Magnes Res* 3(3): 197–215, 1990.

Shojania, A.M., Hornady, G., and Barnes, P.H. Oral contraceptives and serum-folate level. *Lancet* 1: 1376–77, 1968.

Terry, P., Wolk, A., Persson, I., Magnusson, C. Brassica vegetables and breast cancer risk. *JAMA* 2001;285:2975–77.

Van Damme, L. Advances in topical microbicides. Presented at the XIII International AIDS Conference, July 9–14, 2000, Durban, South Africa.

Whitehead, N. et al. Megaloblastic changes in the cervical epithelium. Assn with oral contracep and reversal with folic acid. *JAMA* 226: 14

www.cdc.gov, Centers for Disease Control

www.johnleemd.com, Dr. John R. Lee Information Source for Hormone Balance

www.plannedparenthood.org

Wynn, V. Vitamins and oral contraceptive use. *Lancet* 1: 561–64, 1975.

Chapter 12: Monthly Madness: Cramps, Crankiness, and Other Hormonal Highs & Lows

Benton, D., Cook, R. The impact of selenium supplementation on mood. *Biol Psychiatry* 1991;29:1092–98.

Chen, I., Mcdougal, A., Wang, F., Safe, S. Antiestrogenic and anti-turmorigenic act of di-indolylmethane. *Carcinogenesis* 1998;19:1631–39.

Chinni, S.R., Li, Y., Upadhyay, S. et al. Indole–3-carbinol (I3C) induced cell growth inhibition, G1 cell cycle arrest and apoptosis in prostate cancer cells. *Oncogene* 2001;20:2927–36.

Colditz, G.A., Hankinson, S.E., Hunter, D.J. et al. The use of estrogens and progestins and the risk of breast cancer in postmenopausal women. *NEJM*. 1995 Jun 15;332(24):1589–93.

Docherty, J.P., Sack, D.A., Roffman, M., Finch, M., Komorowski, J.R. *Journal of Psychiatric Practice* September 2005, 11(5):302–14.

Frydoonfar, H.R., et al. The effect of indole-3-carbinol and sulforaphane on a prostate cancer cell line. *ANZ J Surg* 2003 73:154–56.

Hsieh, C.C., and Trichopoulos, D. Breast size, handedness and breast cancer risk. *Eur. J. Cancer* 27:131–35, 1991.

Huang et al. *Br J Cancer* 1999, 80:1838.

Lee, John R., MD, Jesse Hanley, MD, and Virginia Hopkins. *What Your Doctor May Not Tell You About Premenopause.* (Warner Books, 1999)

Leonetti, H.B., Wilson, K.J., Anasti, J.N. Topical progesterone cream has an antiproliferative effect on estrogen-stimulated endometrium. *Fertil Steril*. 2003 Jan;79(1):221–22.

NEJM 2005; 353:2747–57. Long-term use of Aromatase inh produces Better Results.

Milligan, S.R., Balasubramanian, A.V., Kalita, J.C. Relative potency of xenobiotic estrogens in vivo mammalian assay. *Environ Health Perspect*. 1998 Jan; 106(1):23–26.

Rossouw, J.E., Anderson, G.L., Prentice, R.L. et al. Risks and benefits of estrogen plus progestin in healthy postmenopausal women: principal results from the Women's Health Initiative randomized controlled trial. *JAMA* 2002 Jul 17;288(3):321–33.

www.johnleemd.com, Dr. John R. Lee Information Source for Hormone Balance

Yuan, F., Chen, D.Z., Sepkovic, D.W. et al. Anti-estrogenic activities of indole–3-carbinol in cervical cells. *Anticancer Res* 1999;19:1673–80.

Chapter 13: Surge Protection for Your Hot Flashes

Chi-Ling, Chen et al. *Hormone Replacement Therapy in Relation to Breast Cancer JAMA.* 2002;287:734–41.

Colditz, G.A., Hankinson, S.E., Hunter, D.J. et al. The use of estrogens and progestins and risk of breast cancer. *NEJM.* 1995 Jun 15;332(24):1589–93.

Dixon-Shanies, D., Shaikh, N. Growth inhibition of human breast cancer cells by herbs and phytoestrogens. *Oncology Reports* 6: 1383–87, 1999.

Duke, J.A. *Handbook of Medicinal Herbs.* (FL: CRC Press, 2001) pages 120–21

Einer-Jensen, N. et al. Cimicifuga and Melbrosia lack oestrogenic effects in mice and rats. *Maturitas* (The European Menopause Journal) 25: 149–53, 1996.

Evans, Nancy. "State of the Evidence: What is the Connection between the Environment and Breast Cancer." 2004.

Freudenstein, J. et al. Lack of promotion of estrogen-dep mammary gland tumors in vivo by Cim racemosa extract. *Cancer Research* 62: 3448–52, 2002.

Grady, D., Herrington, D., Bittner, V. et al. Cardiovascular disease outcomes during 6.8 years of hormone therapy. Heart and Estrogen-progestin Replacement therapy follow-up (HERS II). *JAMA.* 2002;288:49–66.

Hendrix, Susan, DO et al. *Effects of Estrogen With and Without Progestin on Urinary Incontinence. JAMA.* 2005;293:935–48.

Humphrey, L. et al. Postmenopausal Hormone Replacement Therapy and the Primary Prevention of Cardiovascular Disease. *Ann Intern Med* 2002. 137: 273–84.

Leonetti, H.B., Longo, S., Anasti, J.N. Transdermal progesterone cream for vasomotor symptoms and postmenopausal bone loss. *Obstet Gynecol.* 1999 Aug; 94(2):225–28.

Stoll, W. Phytotherapy influences atrophic vaginal epithelium: Double-blind study of Cimicifuga vs. estrogenic substances (in German). *Therapeutikon* 1:23–31, 1987.

The Women's Health Initiative Steering Committee. The Women's Health Initiative Randomized Controlled Trial. *JAMA* 2004; 291: 1701–12.

The Writing Group for the WHI Investigators. Risks and benefits of estrogen plus progestin in healthy post-menopausal women. *JAMA* 2002;288(3):321–33.

Zava, David T. et al. Estrogen and progestin bioactivity of foods, herbs, and spices. Proceedings of the Society for Experimental Biology and Medicine 217: 369–78, 1998.

Part IV: And Everything in Between
Chapter 14: Lose Fat While You Sleep . . .
When Pink Elephants Fly!

Attele, A.S. et al. Anti-diabetic Effects of Panax ginseng Berry Extract and the Identification of an Effective Component. *Diabetes.* Jun 2002;51(6):1851–58.

Avula, B., Wang, Y.H., Pawar R.S. et al. Determination of the appetite suppressant P57 in Hoodia gordonii plant extracts and dietary supplements by liquid chromatography/ electrospray ionization mass spectrometry (LC-MSD-TOF) and LC-UV methods. J AOAC Int . 2006;89:606-11.

Federal Trade Commission. WebMD Feature: "Quick Weight Loss or Quackery?"

Flegal, K.M., Carroll, M.D., Ogden, C.L., Johnson, C.L. Prevalence and trends in obesity among U.S. adults, 1999–2000. *JAMA* 2002;288:1723–27.

J AOAC Int. 2006 May-Jun;89(3):606–11.

Kelly, G.S. L-Carnitine: Therapeutic Applications of a Conditionally-Essential Amino Acid. *Alternative Medicine Review*, Volume 3, number 5. 1998

Leptin corrects increased gene expression of renal 25-hydroxyvitamin D3–1 alpha-hydroxylase and–24-hydroxylase in leptin-deficient, ob/ob mice. *Endocrinology.* 2004 Mar;145(3):1367–75. Epub 2003 Dec 4.

Maahs, D., de Serna, D.G., Kolotkin, R.L., Ralston, S., Sandate, J., Qualls, C., Schade, D.S. Randomized, double-blind, placebo-controlled trial of orlistat for weight loss in adolescents. 2006-01, *Endocr Pract.* 12(1):18–28.

Menendez, C. et al. Retinoic acid and vitamin D(3) powerfully inhibit in vitro leptin secretion by human adipose tissue. *J Endocrinol.* 2001 Aug;170(2):425–31.

Smart Souce Advertisement May 8, 2004

Szapary, P.O., Wolfe, M.L., Bloedon, L.T., et al. Guggulipid for the treatment of hypercholesterolemia. *JAMA* 2003; 290:765–72.

Urizar, N.L., Moore, D.D. Guggulipid: a natural cholesterol-lowering agent. *Ann Rev Nutr.* 2003; 23:303–13.

WebMD Feature Quack Diet Red Flags

www.dietfraud.com/main.html

www.eatright.org, The American Dietetic Association

www.sbmgiga.com

Chapter 15: Botox and Other Ways to Cheat Father Time

Alternative medicine Review, Volume 1, Monographs

Biagi, P.L., Bordoni, A., Masi, M., Ricci, G., Fanelli, C., Patrizi, A., Ceccolini, E. A long-term study on the use of evening primrose oil (Efamol) in atopic children. *Drugs Exp Clin Res.* 1988; 14(4):285–90.

Businco, L., Ioppi, M., Morse, N.L., Nisini, R., Wright, S. Breast milk from mothers of children with newly developed atopic eczema has low levels of long chain polyunsaturated fatty acids. *J Allergy Clin Immunol.* 1993; 91(6):1134–39.

Environmental Protection Agency (EPA). 1990. *Integrated Risk Information System.* Dibutyl phthalate, CASRN 84–74–2. October 1990.

Kagan, V., Khan, S., Swanson, C. et al. Antioxidant action of thioctic acid and dihydrolipoic acid. *Free Radic Biol Med* 1990;9S:15.

Kagan, V., Serbinova, E., Packer, L. Antioxidant effects of ubiquinones in microsomes and mitochondria are mediated by tocopherol recycling. *Biochem Biophys Res Commun* 1990;169:851–57.

Kaufmann, Klaus. *Silica—The Forgotten Nutrient.* (Alive Books, 1993)

Leibold, Gerhard, N.D. *Silica: The Universal Mineral.*

Lykkesfeldt, J., Hagen, T.M., Vinarsky, V., Ames, B.N. Age-associated decline in ascorbic acid concentration, recycling, and biosynthesis in rat hepatocytes-reversal with (R)-alpha-lipoic acid supplementation. *FASEB J* 1998;12:1183–89.

Mylchreest, E. Disruption of androgen-regulated male reproductive development by di(n-butyl) phthalate. *Toxicol Appl Pharmacol* 1999;156:81–95(1999).

Nichols, T.W. Jr. Alpha-lipoic acid: biological effects and clinical implications. *Altern Med Rev* 1997;2:177–83 [review].

Packer, L., Witt, E.H., Tritschler, H.J. Alpha-lipoic acid as a biological antioxidant. *Free Radic Biol Med* 1995;19:227–50 [review].

www.ewg.org/reports/skindeep2/index.php, The Skin Deep Website

www.safecosmetics.org, The Campaign for Safe Cosmetics

Chapter 17: More Jiggle, Less Joint Pain: What You Can Do About Arthritis

Ambrus, J.L. et al. Absorption of exogenous and endogenous proteolytic enzymes. *Clin Pharmacol Therap* 1967;8:362–68.

Caughey, D.E., Grigor, R.R., Caughey, E.B. et al. *Perna canaliculus* in the treatment of rheumatoid arthritis. *Eur J Rheumatol Inflamm* 1983;6:197–200.

Clegg, D.O. et al. Glucosamine, chondroitin sulfate, and the two in combination for painful knee osteoarthritis. *NEJM* 354:795–808, 2006.

Gibson, R.G., Gibson, S.L. Green-lipped mussel extract in arthritis. *Lancet* 1981;1:439.

Hong, S.J. et al. Bee venom induces apoptosis in synovial fibroblasts of patients with rheumatoid arthritis. *Toxicon.* 2005 Jul;46(1):39–45.

Jacob, R. Fresh cherries may help arthritis sufferers. *Agricultural Research* May 2004, http://www.ars.usda.gov/is/AR/archive/may04/cherry0504.htm.

Kabil, S.M., Stauder, G. Oral enzyme therapy in hepatitis C patients. *Int J Tiss React* 1997;19:97–98.

McAlindon, T.E. et al. Glucosamine and chondroitin for treatment of osteoarthritis. Meta-analysis *JAMA* 283:1469–75, 2000.

Park, H.J. et al. Anti-arthritic effect of bee venom: *Arthritis Rheum.* 2004 Nov;50(11):3504–15.

Ransberger, K. Enzyme treatment of immune complex diseases. *Arthritis Rheuma* 1986;8:16–19.

Reginster, J.Y. et al. Long-term effects of glucosamine sulfate on osteoarthritis progression: a randomized, placebo-controlled trial. *Lancet* 357:251–56, 2001.

Soeken, K.L., Lee, W.L., Bausell, R.B., et al. Safety and efficacy of S-adenosylmethionine (SAMe) for osteoarthritis. A meta-analysis. *J Fam Pract* 2002; 51:425–30.

Chapter 18: Go Blow Your Nose—Just Not Near Me!: Bedtime Stories That Will Boost Your Immunity

Choi, E.M., Kim, A.J., Kim, Y.O., Hwang, J.K. Immunomodulating activity of arabinogalactan and fucoidan in vitro. *J Med Food.* 2005 Winter;8(4):446–53.

Chu, K.K., Ho, S.S., Chow, A.H. Coriolus versicolor: a medicinal mushroom with promising immunotherapeutic values. *J Clin Pharmacol.* 2002 Sep;42(9):976–84.

Developmental Therapeutics Program, National Cancer Institute. In-vitro anti-HIV drug screening results. NSC: F195001, Jan 1992.

Kidd, P.M. The use of mushroom glucans and proteoglycans in cancer treatment. *Altern Med Rev.* 2000 Feb;5(1):4–27. Review.

Meadows, Michelle. Beat the Winter Bugs: How to hold your own against colds and flu. www.fda.gov/fdac/features/2001/601_flu.html

Nantz, M.P. et al. Immunity and antioxidant capacity in humans enhanced by consumption of dried, encaps fruit and veg juice conc. *J Nutr.* 2006 Oct;136(10):2606–10.

Rybacki, J., PharmD. *Essential Guide to Prescription Drugs 2006.* (Collins, 2006)

Vickers, A.J., Smith, C. Homoeopathic Oscillococcinum for preventing and treating influenza. *Cochrane Database Syst Rev.* 2004;(1):CD001957.

Wu, X.M., Gao, X.M., Tsim, K.W., Tu, P.F. An arabinogalactan isolated from Cistanche deserticola induces proliferation. *J Biol Macromol.* 37(5): 278–82, 2005.

Chapter 19: Toenail Crud and Other Really Icky, Weird Stuff

Balch, Phyllis A., CNC. *Prescription for Nutritional Healing*, 4th Ed. (Avery, 2006)

Brodin, Michael, MD. *The Over the Counter Drug Book.* (Pocket, 1998)

Green, Joey. *Amazing Kitchen Cures.* (Rodale, 2002)

Lust, John. *The HerbBook.* (Benedict Lust Publications, 2005)

Medline Plus: www.nlm.nih.gov/medlineplus/druginformation.html

Seltzer, A.P. Minimizing post-operative edema and ecchymoses by the use of an oral enzyme preparation (bromelain): a controlled study of 53 rhinoplasty cases. *Eve Ear Nose Throat Mon* 1962;41:813–17.

www.consumerlabs.com

www.earthclinic.com, Folk Remedies and Holistic Cures

Part V: Think Outside the Pill
Chapter 20: Plant Extracts and Vitamins

Boyle, P. et al. Meta-analysis of Serenoa repens extract in BPH. *British Journal of Urology Int.* 2004 Apr;93(6):751–56.

Endo 2002: Abstracts P3–333, P3–317. June 21, 2002. Presentation 84th Annual Meeting of the Endocrine Society.

FDA Talk Paper Announcing the GMP Final Rule, October 1996

Federal GMPs Still "Hurry Up and Wait"

Is Your Vitamin Pill Worth it or Worthless? Six Rules to Guarantee Quality.

TGA Certificate of Listed Product and Certificate of Pharmaceutical Product.

Warnecke, G. Influencing of menopausal complaints with a phytodrug: successful therapy with Cimicifuga monoextract (in German). *Medizinische Welt* 36: 871–74, 1985.

www.consumerlabs.com, Consumer Labs

www.naturalproductsinsider.com/articles/152gmp1.html

www.ncbi.nlm.nih.gov, National Center for Biotechnology Information

www.tga.gov.au/impexp/commercial.htm

Chapter 21: Placebos and Healing Treats

Evans, Dylan. *Placebo: Mind over Matter in Modern Medicine.* (Oxford Press, 2004)

Gordon, Richard. *Quantum Healing: The Power to Heal*, 2nd Ed (North Atlantic Books, 2002)

Harrington, Anne. *The Placebo Effect: An Interdisciplinary Exploration.* (Harvard University Press, 1999)

Katptchuk, Ted J. "Intentional Ignorance: A History of Blind Assessment and Placebo Controls in Medicine." *Bulletin of the History of Medicine* 72, no. 3 (1998):389–433.

Shapiro, Arthur K. and Elaine Shapiro. *The Powerful Placebo: From Ancient Priest to Modern Physician.* (Johns Hopkins University Press, 1997)

Chapter 26: Drug Mugger

Pelton, Ross, RPh, PhD, CCN, and James B. LaValle, RPh, DHM, NMD, CCN, Ernest B. Hawkings, RPh, MS, and Daniel L. Krinsky, RPh, MS. *Drug-Induced Nutrient Depletion Handbook*, 2nd Ed. (Lexi-comp, 2001)

www.clinicalpharmacology.com

Index

Underscored page references indicate sidebars.